PHYSICIAN ASSISTANTS

POLICY AND PRACTICE

FOURTH EDITION

PHYSICIAN ASSISTANTS

POLICY AND PRACTICE

FOURTH EDITION

Roderick S. Hooker, PhD, MBA, PA

Health Policy Consultant
Adjunct Professor
Northern Arizona University
Flagstaff, Arizona

James F. Cawley, MPH, PA-C, DHL (Hon)

Professor, Department of Prevention and Community Health
Milken Institute, School of Public Health
Professor of Physician Assistant Studies
School of Medicine and Health Sciences
The George Washington University
Washington, D.C.

Christine M. Everett, PhD, MPH, PA-C

Assistant Professor
Physician Assistant Program
Department of Community and Family Medicine
Duke University
Durham, NC

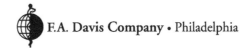
F.A. Davis Company • Philadelphia

F. A. Davis Company
1915 Arch Street
Philadelphia, PA 19103
www.fadavis.com

Printed in the United States of America

Last digit indicates print number: 10 9 8 7 6 5 4 3 2 1

Senior Acquisitions Editor: Andy McPhee
Director of Content Development: George W. Lang
Developmental Editor: Jaime Buss
Art and Design Manager: Carolyn O'Brien

As new scientific information becomes available through basic and clinical research, recommended treatments and drug therapies undergo changes. The author(s) and publisher have done everything possible to make this book accurate, up to date, and in accord with accepted standards at the time of publication. The author(s), editors, and publisher are not responsible for errors or omissions or for consequences from application of the book, and make no warranty, expressed or implied, in regard to the contents of the book. Any practice described in this book should be applied by the reader in accordance with professional standards of care used in regard to the unique circumstances that may apply in each situation. The reader is advised always to check product information (package inserts) for changes and new information regarding dose and contraindications before administering any drug. Caution is especially urged when using new or infrequently ordered drugs.

Library of Congress Cataloging-in-Publication Data

Names: Hooker, Roderick S., author. | Cawley, James F., author. | Everett,
   Christine M., author.
Title: Physician assistants : policy and practice / Roderick S. Hooker, James
   F. Cawley, Christine M. Everett.
Description: Fourth edition. | Philadelphia, PA : F.A. Davis Company, [2017]
   | Includes bibliographical references and index.
Identifiers: LCCN 2016048599 | ISBN 9780803643703
Subjects: | MESH: Physician Assistants | Professional Role |
   Interprofessional Relations | United States
Classification: LCC R697.P45 | NLM W 21.5 | DDC 610.73/72069—dc23 LC record available at
https://lccn.loc.gov/2016048599

FOREWORD

The physician assistant (PA) was a concept created by physicians in the 1960s as a response to the shortage and uneven distribution of generalist doctors and was intended to increase the public's access to healthcare. Before the creation of the PA, the domain of the doctor was sacrosanct, and, with few exceptions, the laws and policies for medical practice restricted the practice of medicine to physicians. But as the practice of medicine evolved and became more complex and specialized, other professions responded.

One of those responses was the PA movement, which began in 1965—a half century ago—at Duke University. It started with four former Navy corpsmen and a Duke University professor of medicine, who had the audacious idea that an abbreviated medical school education could create a flexible healthcare professional who could practice in collaboration with physicians. Others across the country had similar ideas, and thus the PA was born at Duke as well as at the University of Washington and the University of Colorado under the leadership of three charismatic and well-respected physicians. Concurrently it started in Liberia and Ghana as well.

Why did the PA movement start? Part of the reason lies in the realm of policy. In the 5 years preceding the Duke initiative, the American Congress enacted 64 major pieces of legislation; 21 dealt with health. It was indicative of the executive and legislative moods that 12 major health laws were passed in 1965, the first full year of the Johnson administration. Not only was the blueprint bold, but President Johnson, as a former leader in Congress, was exceptionally well qualified to design and implement legislative strategy. The administration's agenda for the Great Society, combined with its War on Poverty, meant that the federal government would take a far greater role in national affairs than ever had been the case in U.S. history. At the same time, the tragic Vietnam War was underway. Many tested corpsmen and medics were returning with unique skills and no outlet for using them. Between the changing policy environment, the availability of corpsmen, and three charismatic and well-respected physicians, academic health centers became the testing ground for another new idea in medicine: the generalist PA.

Five decades later, the PA profession has become a mature component of the medical workforce in the United States, and it is growing in other countries. There are now over 100,000 clinically active PAs in the U.S. workforce, with more than 200 accredited educational programs and 60 more in development. PAs are trained in the generalist model, and are employed in primary care as well as in specialty and subspecialty medicine. They work in close collaboration with physicians in almost every clinical practice setting.

The PA story has always been about exceptional individuals, and three highly respected PA scientists—ones who I know and have admired for their body of work—authored this book. Together, they span more than 75 years of collective research, analysis, and introspection of the health workforce literature. All three began their careers as PA clinicians and remain well-respected academics, two at the apex of their careers and the third rapidly rising. It would be hard to imagine who could better portray this movement than Professors Hooker, Cawley, and Everett. I hope you enjoy the remarkable story and journey of the PA movement.

Lloyd Michener, MD
Professor and Chair
Department of Community and Family Medicine
Duke University School of Medicine

PREFACE

This book is written for PAs by PAs. It is also written for academics, scholars, policy analysts, historians, sociologists, economists, and students—to name a few. It is written with one foot firmly planted in the historical development and the other in the future of an innovative profession. Because the authors wear the hats of academics, analysts, historians, clinicians, futurists, educators, and lifetime learners, this book is fashioned for the global audience of today and tomorrow. Finally, the authors hope that PA students and their faculties find this book useful in pursuing medical workforce and organizational research.

The chapters of the book are written as stand-alone reports, and each can be referenced separately. At the same time, each chapter follows the other in a logical manner. This book was written to be fluid and subject to modifications and change, recognizing that the moment it went to press, it was outdated.

Chapter 1: Introduction and Overview of the Profession
The introduction is an overview of PAs and sets the stage for all other chapters to unfold. It prepares the reader for the rest of the book. Even if you read no other chapter, you will still have a sense of what this book intends to reveal by reading Chapter 1.

Chapter 2: Development of the Profession
All entities have a beginning; this entity is no exception. The historical roots of the PA profession are recorded with an eye on preserving it. For this endeavor, the authors identified the national and sociocultural trends that led to the emergence of the PA profession in the United States, Ghana, Liberia, and elsewhere.

Chapter 3: Current Status: A Profile of the Physician Assistant Profession
This chapter provides a broad update and overview of the contemporary PA profession, including where PAs work, what they do, how well they do it, and how they are part of financing policies, the public domain, and private enterprises.

Chapter 4: Physician Assistant Education
The origins of PA education and its evolution are detailed in this chapter. Creative use of the classroom and the effectiveness of curricula set the stage for the deployment strategies used for PAs. A major practice role for the PA has been—and continues to be—primary care; the educational origins of this philosophy are probed. A profile of PA programs, students, graduates, and faculty is included. Also covered is the development of postgraduate training programs.

Chapter 5: Physician Assistants in Primary Care
Chapter 5 examines the bedrock of PA education: primary care. The United States and most other countries have selected primary healthcare as the foundation for PA education. It is the generalist model that is largely thought to be one of the key factors for their success. This chapter describes PAs' accomplishments and activities in various primary care settings.

Chapter 6: Physician Assistant Specialization: Non–Primary Care
After 4 decades of role delineation, the PA is slowly evolving away from primary care and into non–primary care roles. The diversity of roles is as broad as the types of doctors today.

Most of the major specialties and subspecialties are examined.

Chapter 7: Physician Assistants in Hospital Settings

Another key practice area for PAs is in the hospital setting. Upwards of 40% of PAs are either employed by hospitals or do part of their work in hospitals. This chapter describes the multiple roles that continue to evolve for PAs in inpatient settings in the United States, The Netherlands, and elsewhere.

Chapter 8: Physician Assistants in Rural Health

All countries have populations that live outside urban areas. Many define these areas as *rural*. The authors created a chapter for this body of knowledge knowing that PAs are providing care in underserved and less urbanized areas throughout the world.

Chapter 9: Economic Assessment of Physician Assistants

If PAs were not, in part, an economical alternative to doctors, then they probably would not survive. This chapter discusses the way in which PAs produce a cost-effective benefit to society through efficient educational strategies and the role of economics in PA development and success.

Chapter 10: Legal Aspects of Physician Assistant Practice

The legal basis of the PA profession in the United States is grounded in practice and codified in laws. Such laws that address the conduct of doctors and other health professionals are evolutionary, and their historical roots are anchored over a period of 100 years. This body of laws spells out what a doctor may do and to whom he or she may delegate medical authority. All 50 states enable PAs to work, prescribe, and be reimbursed for their services. That accomplishment came about through legal activism, concern for public safety, coordinated political action, and professionalism. This chapter discusses the legal basis of and liabilities involved in PA practice. Common legal issues, such as malpractice and tort reform, are also addressed.

Chapter 11: Professional and Workforce Issues

Issues related to the professional practice of medicine as a PA and the practice dynamics associated with the workforce tend to shape policy and governance. Factors that affect the culture and environment of the PA's practice have the potential to influence core issues, such as job satisfaction, scope of practice, and role delineation. Although these professional and workforce issues may be viewed as peripheral to the clinical practice of medicine, they do influence the behavior of PAs.

Chapter 12: Physician Assistants on Multidisciplinary Teams

Rarely do PAs function without some relationship in the collective care of the patient. How team members relate to each other and the role the PA plays in this activity is described. Team-based care is often described as "the future of medicine."

Chapter 13: Future Directions of the Physician Assistant Profession

In the concluding chapter, we gaze into the future and analyze the likely trends and forces that will influence the future direction of PAs. The PA is also no longer an American product, and the world has improved on this entity.

This book begins with an overview of what has occurred and ends with what the future holds. The authors have tried to be broad in their vision and seek scholarly views to be informative and produce the most contemporary information about this novel movement. However, they suffer the frailties of being human and encumbered with inherent biases. Their hope is that this book makes a small contribution to the scholarship of a rapidly evolving labor body. The PA profession is a lively one that could not have been foreseen even a few years ago; we are privileged viewers.

Roderick S. Hooker, PhD, MBA, PA

James F. Cawley, MPH, PA-C, DHL (Hon)

Christine M. Everett, PhD, MPH, PA-C

ABOUT THE AUTHORS

Roderick S. Hooker, PhD, PA, MBA, is a health policy consultant. His health career began in the 1960s as a hospital corpsman in the U.S. Navy. This period was followed by time as a civilian emergency department technician before graduating from the University of Missouri with a degree in biology and briefly pursuing a career as a tropical biologist. After working as a research assistant in Costa Rica, he joined the Peace Corps and spent $2^1/_2$ years as a volunteer in the Kingdom of Tonga working as a biologist, teacher, and health worker. After a brief period on the Peace Corps staff, he enrolled in the St. Louis University physician assistant program in the mid-1970s. Upon graduating as a PA, Hooker joined Kaiser Permanente in Portland, Oregon, where he worked clinically in rheumatology and socially as a health services researcher with the Kaiser Permanente Center for Health Research. During his 2 decades in Portland, Hooker obtained a master of business administration degree in healthcare organization and a doctorate in health policy from the Mark O. Hatfield School of Public Administration and Policy at Portland State University. He also was a PA officer in the U.S. Coast Guard Reserves and retired after 24 combined years of active and reserve duty. In the late 1990s, Hooker helped inaugurate, as well as teach at, the Pacific University School of Physician Assistant Studies as an adjunct faculty. In 2000 he joined the Department of Physician Assistant Studies at the University of Texas Southwestern Medical Center in Dallas to develop their Division of Health Services Research, and in 2003, he joined the Dallas VA Medical Center to organize a rheumatology research division and launch a postgraduate program for PAs in rheumatology. Rod completed his career as a Senior Director of The Lewin Group, a healthcare-consulting firm in Falls Church, VA. He now resides in southwest Washington state.

Hooker likes to think of himself as a health services researcher, examining the role of PAs, NPs, doctors, and others in an effort to understand how a mix of occupations can improve healthcare organization and delivery. This work has expanded overseas, being a codeveloper of the International Health Workforce Collaborative, an organization that exchanges information on how healthcare can be better managed globally. He consulted in Taiwan, Canada, Scotland, The Netherlands, and Australia. At various times, he held visiting professor positions at the University of Manitoba, University of Queensland, and James Cook University. This broad portfolio permits views of how medicine is organized in various settings and modeling health professions supply and demand. In the end, though, he regards himself as an amateur sculptor who finds himself, through force of circumstances, trying to shape health services rather than clay.

James F. Cawley, MPH, PA-C, DHL (Hon), is Professor and past Chair of Prevention and Community Health in the Milken Institute School of Public Health and Professor of Physician Assistant Studies in the School of Medicine and Health Sciences at The George Washington University. He is also Director of the joint Physician Assistant/Master of Public Health Program at The George Washington University and serves as Senior Research Fellow at the American Academy of Physician Assistants. A PA since 1974, Cawley has held faculty appointments at The Johns Hopkins University, the State University at Stony Brook, and Yale University. He has been on the faculty at The George Washington University since 1982.

Cawley has coauthored four books on PAs and published extensively in the areas of the PA profession, preventive medicine, non-physician health providers, and health workforce policy. He has authored more than 100 peer-reviewed articles, published in such journals as *Journal of Health Services and Research Policy, Health Affairs, Annals of Internal Medicine, Journal of the American Academy of Physician Assistants, Academic Medicine,* and *British Medical Journal.* As an editor and columnist, he has authored more than 250 columns over the past 25 years and his commentaries have been timely, informative, and challenging. A certified physician assistant for over 40 years, he practiced as a PA in primary care at The Johns Hopkins Hospital, earned his MPH in infectious disease epidemiology from The Johns Hopkins Bloomberg School of Public Health, and has held faculty appointments in the PA programs at Johns Hopkins, SUNY@ Stony Brook, and Yale University School of Medicine. In 1988, he was a fellow in the Epidemiology Program Office of the Centers for Disease Control and Prevention. Cawley has also served as HRSA Primary Care Health Policy Fellow and was a member of the Federal Advisory Committee on Training in Primary Care Medicine and Dentistry (ACTPCMD). He has presented on many occasions to state and national audiences of PAs, public health practitioners, and the public. In addition to this book, he is the coauthor of *Physician Assistants in a Changing Healthcare Environment.*

Cawley is a former Chair of the Research Advisory Workgroup of the American Academy of Physician Assistants (AAPA) and in 2011 received the prestigious Eugene A. Stead Award of Achievement from the AAPA. This award of excellence focused on his pivotal role in moving the PA field forward throughout his distinguished career. He served as President of the Physician Assistant Education Association and of the Physician Assistant Foundation. In 2013, he was awarded an honorary Doctor of Humane Letters degree by the Philadelphia College of Osteopathic Medicine.

Christine M. Everett, PhD, MPH, PA-C, is an Assistant Professor at the Duke University Physician Assistant Program in the Department of Community and Family Medicine. She completed her MPH at Johns Hopkins and her doctoral and postdoctoral training in population health and health services research at the University of Wisconsin—Madison. At Duke University, she teaches evidence-based medicine and provides primary care at a residential facility for patients recovering from addiction. Everett is the first PA faculty to be hired to a predominantly research position. Before joining the faculty, Christine worked clinically in emergency departments in rural Wisconsin; before becoming a physician assistant, Christine worked in research at the National Institutes of Health and in public health policy at the U.S. Food and Drug Administration.

Christine's current research initiatives focus on healthcare team design and the impact on patient, provider, and organizational outcomes. Her work has been published in a variety of journals, including *Healthcare, Journal of Rural Health,* and *Medical Care Research and Review.* Her recent work has focused on understanding the roles of primary care PAs and nurse practitioners and the way in which those roles relate to outcomes for patients with diabetes. She recently completed the first comparative effectiveness study of primary care PAs and NPs, which was published in *Health Affairs.*

Christine has served on a variety of committees, including the Research Advisory Committee of the American Academy of Physician Assistants and the Agency for Healthcare Research and Quality's Workgroup on Primary Care Team Workforce Models. She is a member of the U.S. delegation to the International Health Workforce Collaborative. Christine can't sculpt anything to save her life, but instead is working hard to influence the healthcare delivery system. She recently became the first PA faculty to receive funding from the National Institutes of Health for her research.

REVIEWERS

Renee Andreeff, EdD, PA-C, DFAAPA
Physician Assistant
D'Youville College
Buffalo NY

Sandra Beysolow, MS, PA-C, DFAAPA
PPHP
St. John's University
Fresh Meadows, NY

Darci Brown, MSPAS, PA-C
Physician Assistant Studies
Misericordia University
Dallas, PA

Jennifer Eames, DHSc, PA-C
Physician Assistant Studies
University of Texas Medical Branch
Galveston, TX

Kathleen L. Ehrhardt, MMS, PA-C, DFAAPA
Physician Assistant Program
DeSales University
Center Valley, PA

Walter A. Eisenhauer, Med, MMSc, PA-C, DFAAPA
Department of Physician Assistant Studies
Lock Haven University
Lock Haven, PA

Stephanie Joseph Gilkey, MS, PA-C, DFAAPA
Physician Assistant Studies
Wayne State University
Detroit, MI

Christopher Hanifin, MS, PA-C
Department of Physician Assistant
Seton Hall University
South Orange, NJ

Zachary Hartsell, MHA, PA-C
Wake Forest Baptist Medical Center
Winston-Salem, NC

Ian W. Jones, MPAS, PA-C, CCPA, DFAAPA
Office of Physician Assistant Studies
College of Medicine University of Manitoba
Winnipeg, Manitoba, Canada

Jolene R. Kelly, MPAS, PA-C
Physician Assistant
Des Moines University
Des Moines, IA

Wilton C. Kennedy, DHSc, PA-C
Physician Assistant
Jefferson College of Health Sciences
Roanoke, VA

Pat Kenney-Moore, EdD, PA-C
School of Medicine Division of Physician Assistant
Education
Oregon Health & Science University
Portland, Oregon

Luppo Kuilman, MPA, PhD (cand.)
Master Physician Assistant Program, School
of Healthcare Studies
Hanze University of Applied Sciences, Groningen
Groningen, The Netherlands

Jeanie McHugo, PhD, PA-C
Department of Physician Assistant Studies
University of North Dakota
Grand Forks, ND

Debra S. Munsell, DHSc, PA-C, DFAAPA
Interdisciplinary Human Studies
Louisiana State University Health Sciences
Center–New Orleans
New Orleans, LA

Ron W. Perry, MS, MPAS, MEd, PA-C
Interservice Physician Assistant Program
Army Medical Department Center & School
Fort Sam Houston, TX

Giuseppe A. Screnci, MS, PA-C
Physician Assistant
Thomas Jefferson University
Philadelphia, PA

Justine Strand de Oliveira, DrPH, PA-C
Community and Family Medicine
Duke University Medical Center
Durham, NC

Laura Witte, PhD, PA-C
Physician Assistant
A.T. Still University
Mesa, AZ

CONTENTS

A TIMELINE OF THE PHYSICIAN ASSISTANT PROFESSION

1650 *Feldshers,* originally German military medical assistants, are introduced into Russian armies by Peter the Great in the 17th century.

1778 Congress provides for a number of hospital mates to assist physicians in the provision of patient care modeled after the "loblolly boys" of the British Royal Navy.

1803 *Officiers de santé* are introduced in France by René Fourcroy to help alleviate health personnel shortages in the military and civilian sectors. They are phased out in 1892.

1891 First company for "medic" instruction is established at Fort Riley, Kansas.

1898 The *Practicante* is introduced in Puerto Rico (circa). The role is phased out in 1931.

1930 The first "physician assistant" (PA) in the United States at Cleveland Clinic (urology) is described in the literature.

1940 Community health aids are introduced in Alaska to improve the village health status of Eskimos and other Native Americans.

1959 U.S. Surgeon General identifies a shortage of medically trained personnel.

1961 Charles Hudson, in an editorial in the *Journal of the American Medical Association,* calls for a "midlevel" provider from the ranks of former military corpsmen.

World Health Organization begins introducing and promoting healthcare workers in developing countries (e.g., *médecin africain,* dresser, assistant medical officer, and rural health technician).

1962 Dr. Henry McIntosh, a cardiologist at Duke University, trains local firemen in emergency procedures for the community; in exchange, off-duty firemen staff the cardiac catheterization laboratory. Former Navy hospital corpsmen are hired for similar roles and are classified as *physician's assistants* by Duke's payroll department, which is considered the first formally recognized use of the name.

1965 White House Conference on Health discusses the use of former military corpsmen/medics as *assistant medical officers.* Dr. Eugene A. Stead, Jr., announces the Duke PA program at the conference.

First PA class enters Duke University.

The PA movement is born.

1966 Barefoot doctors in China arise in response to Chairman Mao's purge of the elite and intellectuals. This action sent many physicians into the fields to work, leaving peasants without medical personnel.

The child health associate program begins at the University of Colorado, which serves as the origin of the nurse practitioner (NP) profession and PA specialty.

Allied Health Professions Personnel Act (Public Law 751) promotes the development of programs to train new types of primary care providers.

1967 First PA class graduates from Duke University.

1968 American Academy of Physician Assistants (AAPA) is established.

Health Manpower Act (Public Law 90-490) funds the training of a variety of healthcare providers.

Physician Assistants, Volume 1, the first journal for PAs, is published.

First conference on PA education is held at Duke University.

The Association of Physician Assistant Programs (APAP) is formed.

1969 First class graduates from the University of Colorado's Child Health Associate PA program.

1970 Kaiser Permanente becomes the first health maintenance organization (HMO) to employ a PA.

First class graduates from the MEDEX Northwest PA program at the University of Washington.

American Registry of Physician's Assistants is founded by Robert Howard, MD, at Duke University.

1971 American Medical Association (AMA) recognizes the PA profession and begins work on national certification and codification of its practice characteristics.

Comprehensive Health Manpower Training Act (Public Law 92-157) contracts for PA education and deployment. Congress includes $4 million for establishing new PA educational programs in 1972 (Health Manpower Educational Initiative Awards).

Essentials of an Accredited Educational Program for the Assistant to the Primary Care Physician, the minimum standards for PA program accreditation, are adopted by the AMA.

1972 Association of Physician Assistant Programs (APAP) is established.

Alderson-Broaddus College's first 4-year program graduates its first class.

"The Essentials" accreditation standards for PA programs are adopted, and the Joint Review Committee on Education Programs for the Physician Assistant (JRC-PA) is formed to evaluate compliance with the standards.

Health Resources Administration enacts federal support for PA education.

The Medex Group is established at the University of Hawaii by Richard Smith.

International PA-type programs in the Pacific, Asia, Africa, and South America begin development.

1973 First AAPA Annual Conference is held at Sheppard Air Force Base, Texas, with 275 attendees.

AAPA and APAP establish a joint national office in Washington, DC.

National Commission on Certification of Physician Assistants (NCCPA) is established.

National Board of Medical Examiners administers the first certifying examinations for primary care PAs.

First postgraduate program for PAs is started at Montefiore Hospital by Richard Rosen, MD.

1974 AAPA becomes an official organization of the JRC-PA. The committee reviews PA and surgeon assistant programs and makes accreditation recommendations to the Committee on Allied Health Education and Accreditation.

American College of Surgeons becomes a sponsoring organization of the JRC-PA.

From 1974 to 1977, 150 PAs are recruited to work on the Alaska pipeline—the largest scale employment of PAs in the private sector.

1975 *The Physician Assistant: A National and Local Analysis,* by Ann Suter Ford, is the first book published on the PA profession.

1976 Federal support of PA education continues under grants from the Health Professions Educational Assistance Act (Public Law 94-484).

1977 *The New Health Professionals: Nurse Practitioners and Physician's Assistants,* by Ann Bliss and Eva Cohen, is published.

The Physician's Assistant: A Baccalaureate Curriculum, by Hu Myers, is published.

AAPA Education and Research Foundation (later renamed Physician Assistant Foundation) is incorporated to recruit public and private contributions for student financial assistance and to support research on the PA profession.

Rural Health Clinic Services Act (Public Law 95-210) is passed by Congress, providing Medicare reimbursement of PA and NP services in rural clinics.

Health Practitioner (later renamed *Physician Assistant*) journal begins publication; the publication is later distributed to all PAs as the official AAPA publication.

1978 *The Physician's Assistant: Innovation in the Medical Division of Labor*, by Eugene Schneller, is published.

AAPA House of Delegates becomes the policy-making legislative body of the academy.

U.S. Air Force begins appointing PAs as commissioned officers.

1979 Graduate Medical Education National Advisory Council estimates a surplus of physicians and nonphysician providers in the near future.

1980 AAPA Political Action Committee is established to support candidates for federal office who support the PA profession.

The Veteran's Caucus of the AAPA is formed.

1981 *Staffing Primary Care in 1990: Physician Replacement and Cost Savings*, by Jane Cassels Record, documents that PAs in HMO settings provide 79% of the care of a primary care physician, at 50% of the cost.

1982 *Physician Assistants: Their Contribution to Healthcare,* by Henry Perry and Bena Breitner, is published.

1984 *First Annual Report on Physician Assistant Educational Programs in the United States*, by Denis Oliver, PhD, and the APAP, is published.

Alternatives in Healthcare Delivery: Emerging Roles of Physician Assistants, by Reginal D. Carter, is published.

1985 AAPA's first Burroughs Wellcome Health Policy Fellowship for PAs is created.

Membership of the AAPA surpasses the 10,000 mark. Membership categories are expanded to include physicians, affiliates, and sustaining members.

University of Colorado PA program awards a master's degree to their graduates, the first graduate for PA education.

1986 AAPA succeeds in legislative drive for coverage of PA services in hospitals and nursing homes and for coverage of assisting in surgery under Medicare Part B (Omnibus Budget Reconciliation Act [Public Law 99-210]).

1987 National PA Day, October 6, is established, coinciding with the anniversary of the first graduating class of PAs from the Duke University PA program 20 years earlier.

AAPA national headquarters in Alexandria, Virginia, is dedicated.

AAPA publishes the *Journal of the American Academy of Physician Assistants (JAAPA)*.

Additional Medicare coverage of PA services (in rural underserved areas) is approved by Congress.

1991 U.S. Navy PAs are commissioned.

AAPA assumes administrative responsibility of the Accreditation Review Committee on Education for the Physician Assistant (ARC-PA) (formerly the JRC-PA).

Clinician Reviews debuts, the first clinical journal to target PAs and NPs. The publication is created, owned, and managed by PAs.

1992 U.S. Army and Coast Guard PAs are commissioned.

Canadian National Forces inaugurates a Canadian PA education program in Ontario.

1993 A total of 24,600 PAs are in active practice in 50 states, territories, and the District of Columbia.

1995 *Physician Assistants in the Health Workforce, 1994* (report of the Advisory Group on Physician Assistants and the Workforce), which develops a definition of the PA, is published.

1996 AMA grants observer status to the AAPA in the AMA House of Delegates.

1997 Passage of the Balanced Budget Act of 1997 (Public Law 105-33) changes the level of reimbursement of PA services under Medicare and Medicaid.

1998 Mississippi is the last state to pass PA enabling legislation.

APAP Research Institute is founded.

1999 *Perspectives on Physician Assistant Education* becomes a peer-reviewed indexed journal.

Manitoba creates the first provincial legislation for the introduction of PAs. First providence to do so.

2000 The APAP determines that the master's degree is the appropriate degree for PA education.

ARC-PA becomes an independent accrediting agency for PA educational programs.

Louisiana is the 47th state to pass PA prescribing legislation.

NCCPA converts the Physician Assistant National Certification Examination (PANCE) and the Physician Assistant National Recertification Examination to computer-based administration.

2001 A record 4,267 PAs sit for the PANCE (91.5% pass rate).

2002 The 35th anniversary of the first graduation of PAs is chronicled in a special edition of *JAAPA*.

AAPA celebrates its 30th anniversary. Approximately 45,000 PAs are clinically active in American medicine. Number of accredited PA programs is 134.

2003 PAs are introduced in England.

Centers for Medicare and Medicaid Services (CMS) expands the ability of PAs to have an ownership interest in a practice under the Medicare program.

A PA program at Base Borden in Ontario becomes the first accredited PA program in Canada.

Three PA programs are established in The Netherlands (a fourth is added later).

2004 The number of clinically practicing PAs in the United States reaches 50,121.

Two PAs, Karen Bass of California and Mark Hollo of North Carolina, become the first PAs to be elected to state legislatures.

PA organizations draft shared definition of PA competencies. The participating organizations are the AAPA, APAP, ARC-PA, and NCCPA.

The 33rd annual PA Conference in Las Vegas, Nevada, boasts the largest attendance to date, with a total attendance of more than 10,500.

2005 The Association of Physician Assistant Programs (APAP) changes its name to the Physician Assistant Education Association (PAEA) and relocates to offices separate from the AAPA in Alexandria, Virginia.

The Netherlands graduates its first class of PAs.

University of Hertfordshire, England, inaugurates the first PA program in the United Kingdom.

Eugene A. Stead, Jr., MD, a founder of the PA profession, dies at age 96. The first PA program in India is started by two surgeons.

2006 Rear Admiral Mike Milner becomes the first PA flag officer.

ARC-PA issues the third edition of its accreditation standards.

State of Ohio passes legislation that allows PAs to prescribe—meaning 49 states, the District of Columbia, and Guam allow PAs to prescribe.

Scotland introduces 12 PAs as a pilot program.

2007 United States celebrates the 40th anniversary of the U.S. PA movement. An estimated 65,000 U.S. PAs are clinically active.

PAEA celebrates its 35th anniversary.

Society for the Preservation of Physician Assistant History, Inc., becomes a supporting organization of the AAPA.

HealthForceOntario, an initiative by the Ontario Ministry of Health, begins a pilot program introducing PAs in the province.

Indiana passes legislation allowing PAs to prescribe—all 50 states, the District of Columbia, and Guam now allow PAs to prescribe.

AAPA, PAEA, NCCPA, and ARC-PA join representatives from the National Human Genome Research

Institute and other genomics experts to define how PAs could introduce genomics in patient care.

2008   Manitoba begins the first civilian Canadian PA program.

ARC-PA awards initial accreditation to its first two postgraduate PA programs—the University of Texas M.D. Anderson Cancer Center PA Postgraduate Program in Oncology (Houston) and the Johns Hopkins Hospital Postgraduate Surgical Residency for PAs (Baltimore).

Bureau of Labor Statistics identifies the PA profession as one of 30 occupations expected to grow fast over the next decade.

Number of PAs in active practice in the United States exceeds 70,000.

2009   The number of new U.S. PA graduates is approximately 5,640.

AAPA and the PAEA hold a Summit Meeting on the PA clinical doctorate and declare their opposition to the entry-level doctorate degree for PA education.

Australia begins the first PA program at the University of Queensland.

The number of PA programs in the world totals 160: 145 in the United States, 1 in Australia, 4 in England, 3 in Canada, 4 in The Netherlands, and 3 in South Africa.

2010   The estimated number of clinically active PAs is United States, 75,000; Australia, 15; Canada, 100; Great Britain, 80; The Netherlands, 200.

2014   The United States has 190 accredited PA programs; more than 60 U.S. institutions have requested provisional accreditation.

Karen Bass, PA, is elected to Congress from the 37th District in California.

Approximately 7,000 PAs graduate. Statewide distribution per capita is 26.8 PAs per 100,000.

2015   The contemporary PA movement celebrates its 50th anniversary.

United States has an estimated 94,000 PAs in clinical practice.

PAs are working in Canada, Australia, Great Britain (including Scotland), The Netherlands, South Africa, Ghana, Saudi Arabia, Liberia, Germany, and India.

2016   United States: estimated 100,000 PAs in clinical practice; 17% have dual licenses and 14% claim two or more employers. The mean age is 42 years, and 75% are female.

NCCPA records that approximately 110,000 individuals have ever certified as PAs.

There are 218 accredited U.S. PA programs, with 30 or more in development.

Canada: estimated 540 PAs; 4 PA programs

Australia: 15 clinically active PAs; 1 PA program

The Netherlands: 1,000 PAs; 5 PA programs

United Kingdom: 200 PAs; 4 PA programs (>20 in development)

Liberia: 200 PAs; 2 programs

Ghana: 2,500 PAs; 3 programs

South Africa: 100 PAs, 3 programs

Germany: 1 program

India: 400 PAs, 5 programs

2017   50th anniversary of the first PA graduates – Duke University, Monrovia; Kintampo. The anniversary is celebrated in special editions of JAAPA and JPAE.

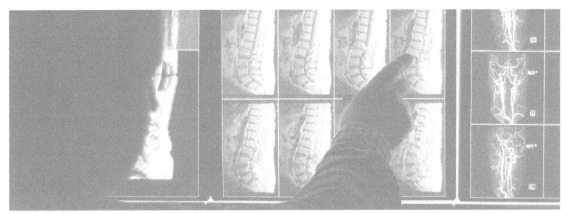

CHAPTER 1

INTRODUCTION AND OVERVIEW OF THE PROFESSION

JAMES F. CAWLEY ▪ RODERICK S. HOOKER ▪ CHRISTINE M. EVERETT

"From each according to his abilities, to each according to his needs."

—*Karl Marx*

The concept of the physician assistant (PA) emerged in the 1960s as a strategy to cope with a shortage of primary care physicians (Cawley, et al., 2012). Giving impetus to idea, what spawned was a handful of graduates and a new profession. From humble beginnings, the new profession struggled to survive, grow, and become recognized. Before the creation of the PA, the domain of the doctor had not been seriously challenged. For more than a century, the laws and policies in place with regard to medical practice and authority favored the doctor over any other professional licensed to practice medicine. But as the practice of medicine evolves, so do the involved professions. The fact that this historical phenomenon occurred at least half a dozen times in the late 1960s suggests that the ground at that time was fertile for almost any seed of change to take root.

With 5 decades of growth, the PA profession is now a mature and capable component of the medical workforce in the United States and other countries as well. It appears that the health systems of the United States and of other countries have come to the conclusion that PAs are an important and effective component of the healthcare workforce. Collectively, the PA profession can claim more than 100,000 US graduates, a strong and stable set of educational programs, and a growing importance within healthcare systems globally. For the United States, in the decades following the origin of the PA profession, there were many debates about the need for PAs and other types of clinicians. These debates came during a predicted surplus of doctors and nurses by the end of the 20th century. Despite the prediction, the PA profession survived and prospered. Why then has this profession flourished, and will its success and growth continue along with the new century? The answers to these and other questions about PAs were less clear when previous editions of this book were written. Now, with roots extending beyond the United States and the concept affirmed in multiple systems, PAs are part of the wide and varied healthcare system that wraps around the world. The labor that went into the planting is bearing fruit in unexpected ways. Continued growth and success are to be expected for this young profession because the demand continues to exceed the supply in a variety of societies that value choice, diversity, quality, and availability. Although looming shortages of doctors and other healthcare workers continue, the US Bureau of Labor Statistics has consistently identified the PA profession as among the fastest growing occupations. Employment of PAs is projected to grow 38% from 2012 to 2022, much faster than the average for all occupations. Increased demand for healthcare services from the growing and aging population and widespread chronic disease, combined with the shortage of physicians, will result in increased demand for alternative healthcare providers, such as PAs. For the foreseeable future, the cost benefits for employers appear to favor the PA over other medical personnel.

EVIDENCE REVIEWED: SUCCESS OF THE CONCEPT

In the mid 1960s, the PA movement began with three students in the US and concurrently a small group in Liberia and Ghana. In 1967, the first three graduate American PAs began their careers. By the end of 2016, the PA profession boasted more than 100,000 US graduates and more than 1,500 graduates in other countries. The United States has more than 215 PA programs; over a dozen PA programs exist in other countries (with more in development). The United States, Canada, Great Britain, Australia, The Netherlands, The Kingdom of Saudi Arabia, India, Liberia, Ghana, and South Africa enable PAs to work in collaboration with doctors. Three-quarters of US PAs are female, the average age is 42 years, and the majority has a graduate degree. Spanning 5 decades, PA education has stayed the course in teaching primary care and general medicine, although the majority of PAs are now employed in specialty and subspecialty practice. Along the way, the role of the PA has

evolved, the educational level has advanced, and professional organizations have become established, indicating the stability and maturity of the profession.

Setting the Stage

The startling growth and success of the PA concept from its origins in the 1960s probably could not have occurred in the absence of ferment and change in the US medical system and in society. The 1960s were a time of transformation in America. A driving force of the change was the existence of social inequities that many members of society believed needed to be addressed, if not fixed. Consumers of healthcare, existing professions, governments, bureaucratic hierarchies, educational institutions, and accrediting bodies were all involved in the transformation. All implicitly, if not explicitly, aided in the process by creating a positive political climate. Cultural revolution was in the air, and a desire to reengineer the social wrongs of the previous 100 years was at hand.

The PA innovation came on the heels of 2 decades of scientific breakthroughs, development of new medical specialties, and growth of hospitals and hospital services. Young doctors, exposed early to this exciting display of technical power, were flocking to academic-based specialties. For the generalist physician, education and training had shrunk after the Korean War. Once the foundation of the medical workforce, the single-year, intern-trained generalist was becoming an anachronism; the new graduates of medical schools were not replacing the general practitioners who were retiring. These new graduates immediately headed into 3 to 5 years of postgraduate education, and from this trend a number of specialties and subspecialties arose. The consequences of this lack of general practitioners were not so obvious in cities with good hospitals and a strong cadre of newly trained specialists. However, in small towns and rural areas, the impact was devastating. Towns that had always enjoyed having their own local doctor suddenly had none.

Thus the stage was set for entry of alternative providers who promised improved access to healthcare for small towns and rural areas.

The country's leaders were aware of inequities in the distribution of medical services, and most were convinced that the problem was one of inadequate numbers of medical care providers. A series of federal and state actions aimed to correct this problem. The most notable ones were the advent of the PA profession, the development of the nurse practitioner (NP), and the reintroduction of the nurse-midwife. However, other actions were undertaken in the 1970s as well:

- Medical schools increased class size.
- New medical schools were established.
- The generalist physician was "revived" in the form of a new general specialty: family medicine.
- Special offices to promote medical practice in underserved areas were created in many states and in the federal government.
- Dispersed medical educational systems (area health education programs) were created.
- Wellness and prevention took on a new dimension with immunization advances, epidemiology, new technology in diagnostics, and safety.

Catalysts for Change

When significant social transformation occurs, it is rarely dependent on one circumstance—an observation made by sociologists, anthropologists, political scientists, and historians. Yet a single, significant catalyst for change can occur and, when coupled with other events, a chain reaction can take place. Explaining why the PA innovation occurred in the United States and elsewhere requires documenting the events and identifying the factors leading up to this change.

One contributing factor was that the war in Southeast Asia was reaching its tragic conclusion in the late 1960s and early 1970s. Yet there was an upside to this conflict: the advancement of trauma management science. Military medical care had significantly improved by using trained medical care teams operating in combat theaters. Physicians, nurses, medics, and corpsmen were returning home with knowledge of these improvements and the key roles played by members of these medical teams. The highly integrated team of doctor, nurse, and corpsman was pivotal in saving lives in forward-positioned battalion aid stations; yet when they resumed their civilian roles, the corpsman was absent from that critical triumvirate because the constraints of the existing healthcare system did not recognize this type of provider in its educational or credentialing systems. Many realized that a highly skilled member was missing.

Another factor was the social climate within the country. The "War on Poverty" had brought to public attention the substandard conditions and deprivation of some people within the bounds of the "richest country on Earth." President Lyndon Johnson's Great Society program brought an optimism that solutions might be found for these chronic social ills. The burden of social inequities had reached a critical point, and righting wrongs was required if Americans were going to be a nation of "*We the people...*."

The White House Conference on Health in 1965 raised the issue of physician shortages and asked if there were no other professionals that could help offset their workload. Some suggestions included military corpsmen and medics, returned Peace Corps volunteers, and public health nurses. One of the conference narrators was Dr. Eugene Stead, and one of the conference organizers was Dr. Richard "Dick" Smith, two of the originators of the American PA movement (Hooker & Cawthon, 2015).

In retrospect, understanding why this era was a favorable time for PAs to enter the health workforce stage has become a bit clearer. State and federal governments were willing to support some of the most far-reaching social programs seen to that time to increase access to healthcare. The fact that this innovation tapped the newly available source of returning military corpsmen was serendipitous.

Intertwined with these circumstances were events more directly related to the PA profession. In 1961, a prominent leader of the American Medical Association (AMA) proposed the idea of using military-trained personnel as assistants to physicians (Hudson, 1961). A White House conference called for a medical auxiliary tapping returned veterans. In the mid-1960s,

Dr. Richard Smith, then a deputy director of the Office of Equal Health Opportunity, moved into a new role in which he proposed the creation of a new source of healthcare providers for rural areas. At this same time, a prominent academic pediatrician, Dr. Henry Silver, with Dr. Loretta Ford, a nurse educator, began to develop a new type of nonphysician practitioner at the University of Colorado.

At Duke University, the first PA program began with four ex-Navy corpsmen under the direction of Dr. Eugene Stead and Dr. E. Harvey Estes, Jr. As an academic physician leader, Dr. Stead recognized the need for new personnel in the medical center and in the rural areas of his state. His previous experience with military personnel convinced him that the training period for assistants in a new program could be much shorter than that for medical students and that close supervision by their physician employers would ensure competence and further development of skills in practice. Dr. Stead noted that a prominent generalist in a rural town had trained a highly skilled assistant. Influenced by this prototype PA, the concept of extending the services of physicians in rural practices emerged. Shortly after the inauguration of the first PA educational track, Dr. E. Harvey Estes, a respected internist and academic at Duke, took the reins and further developed the PA movement.

The specific histories of the University of Colorado program, the Duke program, and the University of Washington Medex program—each a different model of PA education—are discussed in detail in later chapters. At this point, various features of the PA conceptual model bear mentioning. Two have already been discussed: the relatively brief history of the PA concept and the role of the employing physician as supervisor. Additionally, all of the PA programs were patterned after the familiar medical model: a period of basic science education followed by clinical skill development under the supervision of medical instructors. The prospective PA would be trained to take a medical history, document symptoms, examine the patient, develop diagnoses, and take over some medical management tasks. Complicated cases and procedures were to be referred to the supervising physician. Although it was expected that the new personnel might spend more time with patient education and preventive interventions, the activities and skills would be similar to those of the physician, with the assistant assuming many but not all of the physician's tasks (Cawley, 2012).

Another feature of the PA model, as each developer envisioned it, was the clear intention to train a generalist assistant whose training and skill development were adequate to serve as a platform for further education and skill development by the physician employer. The generalist assistant could work with a rural doctor, gaining additional insights and skills with time but could also work with a highly focused specialist who would add another layer of expertise to the general education of the PA.

As might have been predicted, state and federal governmental attention was quickly achieved by three of the model PA programs: Duke University, University of Washington, and University of Colorado. Soon the government developed an interest in the regulation of this new category of healthcare provider. The Department of Health, Education, and Welfare sponsored a study and a series of conferences at Duke University on the regulation of PA practice. This activity, under the direction of Martha Ballenger, JD, and Dr. Estes, resulted in model regulatory laws that were enacted by many states and prepared the way for the 1971 Health Manpower Act. More importantly, such legislation provided funds for medical schools to increase the number of students to meet the perceived shortage of medical personnel. It also included funding for PA training programs. The availability of funding quickly increased the number of training sites, and 50 such programs were active by 1974 (Cawley, 2008).

In 1971, the AMA recognized the new profession and lent its name and resources to the national certification process, accreditation of educational programs, and codification of practice laws. This recognition, however, did not ensure acceptance by all physicians. Even the AMA did not fully endorse the PA concept until the 1990s, and this endorsement was spurred on by the decision of the NP movement to maintain its independence from medicine. (NPs are an extension of nursing and, therefore, fall under the state-specific nurse acts.)

An underappreciated event that signaled acceptance of the PA concept in US medicine was the passage of the Omnibus Budget Reconciliation Act of 1986, which authorized reimbursement for PA services through Medicare. Reimbursement is paid to the employing practice, typically at 85% of the rate paid to physicians for the same service.

Physician Assistants Today

The PA of the new century differs from its predecessor of 5 decades ago. Much of the information on PAs comes from the United States; however, new information is emerging from other countries. Following is an overview of today's PA:

■ **Graduates:** At the beginning of 2017, more than 102,500 PAs were in active clinical practice globally, although the United States dominates with the most practicing PAs and PA graduates (Table 1–1). The stability and dedication of this workforce to

TABLE 1-1
Physician Assistant Movement, 2016

Country	Number of Clinically Active PAs	Number of PA Programs
Australia	20	1
Canada	200	4
Germany	Unknown	2
Ghana	200	3
India	800	3
Ireland	0	1
Liberia	Unknown	3
Netherlands, The	300	5
United Kingdom (Physician Associates)	75	4
Saudi Arabia (Associate Physicians)	120	1
South Africa (Clinical Assistants)	Unknown	3
United States	100,500	218
Total (estimated)	**>100,000**	**248**

the profession are demonstrated by the fact that this number represents almost 88% of all persons formally trained as PAs since the first class graduated in 1967. The annual attrition rate is less than 5%.

■ **PA characteristics:** The mean age of PAs is 42 years, and 66% are women. These statistics reflect the relative youth of the profession and the marked shift in gender. The early predominance of men in the profession (related to the male gender of the former military students of the early years) has gradually changed and transformed the PA profession, as women now represent a majority of the profession (Figure 1–1).

■ **Deployment:** Forty-two percent of US PAs practice in communities with a population smaller than 50,000, and 20% practice in communities with a population smaller than 10,000 (a much higher percentage than physicians). Twelve percent of PAs work in inner-city clinics.

■ **PA educational programs:** Globally, there are almost 250 PA programs in 2016, with more in development. The Accreditation Review Commission on Education for the Physician Assistant (ARC-PA) accredits US programs. Canadian programs are accredited by the Canadian Medical Association Conjoint Commission on Accreditation. The Dutch PA programs are accredited by a governmental agency. "Physician associate" programs in the United Kingdom are accredited by the Department of Health. In the United States, the typical PA program is 26 months long and requires a college degree and some healthcare experience before admission. As the *29th Annual Report on PA Educational Programs in the United States, 2012–2013* reports, more than 90% of US programs award a master's degree, a number that continues to increase.

■ **Students:** In the United States, more than 15,000 students are enrolled in PA programs at any one time. In 2016, approximately 7,500 new graduates passed the national certification examination and became eligible to practice.

FIGURE 1-1
PA Profession by Age and Gender, 2013

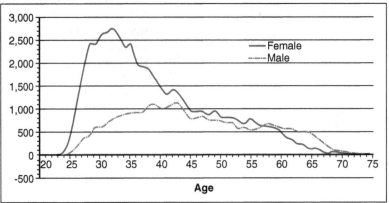

- **Legislation:** All 50 US states, the District of Columbia, and the US territories (except Puerto Rico) have enacted laws that recognize PA practice. All US jurisdictions require graduation from an accredited PA program as well as national certification. The Canadian provinces, Australian states, and central governments of other countries are working to define accreditation, registration, and certification requirements for PA students and graduates.
- **Prescribing:** All 50 US states, the District of Columbia, and the US territories (except Puerto Rico) have enacted laws that authorize PA prescribing. Prescribing legislation is under development in other countries.
- **Income:** In 2013, the median wage from the main employer for PAs in all specialties who are not employed by the federal government, who are not self-employed, and who work full time (at least 32 hours per week) was $44.70 per hour. The median annual wage (40 hours per week × 52 weeks = 2,080 hours) was $92,970, with a range of $62,030 to $130,620 (Quella et al., 2015). Overtime, shift differential, bonus, and other prerequisites can add up to 30% more to an annual compensation.
- **Certification:** US PAs receive their national certification from the National Commission on Certification of Physician Assistants (NCCPA). All states require this certification for licensure. A commission involving the Canadian Association of Physician Assistants certifies Canadian PAs.
- **Ethnicity:** According to 2016 data from the National Commission on the Certification of Physician Assistants (NCCPA), 13% of members of the US PA profession are from underrepresented groups. Of those in active clinical practice, 3.9% are African American, 6.2% are Hispanic/Latino, 0.4% are Asian/Pacific Islander, and 0.4% are American Indian/Alaskan Native. The remaining 87% are white or do not choose to identify their racial/ethnic origin.
- **Practice settings:** PAs practice in all the types of clinical settings where physician services are traditionally offered: urban neighborhoods, rural communities, hospitals, and public and private medical offices. They serve as commissioned officers in all US and Canadian military branches and in the US Public Health Service. In clinical practice, most PAs spend their time in medical offices or clinic settings, but some work in hospitals and divide their time among the wards and the operating and delivery rooms.

During the formative years of the profession, the distribution of PAs reflected the federal and state initiatives and the interest of the medical profession in extending primary care into areas of need. Early recruits were individuals with experience that enabled them to practice with minimal supervision. As the capability of PAs to fit into specialties outside primary care has become known and as their ability and productivity have been confirmed, physicians in these specialties have attracted more and more PAs. The trend of PA specialization has become most pronounced in the first decade of the 21st century, with now more than 66% of all PAs practicing in specialties and subspecialties (Table 1–2). PAs can be found in most non–primary care specialties. However, they are underrepresented in nursing home care, home healthcare, pathology, radiology, behavioral health, and some of the surgical and medical subspecialties.

The medical model of PA education has been confirmed by the adaptability of PAs to new roles in the medical and surgical specialties. In primary care and the specialty care roles, the relationship between the PA and the supervising doctor remains constant—a functional team. This relationship has been characterized as "negotiated performance autonomy," reflecting the continually evolving delegation of medical tasks from physician to PA based on a mutual understanding and trust in their respective professional roles. Schneller (1978) proposed that this mutual evolution was a major determinant of the PA's clinical practice effectiveness and was advantageous to both types of providers.

The recognition and acceptance of this association is key to understanding the durability between the PA and physician. It is also key to understanding the official stance of the profession: that it does *not* desire autonomy from physician supervision. The creators' early recognition of this principle is reflected in their prediction that PAs would gain greater freedom and growth from delegation by wise physician supervisors who share the benefits of this growth than they would from legislated autonomy. Further proof of the beauty of this concept

TABLE 1-2
US Physician Assistant Roles Per Year

Specialty	1984	1989	1990	1992	1994	1996	2000	2002	2009	2013
Primary Care[†]	55.8	49.3	45.9	472.8	45.2	50.8	47.9	43.1	34.2	32
Family Medicine	54.5	37.9	33.0	31.4	33.7	39.8	36.5	32.1	24.9	23
General Internal Medicine	9.2	7.8	9.0	8.9	9.2	8.3	8.8	8.4	6.9	7.8
Pediatrics	4.1	3.6	3.0	2.5	2.3	2.7	2.6	2.6	2.4	2.0
Non–Primary Care[‡]	44.2	50.7	55.0	57.2	48.5	49.2	52.1	56.9	57.6	68
Obstetrics/ Gynecology	3.1	4.6	4.0	3.3	2.9	3.0	2.7	2.7	2.4	3
Surgical Subspecialties	9.0	7.5	9.0	9.8	10.5	8.8	10.4	10.0	19.5	24
General Surgery	9.2	7.9	8.0	8.0	7.7	3.1	2.7	2.5	2.5	2
Internal Medicine Subspecialties	4.8	3.8	6.0	7.1	6.3	5.8	8.1	9.4	11.3	11
Pediatric Subspecialties	0.0	1.0	2.0	1.2	1.2	2.1	1.5	1.5	1.6	—
Emergency Medicine	6.4	6.2	7.0	8.0	8.7	7.0	9.7	10.2	8.7	10.6
Orthopedics	4.1	5.6	6.0	7.6	7.8	6.9	7.3	9.2	9.5	11
Occupational Medicine	4.1	5.8	5.0	3.9	3.4	3.0	3.4	3.0	2.1	2
Other Specialties[§]	3.5	10.3	8.0	8.3	6.3	9.5	6.3	8.4	—	4

Data from authors and from the American Academy of Physician Assistants, Alexandria, VA.
[†]Primary care includes family medicine, general internal medicine, and general pediatrics.

that allows PAs to have functional autonomy within the dependent role is the high degree of job and career satisfaction.

Delegation of tasks from doctors to PAs is also contained in the basis of the legal and regulatory authority granted to PAs in most state laws. Model legislation proposed as a result of the Duke conferences on this topic in the late 1960s permitted PAs to work in the full range of clinical practice areas: offices, clinics, hospitals, nursing homes, and patients' homes. This wide latitude was considered essential for a full range of services and effectiveness. The model legislation recognized the authority of physicians to delegate medical tasks to qualified PAs while holding them legally responsible through the doctrine of "respondeat superior." North Carolina, Colorado, and Oklahoma were among the first states to amend their medical practice acts, and Mississippi was the last.

Developed state by state over more than 40 years, these practice regulations and the supervisory relationship has led to the striking versatility among the practice roles of PAs. As a result, PAs are permitted to assist physicians in any task or function within the scope of a physician's practice but with the recognition that the responsibility and legal liability for this delegation remain with the physician. This delegation is not limited to the immediate presence of the physician, but it can be extended to locations from which the supervising physician can be readily contacted for consultation and assistance, such as through various means of telecommunication.

Although the demand for PAs and acceptance of their roles has steadily increased, added emphasis on cost-effectiveness has greatly augmented the importance of the profession in health delivery. Managed care organizations quickly found PAs to be capable of providing primary care at a lower cost than physicians and to be willing to move into areas in which it would not be cost-effective to place a doctor. Later, physicians, particularly those in specialty groups, recognized the favorable economic advantages that PAs brought to private practices and hospitals. The development and demand for PAs in these settings have caused a shift of PAs away from primary care. In addition, to some degree, PAs have been willing to move into various other settings that have not been popular with physicians, such as correctional health systems, substance abuse clinics, occupational health clinics, and geriatric institutions. Patient acceptance has remained high, disproving critics who predicted patient rejection.

THE PHYSICIAN ASSISTANT DEFINED

The benefits of using generalist assistants capable of mastering new skills and enlarging their roles under responsible supervision of a physician partner continues to be confirmed. In fact, the original PA concept has been modified and enlarged so much that the AAPA has periodically developed new definitions of the profession. The AAPA House of Delegates adopted the current definition in 1995. This definition addresses the versatility of the profession, its distribution in all geographic locations, and the various nonclinical roles that PAs might pursue:

PAs are health professionals licensed to practice medicine with physician supervision. PAs are qualified by graduation from an accredited PA educational program and/or certification by the National Commission on the Certification of Physician Assistants. Within the physician–PA relationship, PAs exercise autonomy in medical decision-making and provide a broad range of diagnostic and therapeutic services. The clinical role of PAs includes primary and specialty care in medical and surgical practice settings in rural and urban areas. PA practice is centered on patient care and may include educational, research, and administrative activities.

Some interpretation of this definition of PAs may be required. The Professional Practices Council of the AAPA provides the explanations that follow.

Physician assistants are health professionals …

This statement recognizes the scope of PA practice, the advanced knowledge required to be a PA, the PA's use of discretion and judgment in providing care, the PA's use of ethical standards, and the PA's orientation toward service.

… licensed to practice medicine with physician supervision.

This part of the definition may be of concern to PAs accustomed to the terms *certified* and *registered*. Examination of accepted definitions of occupational regulation, however, reveals that PAs are subject to *de facto* licensure regardless of terminology used by the state.

Registration is the least restrictive form of regulation. It is the process of creating an official record or list of persons—for example, voter registration. The main purpose of registration is not to ensure the public of quality but to serve as a record-keeping function.

Under a certification system, practice of an activity or occupation is not directly restricted, but limits are placed on the use of certain occupational titles. The label *certified* publicly identifies persons who have met certain standards but does not prevent uncertified practitioners from engaging in the activity.

Under licensure, which is the most restrictive method of regulation, persons have no right to engage in a particular activity without permission to do so by the state. Such permission is generally conditioned on stringent requirements, such as certain educational qualifications and passage of an examination.

Because PAs must meet such standards and may not practice without state approval, *licensed* is the most appropriate way to describe the control exercised by states over PA practice. PAs are qualified to practice by graduating from an accredited PA educational program and/or by certification by the NCCPA.

Within the physician–PA relationship ...

Within the physician–PA relationship, PAs exercise autonomy in medical decision making and provide a broad range of diagnostic and therapeutic services. This term reinforces the concept of team practice while emphasizing the ability of PAs to think independently when making diagnoses and clinical decisions.

The clinical role of PAs includes primary and specialty care in medical and surgical practice settings in rural and urban areas. PA practice is centered on patient care and may include educational, research, and administrative activities.

The clinical role of PAs is varied depending on the clinical specialty and practice setting in which they work. This concept is integrated into the PA definition and also serves as a guiding notion throughout this book, which addresses the versatility of the PA profession, the distribution of the profession in all geographic regions, and the nonclinical roles that PAs may pursue.

What has emerged from defining the role of the PA is a template for a PA body to move within the tangles of state, provincial, and federal government rules and regulations. Not all countries have the same definition of a PA, but those who have a PA-like entity have crafted an assistant that stands alongside the doctor employer or doctor in charge as a colleague. New PA definitions are emerging, and new policies have been created for the governance of PAs in all countries. However, these policies are created with the interests of society in mind. What is significant in these instances is that these other countries have adopted the concept of the PA.

PHYSICIAN ASSISTANT: THE NAME

The name *physician assistant* has a historical base, and this history is outlined in Chapter 2. The name has been used since the concept originated but has not always been embraced. It is not embraced today because the title contains "assistant," a term that undervalues the role and level of function of PAs and is often misconstrued with medical assistants. Adding to the difficulty is the fact that the word *physician* means different things in different countries. *Physician* in the United Kingdom refers to an internal medical specialist—an internist. This notion was ignored when US doctors coined the name. Many speculate what the term should be and what it would have been had PAs themselves been asked. The United Kingdom changed the name to *physician associate* in 2014.

The original PA concept was of an assistant who would be able to handle many aspects of a doctor's work. Initially, the focus was on the education process, not the name. PA was not a copyrighted term, such as *physical therapist* or *psychologist*, but it generally conveyed what US doctors thought should be conveyed. Other names were proposed and continue to be proposed. For example, the term *medical care practitioner* was initially considered in England because of the inaccuracy of the word *physician;* however, the term *physician associate* has now been selected for use there. It was evident that the PA's role filled a healthcare delivery need, but before long, the movement was growing and taking on new dimensions. However, confusion arose about the label *PA,* which, after coming to public attention, was sometimes misused to describe a variety of individuals, including support personnel from physicians' offices.

The title *PA* is not a legally recognized term either nationally or internationally. However, National PA Day (October 6) is observed in most states. It is up to the states to protect the public's health, safety, and welfare by determining how the term *PA* is used. Generally, this means setting minimum standards and regulations to practice using a certain health profession or occupation. In the United States, state statutes and regulations define PAs as individuals who have graduated from an accredited program and passed the NCCPA examination. Although these statutes and regulations have not prevented some imposters from occasionally emerging, the known incidences are rare, and the checks and safeguards in place in most states seem sound.

An abundance of diminutive and unflattering names has been interchangeably used in both medical literature and the media with *physician assistant,* including midlevel provider, nonphysician provider, physician extender, allied health professional, healthcare practitioner, and advanced practice provider. However, AAPA's policy affirms that "physician assistant" is the official title of the profession. AAPA policy also provides that, whenever feasible, PAs should be referred to as *physician assistants* and not included with other providers in comprehensive general terms, such as *midlevel practitioner.* The official name of the profession has been fervently debated throughout its almost 50-year history.

From a historical standpoint, PAs themselves did not determine the title by which they would be known. Instead, educators, physicians, regulators, and advocates of the concept made the first suggestions for a name. Later, PAs exerted some influence in the drive toward

title uniformity when state laws were being enacted, accreditation and certification mechanisms were being established, and professional organizations were being founded. It was at this point that Eugene Stead observed, "The time has come to consider a new name for the product produced by Duke and other similar programs." Although he favored the title *physician's associate,* Stead (1971) concluded, "Agreeing on a name is the important step. What name is adopted is secondary." A number of names were advanced, including *Medex,* coined by Dr. Richard Smith at the Medex Northwest Physician Assistant Program at the University of Washington (Box 1–1).

Although *PA* has become the dominant title, proponents of changing it argue that it is not universally recognized and understood, which leads to problems with insurers, employers, and others.

Another argument for changing the title is that the term *physician assistant* does not accurately describe what PAs do. The AAPA describes PAs as "practicing medicine with physician supervision." However, as PAs have taken on more responsibilities for patient care, their role has evolved into more than that of an

BOX 1-1
Historic List of Proposed Names for Assistants to Physicians

Physician assistant (PA)
Physician's assistant, physicians' assistant
Physician associate, physician's associate
Medex (Mx)
Child health associate (CHA)
Surgeon's assistant (SA)
Anesthesia assistant and associate
Clinical associate
Community health aide
Community health medic
Medical services assistant
Medical care practitioner
Ophthalmic assistant
Orthopedic physician's assistant
Pathologist's assistant
Primex (Px)
Radiology physician's assistant
Syniatrist
Urologic physician's assistant
Flexner
Osler

"assistant." The scope of the medical services and level of care that PAs provide go beyond assisting physicians. In many underserved areas, PAs are the main primary providers of healthcare. Even if the term at one time appropriately described PA practice, some argue that it is no longer accurate.

In an era when consumers and patients are demanding more transparency, proponents of a title change also contend that the title is not readily understood. They argue that the title *assistant* is demeaning, deceptive, and inconsistent with the level of responsibility and autonomy involved in the role. It is associated with entry-level knowledge, on-the-job training, or trade-school education and implies that PAs are mere helpers or auxiliary personnel who facilitate the work of their superiors or function in subordinate positions. Those in favor of a name change believe the current title virtually ensures that PAs will be mistaken for medical assistants. This perception leads patients to conclude that they are receiving lower level care or that a physician will subsequently evaluate them. In some cases, patients have asked PAs when they plan to attend medical school. This confusion is demeaning to some PAs because it fails to credit the substantial clinical and didactic education they have received and disregards the fact that many have earned graduate degrees. The confusion brought on by the PA nomenclature is not limited to patients. Other healthcare providers, such as nurses, sometimes resist taking orders from PAs because they do not understand their role. Although such occurrences are becoming increasingly less common, proponents of a name change argue that they would never occur if the PA title accurately reflected the level of practice and expertise of the profession.

Some proponents of a name change favor the term *physician associate* because they believe it more accurately reflects the PA–physician relationship, avoids comparison with medical assistants, and is less confusing to the public. They also contend that such a change is reasonable given that, in the early days of the profession, some of the country's most prominent PA programs were "physician associate programs." In other parts of the world, *doctor's assistant, clinical assistants,* and *physician's assistant* are well-defined terms for people who support general practitioners. Advocates point to the change from *Medex* to *PA* that occurred easily and say a change could occur again, given the relative simplicity of changing the word from *assistant* to *associate*. Respect and self-esteem are gained by practicing with excellence and skill and by providing the best possible medical care to patients. These defenders find little or no dissatisfaction with the current title. For them, the title correctly conveys the dependent nature of the relationship with their supervising physicians.

For some, the issue is one of semantics. Clerks and telemarketers may be called *sales associates,* whereas high government officials hold the title *special assistant to the president;* in academics, assistant professors are still referred to as *professors.* Supporters of the current name say that time and growth, not a new name, will produce more recognition. The lack of universal recognition occurs because the profession is small and has a relatively brief history, but this situation is changing. The profession has already made an enormous investment in educating the patients and the public about the true meaning of the title *PA.* The title *physician assistant* is now familiar to most individuals in the healthcare sector and the public. A 2008 public opinion poll conducted by the AAPA revealed that two-thirds of all Americans were familiar with (had heard of) the term *PA.* Furthermore, state laws define the qualifications of those who use a particular title, and once the profession abandons the title *PA,* it could be awarded to another category of healthcare provider, such as unlicensed medical graduates.

Another important observation is that the laws of all legislative jurisdictions and the federal government could not be changed simultaneously. A period of years would pass, during which many different individuals would reap the benefits achieved by the PA profession by assuming the name and calling themselves PAs. In addition to the changes required by the state legislatures, licensing boards, and the federal government, other agencies would be required to make changes. Educational institutions, state and national

PA organizations, and the accrediting and certifying agencies would need to be persuaded to change. Many of these organizations would have to bear significant administrative and financial costs to make the change.

The argument most strongly expressed by opponents of change is that this debate draws time and effort away from issues that demand urgent attention. The PA profession is at a crossroads and is faced with unprecedented opportunities to define and influence its future. The name has been adopted in some countries; in others, a euphemism for PA has been derided. The options are varied. One observer says, "it is time for PAs to dedicate themselves to achieving the greatest benefit for the greatest number of people by becoming advocates for health promotion and preventive medicine."

Physician Assistant–Certified

US PAs who have passed the Physician Assistant National Certification Examination (PANCE) have the option of putting the word *certified* behind the title *PA*: PA-certified (PA-C). The intent of using *PA-C* is to distinguish formally trained PAs who are nationally certified from PAs who are informally trained and not eligible to sit for the PANCE. In the 1970s and 1980s, this distinction was thought to be important because the percentage of noncertified PAs was small but significant, and formally trained PAs felt they should have some way to show the public the difference. However, the certification is not recognized across all states and is considered superfluous by some. As the profession grows more global, this designation may be cast aside.

Generic Terms for Nonphysician Providers

One of the more confusing evolutions of names has been the effort on the part of health services workers and medical sociologists to develop a generic term that encompasses PAs and other workers who fill traditional physician roles, such as NPs and certified nurse-midwives (CNMs). One term used in the early 1970s was *new health professionals*. This was once the most frequently used term for PAs and NPs. Other terms that came into vogue were *physician extenders* and *midlevel practitioners*. These terms were never defined and remain largely meaningless: midlevel between whom? What does it mean to extend a physician? Another term carelessly used is *allied health*. *Allied health providers* is a term used rather restrictively to indicate only those occupations that are allied with the medical profession through their cooperative scheme of accreditation and certification organizations. This term has a fairly precise definition and is usually reserved for those occupations that support physician services, such as x-ray technicians, physical therapists, and medical laboratory personnel. Most in the PA profession are uncomfortable being lumped under the umbrella term of *allied health professionals*, in part because PAs practice medicine like physicians. Nurses are in an occupation that is not considered part of allied health, so it is not appropriate to refer to advanced practice nurses such as NPs and CNMs as allied health personnel. Similarly, it is not appropriate to refer to PAs as allied health personnel.

THE EVOLVING ROLE

During the formative years of the PA profession, many arguments were put forth about why this new health occupation was not needed or would fail. Among these arguments was the idea that PAs would be frustrated in their role and leave the field for greener pastures. The source of frustration envisioned by these critics was the stress and strain of being an "almost doctor" without the intrinsic or extrinsic rewards that society provides for physicians. For others, the intrinsic rewards of professional autonomy in clinical practice would not be available because of the need for close supervision by a physician.

For nearly 5 decades, the PA occupation has helped to fill a health sector niche with highly skilled professionals. These clinicians are capable of carrying out responsibilities that in the past had been within the physician's domain. Given the degree of formal training involved, the PA profession offers highly challenging and satisfying work.

Job Satisfaction

The demand in the medical sector for PAs continues to exceed the available supply, and this demand has been unabated for more than 20 years (Quella et al., 2015). The legal and bureaucratic obstacles preventing a broader scope of responsibilities in diagnosis and treatment were largely overcome during the first 2 decades. The initial view held by some that PAs would become frustrated because of a narrow and limited professional role is now untenable. The intrinsic rewards are there, and the job satisfaction of PAs remains high.

A career as a PA is an attractive alternative to the years of competition, pressure, long hours, and expense required to enter and complete medical school and to finish residency training. Even 30 years ago, some recognized that a career as a PA was an alternative to the narrower scope of work and lower pay available to the nursing profession (Hooker, Kuilman, & Everett, 2015). The nature of the career affords PAs the opportunity to practice in varied specialties, disciplines, and settings throughout their career, a flexibility not readily available to physicians, NPs, and some other medical professionals.

PAs have the responsibility and independence most could reasonably expect. Role frustration is certainly present but does not appear to be a dominant problem. In fact, PAs have reported high levels of career satisfaction in several recent AAPA surveys, including the latest (AAPA Survey, 2014). PA salary levels and career advancement opportunities have steadily expanded over the last 2 decades. The demand for graduates of PA programs is greater than the number of applicants entering PA education programs (McDaniel, 2015).

The Need for Research

In the first decade of the PA movement (1965 to 1975), there was considerable interest in exploring the characteristics of this new healthcare profession. As the profession matures, renewed vigor for research that will shed light on the understanding of this group of highly motivated, well-trained, compassionate healthcare providers is expected. This work will likely emerge from concentrated efforts around the world. Such research should help the PA profession to become an even more dynamic force in the improvement of the quality and availability of healthcare for all people.

Qualification for Practice and Legal Parameters

Federal, state, and provincial medical practice statutes and regulations define the scope of practice activities, delineate the range of diagnostic and patient management tasks permitted, and set standards for professional conduct. Qualification for entry to practice as a PA in most areas requires that individuals possess a fairly uniform set of characteristics. These requirements usually include a certificate of completion verifying graduation from a PA educational program accredited by some national body and/or proof of having sat for and obtained a passing score on a national examination. In the United States, the PANCE is a standardized test of competence in primary care medicine administered annually by the NCCPA.

The clinical professional activities and scope of practice of PAs are regulated by federal, state, and provincial licensing boards, which are typically boards of medicine; in some instances, however, a separate PA licensing board exists. The PA profession appears to be comfortable with its dependent practice role and has not wavered in that stance since its inception. In contrast, NPs have articulated a position of practice independent from physicians. Statements by professional nursing organizations have stirred debate with physician groups at the national level regarding the turf of primary care and related legal practice barriers and regulations. Although NPs are professionally autonomous in the performance of nursing care functions, most state medical and nursing practice regulations require that NPs work in collaboration with a physician practice, recognizing that their extended roles encompass medical diagnostic and therapeutic tasks. Thus, in providing medical care tasks, most NPs work closely with physicians in a majority of clinical settings.

The legal basis of PA practice is centered on physician supervision. Doctors are ultimately responsible for the actions of the PAs, and state laws typically require that physicians clearly delineate the practice scope and supervisory arrangements of employed PAs. However, wide latitude exists within the physician's practice for the PA to exercise levels of judgment and professional autonomy in medical care decisions (Davis et al., 2015).

It has been noted that the level of acceptance and integration of PAs in American medicine is related to the profession's continued adherence to this position and to the PA's willingness to practice in settings, locations, and clinical care areas that physicians deem to be less preferable. Observers believe that PA use will continue as long as it extends the medical care services of physicians without competing for or challenging physician authority and autonomy.

SUMMARY

Continual evolution and enlargement of the PA, both in development and role, have spanned a half century. As for employment, the 15-year future appears rewarding for new graduates of this profession. What pitfalls the distant future contains can be anticipated but only to a limited degree. A worldwide shortage of doctors and the limited number of medical schools portends permanent shortages for two-thirds of the globe and equally represents a continued need for the PA profession.

References

The following citations are key to supporting this chapter's content. You can find a complete list of citations for all chapters at www.fadavis.com/davisplus, keyword *Hooker*.

American Academy of Physician Assistants. (2014). *2013 AAPA Annual Survey Report.* Alexandria, VA: American Academy of Physician Assistants.

Cawley, J. F. (2008). Physician assistants and Title VII support. *Academic Medicine, 83*(11), 1049–1056.

Cawley, J. F., Cawthon, E., & Hooker, R. S. (2012). Origins of the physician assistant movement in the United States. *Journal of the American Academy of Physician Assistants, 25*, 1–7.

Davis, A., Radix, S., Cawley, J. F., Hooker, R. S, & Walker, C. (2015). Access and innovation in a time of rapid change: Physician assistant scope of practice. *Annals of Health Law, 24*(1), 286–336.

Hooker, R. S., Kuilman, L., & Everett, C. M. (2015). Physician assistant job satisfaction: A narrative review of the empirical research. *Journal of Physician Assistant Education, 26*(4), 176–186.

Hooker R. S., & Cawthon E. A. (2015). The 1965 White House Conference on Health: Inspiring National Policy and the Physician Assistant Movement. *Journal of the American Academy of Physician Assistants, 28*(10). 46-51.

Hudson, C. L. (1961). Expansion of medical professional services with nonprofessional personnel. *Journal of the American Medical Association, 176*, 839–841.

McDaniel, M. J., Hildebrandt, C. A., & Russell, G. B. (2016). Central Application Service for Physician Assistants (CASPA) ten-year data report 2002–2011. *Journal of Physician Assistant Education, 27*(1), 17–23.

Quella, A., Brock, D., & Hooker, R. S. (2015). Physician assistant wages and employment: 2000–2025. *Journal of the American Academy of Physician Assistants, 28*(6), 56–63.

Schneller, E. S. (1978). *The Physician's Assistant: Innovation in the Medical Division of Labor.* Lexington, MA: Lexington Books.

Stead, E. A., Jr. (1971). Use of physicians' assistants in the delivery of medical care. *Annual Review of Medicine, 22*, 273–282.

US Department of Health and Human Services, Health Resources and Services Administration, National Center for Health Workforce Analysis. (2013). *The US Health Workforce Chartbook.* Rockville, MD: US Department of Health and Human Services.

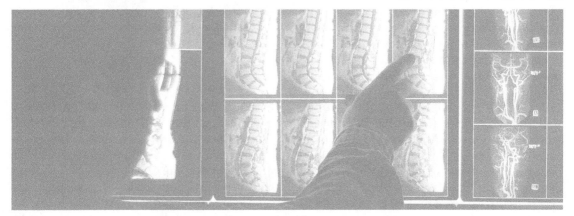

CHAPTER 2

DEVELOPMENT
OF THE PROFESSION

JAMES F. CAWLEY ■ RODERICK S. HOOKER ■ CHRISTINE M. EVERETT

"If you don't know history, then you don't know anything. You are a leaf that doesn't know it is part of a tree."

—Michael Crichton

The 1960s saw a rethinking of healthcare delivery in the United States. The physician assistant (PA) emerged from that reconceptualization, along with two other healthcare professionals: the nurse-midwife and the nurse practitioner (NP). The PA, nurse-midwife, and NP were the products of demand for greater healthcare access, especially for the nation's medically underserved citizens. All three professions benefited from federal activism in health workforce policy. However, the PA had one characteristic not shared with the new nursing professionals: a connection in the public's mind with returning Vietnam War veterans.

Several energetic individuals, notably Harvey Estes, Eugene Stead, Jr., Henry Silver, and Richard Smith, conceived and promoted their particular versions of the PA. Advocates of this new health profession worked through existing medical education programs and federal healthcare initiatives. Their efforts, sometimes informed by models of nonphysician healthcare abroad, received critical support from private philanthropy and eventually gained widespread acceptance. Some accepted the idea of a PA because physicians sanctioned it; other members of the public found that PAs improved access to care in rural and isolated locales or in underserved urban areas. Many physicians seemed comfortable with the idea because the PA was trained in the medical model and the American Medical Association (AMA) offered its stamp of approval. As optimistic as the originators of the PA movement were, even they did not anticipate the critical role that PAs would play in healthcare delivery well into the new century. PAs in the United States continue to influence medical providers in other areas of the world.

DEVELOPMENT OF THE PHYSICIAN ASSISTANT CONCEPT

The establishment of the PA was a remarkable occurrence in American medicine: a voluntary sharing of privileges by one type of medical professional with another. This represented a major transformation in US medical practice. The PA movement in America came about from a convergence of circumstances: increased specialization of physicians, the demise of the general practitioner, advancing technology, returning veterans with medical training, the war on poverty, other federal policies, and charismatic leaders who understood the processes of education and apprenticeship. The public accepted the PA concept because physicians sanctioned it; other members of the public found that PAs improved access to care in rural and isolated locales or in underserved urban areas. Many physicians seemed comfortable with the idea because PAs were trained in the medical model and because the AMA had offered its stamp of approval. In the 1960s, the fledgling PA profession took on tasks from the once sovereign domain of medicine. The empowerment of PAs was facilitated, in part, by relative animosity between organized medicine and organized nursing (Holt, 1998). The failure of these two powerful groups to work together to solve the problem of access to healthcare in the post–World War II decades advanced the concept of an assistant to the physician. Those who envisioned the PA as a force in US medicine were wise in certain specific strategies they employed: initially utilizing veterans, not taking other professionals out of their roles in the healthcare workforce, and creating a dependent practice framework that allowed PAs to function in concert with physicians rather than in competition with them. This construct, termed *negotiated performance autonomy* by one medical sociologist (Schneller, 1978), marks the major difference between PAs and NPs, who seek a more independent stance in practice from physicians.

A factor that contributed to the establishment of US PAs were the models that existed abroad. There was the assistant medical officer in Fiji and Papua, New Guinea; the apothecary in Ceylon; the *behdar* in Iran; the public health worker in Ethiopia; the clinical assistant in Kenya; the barefoot doctor in China; the *practicante* in Puerto Rico; the rural nurse in Cuba; the *officier de santé* in France; and the *feldsher* in the Soviet Union. Some in the United States promoted the generic name "assistant medical officer" (AMO) to describe this type of healthcare worker.

A New Social Climate

One historian famously characterized medicine in the 20th century as a "sovereign profession" (Starr, 1982). The term flowed from the way in which US hospitals assumed greater size and prestige in the late 19th to mid-20th century, and as a result, their close association with physicians grew proportionally. Linkages between physicians, hospitals, and medical education strengthened physicians' power over health affairs. By the middle of the 20th century, physicians had cultural prominence, professional independence, and political influence over the health system.

The AMA was a dominant player in many critical decisions affecting healthcare. It protected the interests of physicians—their income and security as well as their professional stature. Allopathic physicians in the middle of the 1900s embraced discoveries in microbiology, surgery, and diagnostic imaging. The US public perceived that physicians controlled access to those exciting technologies. Medicine also grew more specialized. No longer was it typical for urban physicians to consult with patients, hospitalize them, provide anesthesia, and perform surgery; rather, each of those functions became the purview of a specially trained medical expert.

Given the rise in the US population in the late 1940s to middle 1950s, medical specialization led to another key development among US physicians: a shortage of general practitioners. By 1949, the number of full-time specialists had risen to 62,688 (almost doubling the number of specialists that there had been in 1940), while the number of general practitioners and part-time specialists had dropped by nearly 10,000 from the 1940 level of 120,090. The self-shunting of physicians into specializations meant that access to general medical physicians was decreasing.

One hope for encouraging general practice rested with legislative measures such as the Wagner-Murray-Dingell Bill of 1943. That proposal would have instituted a federal system of compulsory health insurance in the United States along the lines of Great Britain's national health insurance scheme. Rather than pursuing such a course, the federal government instead adopted payment policies that rewarded medical specialist services at higher rates than generalist services. Medical care based in hospitals was especially privileged.

During the 1950s, the AMA insisted that there was an adequate supply of physicians. From outside the medical community, however, came pressure to rectify a perceived shortage of primary care health providers. In 1953, the President's Commission on the Health Needs of the Nation predicted a physician shortage of 59,000 by 1960. Influential studies such as the Bayne-Jones Report of 1958, the Bane Report of 1959, and the Millis Commission Report of 1963 expressed concern about a physician shortage and recommended the establishment of new medical schools. In 1964, the AMA Committee on Medical Education recommended that a new specialty in family practice be established to address the shortage of primary care providers. Such concerns about a lack of physicians, especially in the general medical care setting, continued into the 1970s and persist today in the current decade.

Some people who sought to address the shortage of physicians envisioned a "physician extender" who would perform medical tasks that had previously been reserved only for physicians. Such an adjunct to physicians was supposed to expand the capabilities of physicians in the delivery of primary care, particularly in medically underserved populations. One of the earliest suggestions to create this type of medical provider came in 1961 from Charles Hudson, then president of the National Board of Medical Examiners (NBME). Hudson put forth the notion of "externs" for physicians. The rationale for this new type of healthcare provider was grounded in changing hospital staffing demands and innovations in technology. He planned for the extern to be directly responsible to a physician. Hudson expected that nursing professionals would resist the creation of such a physician adjunct. While Hudson contended that the "goals of nursing would be redefined as part-nursing and part-medicine," he predicted that nurse leaders would frown on "the proposal of a medicine-nursing hybrid."

The First Physician Assistant Programs

Duke University

It was Dr. Eugene A. Stead, Jr., Chairman of Medicine at Duke University, who transformed Hudson's prophecy into reality by developing the first training program for persons who would assist physicians as medical providers (Figure 2–1). Stead had long been interested in breaking down barriers in medical education. While at Emory University, he worked with third- and fourth-year medical students as hospital staff at a time when the intern staff went from 15 to 0, due in part to the WWII draft being extended to physicians in training. Despite their limited training, these medical students gave "superb medical care." Stead envisioned a medical clinician who could be

FIGURE 2-1
Eugene A. Stead, Jr., MD

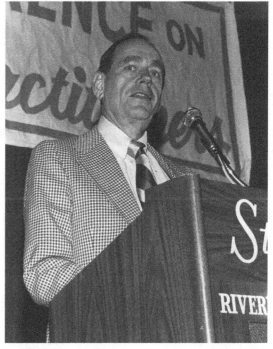

Courtesy of the American Academy of Physician Assistants.

trained in a relatively short time to assist physicians in a broad range of practice settings.

Stead attempted to train nurses to function in the role of assistants to physicians. Thelma Ingles, a nursing leader at Duke who was interested in an advanced medical role for nurses, approached him. Stead and Ingles experimented with training approaches to expand the nursing role in generalist medical care delivery. Stead had great respect for nursing experience in patient care. After creating a prototype advanced medical training program for nurses at Duke, he concluded that nurses "were very intelligent and they learned quickly, and at the end of a year we had produced a superb product, capable of doing more than any nurse I had ever met" (1967).

This program could have initiated the NP movement. The National League of Nursing, however, refused to accredit the proposal on three occasions, with the judgment that delegating medical tasks to nurses was inappropriate. In 1964, Stead, frustrated with his experiment based on the model of the nurse, formulated a plan for the establishment of a program to train assistants to physicians. Increasingly, Stead and others employed the term *physician assistant* to describe the novel healthcare worker they envisioned. Members of an ad hoc committee that Smith charged with developing a proposal for PAs were physician researchers who had worked with Navy hospital corpsmen in the course of their training at the National Institutes of Health and Bethesda Naval Hospital.

Stead, the committee, and others wondered if medics and corpsmen could serve as adjuncts to physicians. Holt (1998) contends that Stead considered Vietnam War veterans to be ideal candidates to assist physicians because they had experience with conflict and controversy. Richard Smith, who played a pivotal role in promoting the same concept through the MEDEX program at the University of Washington, which developed shortly after, recalls reasoning why former military medics were considered ideal for these initiatives: "America could not slam the door on the corpsman," a reference to their hero status (Figure 2–2). Several ex-military personnel were working at

FIGURE 2-2
Richard A. Smith, MD

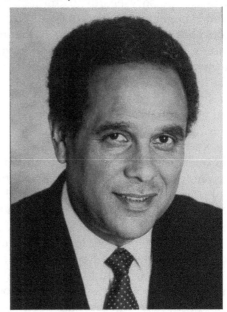

Courtesy of the American Academy of Physician Assistants.

Duke in hyperbaric medicine research. One of Stead's assistants, James Mau, a former Navy fighter pilot, recalled that newly discharged corpsmen often had extensive field medical experience. Some possessed advanced skills in acute injuries, laboratory medicine, x-ray capability, suturing, fracture stabilization, and ventilation therapy.

The war in Vietnam produced a large pool of militarily trained medical personnel. The roughly 6,000 medically trained veterans returning per year in the early 1970s were an ideal substrate for the health workforce experiments of Stead, Smith, Silver, and others. The medic and corpsman clearly were associated in the minds of the public with the PA in the 1960s and 1970s. Indeed, this was the focus of an AMA promotion of the PA concept. Historian and archivist Reginald Carter (2001) points out that an AMA advertisement in *Life* magazine's July 30, 1971, issue depicted a young African American veteran washing windshields. The advertisement proposed that his medic training would be better utilized as a PA. However, the supply of medically trained veterans shrank as

US involvement in the Vietnam War wound down through the 1970s. By 1978, 42% of the 4,500 PAs in practice were ex-military medical corps members. It was also the case in 1978, however, that 51% of PAs had backgrounds as medical technicians or technologists rather than in military service. And despite the tendency to see PAs as male in the 1960s and 1970s, in 1978, nearly one-quarter of PAs were nurses—and, at that time, nursing was an overwhelmingly female-dominated profession.

In 1965, Duke University inaugurated the first formal PA program, consisting of a curriculum based on the traditional medical education model of training. This plan of study was devised and implemented by Drs. Stead and E. Harvey Estes (Figure 2–3). The goal of the 2-year program was to "expose the student to the biology of humans and to learn how

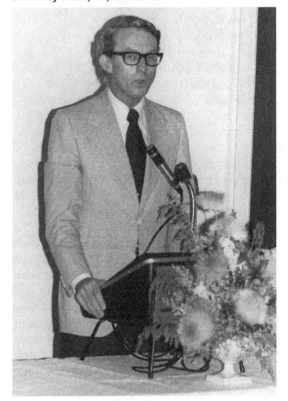

FIGURE 2-3
E. Harvey Estes, Jr., MD

Courtesy of the American Academy of Physician Assistants.

physicians rendered services." By graduation, PAs had learned to perform many tasks previously performed only by licensed physicians and could serve a useful role in many types of practices.

The Duke prototype rapidly expanded. In 1969, Stead retired from active professional duties at Duke. Under Estes's leadership, the Duke program increased its number of students, physical facilities, and scholarship. The audacity of this new program attracted immediate attention far beyond its size. It provided the curricular model for new programs at other institutions.

If the idea of a PA movement was a gleam in the eyes of its creators, its success rested squarely on the shoulders of its first students. The first PA graduates recalled thinking that, if any of them did poorly, it could be the early demise of the movement. Victor Germino, a graduate of the first class, had a background as a surgical technician and a corpsman. He practiced in the hyperbaric unit at Duke for 5 years. Afterward, he joined an adventurous group of PAs who sought to work in occupational medicine on the Alaska pipeline. The Alaska pipeline contributed to the acceptance of PAs among the public. During the mid- to late 1970s, more than 200 PAs accepted pipeline positions. The jobs were based in Fairbanks, Alaska, but the actual practices were located hundreds of miles north near Prudhoe Bay. In such a setting, PAs were the only medical providers. Conditions were rugged, but the pay was very good. These PAs seemed to thrive with little to no direct physician supervision and endeared themselves to a whole generation of laborers. Many PAs traveled to Alaska to serve 6- to 9-month stints, returned to the United States mainland for a time, and then engaged for another period of remote practice (Marzucco, 2013).

University of Washington (Medex Program)
Richard A. ("Dick") Smith ranks alongside Stead and Estes as a pioneer in the PA movement. The MEDEX program, started by Smith at the University of Washington, was an innovative approach to health professions education. A strong sense of social purpose informed

Smith's vision of medical education. Smith's interest in medicine was stimulated in 1951 during a college summer work camp in Cuba in the cane fields, where he observed a nurse running a rural clinic. He decided that he wanted to become a medical missionary and train people to provide basic health services in underserved areas.

Smith attended medical school at Howard University and completed a residency in public health and preventive medicine at the University of Washington. In 1960, he requested that his church's mission board send him overseas as a trainer of new healthcare providers; the request was turned down. Undaunted, he asked England's Archbishop of Canterbury to present his plan to the World Council of Churches meeting in New Delhi, India, in 1961. Once again, his plan to "multiply my hands" by training other healthcare providers on a large scale was declined. He turned to public health.

When Smith joined the US Public Health Service, he was assigned to the Indian Health Service in Arizona in the early 1960s. This assignment was followed by 2 years in the Peace Corps in Nigeria. Some of his ideas were formed as a result of visiting medical missionary Albert Schweitzer at Lambaréné Hospital in Gabon, West Africa. Upon returning to the United States, Smith worked in the US Surgeon General's office from 1965 to 1968, eventually becoming Deputy Director of the Office of International Health. While in the Surgeon General's office, Smith, an African American, was assigned to lead the effort to desegregate hospitals in the South.

In the 1960s, Smith became acquainted with Dr. Amos Johnson from Garland, North Carolina. Johnson employed an assistant, Buddy Treadwell, who figured prominently in the development of the PA profession. Treadwell's ability to take care of routine medical and surgical tasks with minimum supervision and to keep the practice open while Johnson attended medical seminars and meetings were specific reasons cited by Stead for training a "new type of clinical support personnel for physicians." Without Treadwell, Johnson would not have been in a position to lead the American Academy of General Practitioners during watershed moments or to champion the establishment of family medicine as a specialty. Johnson also introduced Dick Smith to the leadership in the AMA.

Smith created the MEDEX concept (a contraction of the two words "*medic*ine" and "*ex*tension"). It was a collaborative model of healthcare development that actively involved health professions schools, local and national medical organizations, rural and urban communities, and overworked practicing physicians. MEDEX aimed to deploy clinicians to rural and remote areas. Smith wanted MEDEX to be more than a demonstration project that was underwritten by the federal government and then forgotten a few years later. He had earned his master's in public health at the University of Washington and, upon leaving the Surgeon General's office, relocated there, trusting that his familiarity with local medicine and politics would be an advantage.

In 1968, the MEDEX Demonstration Project was jointly sponsored by the University of Washington and the Washington State Medical Association and funded by the National Center for Health Services Research. One year later, the first MEDEX class of 15 former military medical veterans began their training; they graduated in 1970. Initially, the program was 1 year long and consisted of 3 months of intensive didactic work in basic and clinical sciences at the university medical center, followed by a preceptorship with a practicing primary care physician for 9 months. Graduates put *Mx* after their names. In 1971, as a result of Smith's work, an amendment to the Washington Medical Practice Act was passed, allowing Mx (PAs) to practice medicine under the supervision of a licensed physician.

The MEDEX program differed from the Duke model in that entering students needed to have considerable health experience. Students received most of their training on the job with selected physicians in rural areas of the Pacific Northwest. Often, these sponsoring physicians became employers. The MEDEX movement caught on: By 1974, eight programs were distributed from the inner city of the Watts district of Los Angeles to rural areas such as Alabama, North Dakota, and Hershey, Pennsylvania.

Programs also emerged at the University of Utah, the University of South Carolina, and Dartmouth College.

Expansion and Early Acceptance of the Concept

The PA concept would not have germinated and become successful had it not been for the overt support of major physician groups. The notion that physicians were able to directly control the activities of the newly created PAs was to a large degree responsible for their acceptance. The AMA contributed substantially to confirming legitimacy along with acceptance of the concept and providing a strong role in the establishment of standards of PA educational program accreditation. The earliest correspondence with the AMA related to the concept of a PA involved Stead and Estes, who convinced organized medicine that this was an idea that would provide benefit to physicians. Stead and several of his colleagues introduced a resolution in the AMA House of Delegates to encourage state medical boards to amend medical practice acts to sanction PA practice. A critical event in the survival of the PA concept was the unexpected endorsement given to it by the AMA in 1969.

Support for the development of the PA profession also came from the American College of Surgeons, the American Academy of Family Physicians, the American Academy of Pediatrics, and other medical groups. Such organizations were involved in the formation of two critical systems that were vital parts of the young profession: the PA program accreditation system and the national certifying examination. The AMA assumed a major role in establishing the program accreditation structure through its Subcommittee of the Council on Medical Education's Advisory Committee on Education for Allied Health Professions and Services in 1971. The Joint Review Committee (JRC) of the AMA was the organization that developed the *Essentials for an Accredited Program for the Assistant to the Primary Care Physician*, the accreditation standards document. The JRC also conducted on-site evaluation visits to programs seeking accreditation status. A similar structure of substantial physician organization involvement was seen in the development of the certifying examination and the certification agency.

Had the PA movement gained momentum in the 1950s, there might not have been adequate support on any front; effective prototypes would have also been lacking. One imagines considerably more resistance during the 1950s to the efforts of African American medical leaders, such as Richard Smith, than occurred just after the passage of the Civil Rights Act of 1964. Moreover, had impetus for development of the PA begun in the 1970s, the family physician and NP movements might have eclipsed the PA.

Holt (1998) contends that the major health profession groups—the AMA and the American Nurses Association (ANA)—played a relatively small role in the earliest conceptual days of the formation of the PA from 1961 through 1965. She notes, however, that there was a good deal of debate about the PA, particularly within the ANA, which denounced the creation of the PA primarily because it was proposed by medicine. Yet once the PA initiatives began at Duke, the University of Washington, and the University of Colorado, with the resultant ripple in other educational institutions, the necessity to involve and gain the approval of the AMA was key.

In the 1960s, the fledgling PA profession took on tasks from the once sovereign domain of medicine. That empowerment of PAs was facilitated, in part, by relative animosity between organized medicine and organized nursing. The failure of these two powerful groups to work together to solve the problem of access to primary healthcare in the post-WWII decades advanced the concept of an assistant to the physician. Those who envisioned the PA as a force in US medicine were wise in certain specific strategies they employed: initially utilizing veterans, not taking other professionals out of their roles in the healthcare workforce, and creating a dependent practice framework that allowed PAs to function in concert with physicians rather than in competition with them. This construct, termed *negotiated performance autonomy* by one medical sociologist, marks the major difference between PAs and NPs, who seek a more independent stance in practice from physicians.

In the 1960s, the originators believed the PA would supplement physicians' work. At the half-century mark, however, PA specialization has become the norm. There is another recent development in the PA movement, especially given the early association between Vietnam-era corpsmen and the PA: the increasing prominence of women in the field.

Specialty Physician Assistance Models

Trends in specialization took place in the late 1960s as well, including a surge of new programs to train nonphysician providers in specific areas of care. Examples include the orthopedic assistant and the urologic PA, 2-year programs designed to train personnel to work directly for specialists. A 4-month "health assistants" training program sponsored by Project Hope in Laredo, Texas, was launched in 1970. The program was intended to improve healthcare among the Hispanic population. The only requirement for entry was that the student had to be 18 years of age. Of the 11 students who entered the first class, eight lacked high school equivalence but were able to earn their General Equivalency Diploma certificate on completion of the program.

Other specialty program areas included gastroenterology, allergy, dermatology, and radiology. In fact, the radiology program at the University of Kentucky and the pathology program at Duke University lasted longer than most specialty programs. By 1971, more than 125 programs in 35 states announced they were training "physician support personnel" (Bureau of Health Manpower Education, 1971). Yet it is interesting to note that the concept of the primary care PA became consolidated in the early years. By 1975, the PA concept was anchored in primary care and survived; at the same time, most of the specialty programs expired (although a few converted to primary care models).

Most primary care–based programs flourished. A number of these programs were sponsored by academic health centers. By 1972, a total of 31 programs were in operation: 21 of the programs were federally supported by agencies such as the Office of Economic Opportunity, the Model Cities Program, the Veterans Administration, the Public Health Service, the Department of Defense, and the Department of Labor, whereas the remainder were financed by private foundations and institutional sources. Throughout the 1970s, private philanthropy from the Robert Wood Johnson Foundation, the Macy Foundation, and the Brunner Foundation provided start-up support for a number of new PA educational programs.

Nursing and the Evolution of the Physician Assistant Concept

In the 1960s, organized nursing was not interested in expanding its role to one that included the medical model. What became the PA concept was less appealing to nurses because organized medicine had suggested it. Beginning with the initial proposal of Stead and Ingles in 1964, and later in 1969 when the AMA suggested the recruitment of nurses to be trained as PAs, the ANA flatly rejected these ideas. The rejection was based on the view that nurses were unwilling to be subordinate to physicians in performing professional duties and served as a reminder to medicine that it is not the prerogative of one profession to speak for another.

Ultimately, the position of the ANA became: "If physicians want additional assistance, they can have it, but nurses should not supply the manpower [sic]." Despite this attitude on nursing's part, Loretta Ford, RN, and Henry Silver, MD, started the first NP program at the University of Colorado. Ironically, when this development occurred, physicians were quick to suggest that NPs were practicing medicine, whereas nursing leaders claimed that NPs had left nursing to become handmaidens to physicians. Later, however, nursing leaders suggested that the NP role had done much to invigorate nursing as a whole.

The AMA proposed the PA profession as an opportunity for nurses to leave their field to gain more responsibility and pay. Referencing the fact that most PAs were men and earned salaries equal to or higher than more formally educated nurses, the ANA retorted by characterizing the new role as a bit of "government-supported male chauvinism." What leaders at the respective organizations did not know was that the PA concept was the result of nearly a decade's work by Stead, Smith, Silver, and others. These leaders were exploring options for training healthcare professionals—nurses among them—for advanced clinical roles. The dialogue between the AMA and ANA on the PA was often characterized by sharp language and strong debate over the new profession. It is becoming axiomatic that miscommunication and misunderstanding between medicine and nursing caused their respective professional organizations to remain at odds rather than promote collaborative endeavors (Holt, 1998).

Stead had great respect for nursing experience in patient care. After creating a prototype advanced medical training program for nurses at Duke, he concluded that nurses "were very intelligent and they learned quickly, and at the end of a year we had produced a superb product, capable of doing more than any nurse I had ever met" (Holt, 1998). This program could have initiated the NP movement but was refused accreditation as an educational program by the National League for Nursing (NLN), the agency for degree-granting nursing programs, because the NLN determined that delegating medical tasks to nurses was inappropriate. This early foray into advanced practice nursing programs was eventually phased out. Ingles left Duke for the Rockefeller Foundation, and Stead was left with a conviction that people with varied backgrounds can deliver high-quality patient care if adequately trained, which led to the historic development of the first PA program at Duke University.

EARLY PROFESSIONAL CHALLENGES

A wide range of challenges faced the new PA profession: deciding on a common name for the new profession; promoting acceptance by physicians, patients, and other health professionals; establishing systems of educational program accreditation; creating a national system of certification; and, perhaps most important, obtaining legal recognition within the medical regulatory system. State health professions regulatory statutes were needed in all US jurisdictions, which would be based on physician dependency and include a scope of practice that would permit PAs to essentially practice medicine (diagnostic and prescriptive authority) but not require independent licensure (Ballenger & Estes, 1971). This process proceeded state-by-state over 3 decades, culminating in 2000 when practice authorization was passed in Mississippi.

Naming the Profession

As the PA profession grew, experimentation to identify a more appropriate title also took place. The title *physician's assistant* was problematic because it incorrectly indicated possession by the physician and was not initially well accepted by physicians and PAs alike.

Silver (1971) suggested a new term, *syniatrist*, from the Greek *syn*, signifying "along with" or "association," and *-iatric*, meaning "relating to medicine" or a "physician." He proposed that the *syniatrist* terminology have a prefix relating to each medical specialty; for example, general practice would be a *general practice syniatrist associate* or a *general practice syniatrist aide*. Smith opted for the term *MEDEX* and saw his graduates placing the letters "Mx" after their names as an appropriate and distinct title. Other proposed titles in lieu of PA included *Osler, Flexner,* and *Cruzer,* in honor of famous figures in American medical history. The intent of these new names was to be neutral, less controversial, and less demeaning than the term *physician's assistant.* Although some professionals preferred the term MEDEX, there were no strong advocates for any one term in particular and none reached prominence enough. Thus, the title "physician assistant" remains.

In 1970, the National Congress on Health Manpower (sponsored by the AMA's Council on Health Manpower) sought to develop uniform terminology for the many emerging PA programs. The congress concluded that the term *physician's assistant* was too general to be adopted as the single generic term because PAs were receiving varied levels of training. They decided that *associate* would be a preferred term for healthcare workers who assume a direct and responsible role in patient care and act as colleagues to physicians rather than as technical assistants. The congress also noted that the PA terminology was often confused and used interchangeably with the established term *medical assistant*, the title for a nonprofessional office helper who functions in a clerical and technical fashion. However, the AMA's House of Delegates rejected the *associate* terminology in the belief that *associate* should be applied only to physicians working in collaboration with other physicians. (This criticism ignores the 's, which denotes that the *associate* is not another physician.) Thus, no consistent position emerged from organized medicine.

In the United States, the new health practitioner concept initially embodied multiple types of healthcare providers, including PAs. Educational curricula designed to train a variety of PA-style healthcare providers were becoming abundant in the late 1960s. In 1970, the Institute of Medicine of the National Academy of Sciences (NAS) unsuccessfully attempted to classify various types of PAs according to the degree of independent function in exercising medical judgment. The board report identified three levels of PAs: Type A assistants, Type B assistants, and Type C assistants:

■ *Type A assistants* were capable of collecting patient history and physical data and organizing and presenting them so the physician could visualize the medical problem and determine appropriate diagnostic or therapeutic steps. The assistant could help the physician by performing diagnostic and therapeutic procedures and coordinating the roles of other more technical assistants. Functioning under the general supervision and responsibility of the physician, the assistant was permitted to practice under defined rules without the immediate surveillance of the physician. The assistant was qualified to integrate and interpret clinical findings on the basis of medical knowledge and to exercise a degree of independent judgment.

■ *Type B assistants*, although not equipped with general knowledge and skills relative to the entire range of medical care, possessed exceptional technical expertise in a clinical specialty or in certain procedures within such a specialty. Within a specialty area, this provider had a degree of skill beyond that of a Type A assistant

and perhaps beyond that normally possessed by physicians who are not engaged in the specialty. Because Type B assistants' knowledge and skill were limited to a particular specialty, they were less qualified for independent action.

■ *Type C assistants* were capable of performing a limited number of medical care tasks under the more direct supervision of a physician. These providers were similar to the Type A assistants in the areas in which they could perform, but they could not exercise the degree of independent synthesis and judgment.

Initially, the NAS classification of PAs using the Type A, B, and C system appeared to help define the nature of the relationship and division of duties between physicians and PAs, but it was soon discarded because it tended to create confusion within the hierarchy of emerging models of PA providers. The leaders of MEDEX programs were unhappy with this concept; their graduates were assigned a Type C rating, whereas Duke graduates were assigned a Type A rating—designations based on perceptions of formal training rather than on past healthcare experience. Although this system was changed and refined, eventually the entire NAS classification scheme lost relevance in attempting to capture the emerging nature of the PA–physician relationship and was abandoned.

Garnering Support of Organized Medicine

Initially, some physicians received the idea of a PA coolly, and only a few were initially willing to engage in the novel experiment of a formally trained assistant for physicians. Ken Ferrell, from the first Duke class, recalls that some of the physicians who would have benefited most from assistants were quite resistant to the idea. They were reluctant to relinquish any of their responsibilities, even though they were overworked.

Ultimately, however, the PA concept would not have germinated and certainly would not have succeeded without the overt support and active involvement of major physician groups. The AMA in particular contributed substantially to confirming legitimacy and acceptance of the concept and had a strong role in the establishment of standards of PA educational program accreditation and professional credentialing organizations. Support for the development and shaping of the infrastructure for the PA profession also came from the American College of Surgeons, the American Academy of Family Physicians, the American Academy of Pediatrics, the American College of Physicians, and other medical groups. These groups worked to build the critical components of the profession's structure, particularly legal and regulatory components. PA practice certification mechanisms were patterned to a large degree on their counterparts in the medical profession. An example of medical collaboration was the creation of the National Commission on Certification of Physician Assistants (NCCPA), the national credentialing agency for the PA profession that administers the Physician Assistant National Certifying Exam (PANCE). Physician and PA groups worked with government agencies, the NBME, the Federation of State Medical Licensing Boards, and members of the public to create the NCCPA, and most of these groups continue to comprise the governance of the organization.

Establishing Federal Policy

The critical role of the federal government in nurturing the development of new healthcare practitioners in general, and the PA in particular, came about through specific legislation. The Comprehensive Health Manpower Training Act called for the Bureau of Health Manpower to provide support for educational programs for PAs and other nonphysicians. This act established the education grants program that was administered by the Bureau of Health Manpower under the Health Resources Administration of the Department of Health, Education, and Welfare, mandated by Section 774a of the Public Health Service Act as Public Law 93-157.

Shortly thereafter, assistance for 24 of the then 31 existing programs and contracts with 16 developing programs was initiated. Federal support represented an investment in health profession programs to test the hypothesis that nonphysician healthcare professionals could provide many physician-equivalent services in primary and continuing care. The bureau's programs were designed to carry out the intent of Congress to relieve problems of geographic and specialty maldistribution of physicians in the healthcare workforce. This intent was reflected in the contract process, which required each PA program to emphasize the following three major objectives in its demonstration:

- Training graduates for delivery of primary care in ambulatory settings
- Placing graduates in medically underserved areas
- Recruiting residents of medically underserved areas, minority groups, and women as students for these programs

Each program was free to devise various curricula and methods of instruction, but the preceding three requirements were held constant to carry out the intent of Congress. This factor contributed to the demise of most Type B and C programs; they either folded in a few years because of lack of funding support or converted into primary care programs. The only survivors are the SA, CHA (which teaches primary care and qualifies graduates for national certification), and pathologist's assistant programs.

PHYSICIAN ASSISTANT ORGANIZATIONS

Once the initial challenges of the PA profession were beginning to be addressed, early leaders recognized the importance of organization of efforts. The American Academy of Physician Assistants (AAPA) was founded by students at Duke University in 1968 (Figure 2–4), and the Association of Physician Assistant Programs (APAP) was founded by physician faculty from major PA educational programs in 1972. These organizations led collective efforts in determining policy direction for the nascent profession in terms of the establishment of certification processes and professional standards and in efforts to obtain federal and state funding for PA program development.

PA programs of all types proliferated between 1965 and 1970. This period of unwieldy growth preceded the development of accreditation standards in 1971 and national certification

FIGURE 2-4
AAPA Leaders with Conference Guest Richard Schweiker, then Secretary of Health and Human Services, Circa 1981 [From left: Peter Rosenstein, Bruce Fichandler, Jarrett Wise, Richard Schweiker, Dee Alexander, Ron Fisher, and Charles Huntington]

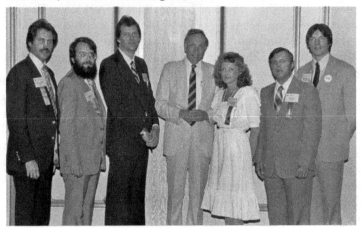

Courtesy of the American Academy of Physician Assistants.

requirements in 1973. Consequently, many of these programs were highly experimental. The curricula for these "generalist" and "specialist" programs ranged in length from a few weeks to more than 4 years, depending on the background of the student and on the role the "new health practitioner" was to play. Programs were located in medical schools, schools of allied health professions, universities, colleges, junior colleges, hospitals, clinics, and federal facilities.

On the state licensure front, the first attempt at professional standards of legal recognition was the American Registry of Physicians' Associates, which was incorporated in North Carolina on May 26, 1970. Robinson O. Everett, Martha D. Ballenger, and D. Robert Howard signed the Articles. The first board of directors included Robert Ewer, MD, University of Texas, Galveston; D. Robert Howard, MD, Duke University; and Leland Powers, MD, Bowman Gray School of Medicine. The purpose of the Registry was to encourage training and to promote and regulate the activities of physicians' associates by determining their competence through examinations and investigative studies. It would grant and issue certificates to graduates of approved educational and training programs and to others who demonstrated by

examination that they possessed the background and experience to perform satisfactorily as graduates of approved programs.

Duke University and several other programs started using the term *associate*, rather than *assistant*, to distinguish their programs from the Type B and C programs, and the term *associate* became embedded into the registry's name. Bylaws were adopted, officers were elected, and other university-based programs soon joined the registry. Graduates of these programs were eligible to apply to the registry and be certified as *registered physicians' associates*. Once registered, the graduates were encouraged to place the initials RPA after their names, wear a lapel pin and patch with the registry's patented insignia on it, and display a signed certificate from the Registry in their offices. From May 1970 until April 1972, Dr. Howard served as the Registry's first appointed and then elected president until Alfred Sadler, MD, of Yale University, assumed the position. Dr. Powers served as secretary treasurer until Susanne Greenberg of Northeastern University assumed this role, keeping minutes and handling the organization's finances.

Although a useful focal point for exchange of ideas, the registry did not meet educators' broader academic needs. In April 1972, at the fourth Duke Conference in Durham, North Carolina, PA educators decided to form the APAP. A meeting of the registry was held after the APAP meeting and the Registry was formally transferred to the AAPA. The academy's first task was to elect new officers of the registry. William Stanhope was elected president, Steven Turnipseed secretary, Jeffery Heinrich treasurer, and Gail Spears member-at-large.

Along with the APAP and AAPA, the registry appeared as a cosponsor on the programs distributed at the first and second National Conference on New Health Practitioners, held in 1973 in Wichita Falls, Texas, and in 1974 in New Orleans, Louisiana. With the administration of a national certifying examination for PAs in 1973 and the development of the National Commission on Certification of Physician Assistants, which became operational in 1975, the need for the registry disappeared and the organization was liquidated by the AAPA soon thereafter. At its peak, the registry included 12 member programs and listed more than 125 graduates as registered physicians' associates.

EVOLUTION OF THE PHYSICIAN ASSISTANT PROFESSION

All social movements have periods of evolution, and the development of the PA profession is no exception. To appreciate the evolution of the PA profession, the history of the PA profession can be divided into six periods. These periods span the first 5 decades of the PA profession. As stages in the evolution of the PA profession, the natural history of other nonphysician professions is shown in Box 2–1.

Period 1: Ideology (1960–1969)

The PA was envisioned as a new type of medical generalist, one whose role would build on previous medical experiences. As such, PAs would be trained in a shorter time than medical students and then be deployed to practice locations in medically needy areas. The concept of an assistant to a primary care physician in rural and underserved areas was idealized during this time. The concept was put into action,

PA programs were inaugurated (independent of each other), and the concept began to gel.

Period 2: Implementation of the Concept (1966–1975)

Charismatic leaders and the federal government provided strong support for the creation and early development of PAs in the healthcare system. Domestic policy in the early 1970s sought to improve citizen access to health services by increasing the development and dispersal of healthcare personnel. Most policymakers believed there was a shortage of physicians overall, with a decreasing proportion in general practice. Because organized medicine had not adequately addressed these issues, a new federal workforce approach was created. This initiation consisted of two major elements:

- Expansion of physician supply by expanding medical education
- Promotion of the introduction of new practitioners whose roles would focus on primary care.

The early 1970s was a period of intense activity and evolution for the PA concept. During this period, the key organizations representing the profession were founded: the AAPA in 1968, the APAP in 1971, and the NCCPA in 1973. Also during this time, the mantle of responsibility for the continuation of the development of the PA profession was passed on to the next cadre of progressive-thinking physician educators who had assumed leadership positions in medical education. These individuals were also leaders in medical and regulatory organizations.

Legal and Regulatory Challenges
The introduction of the PA into the US health system brought with it the necessity to consider appropriate legal and regulatory approaches to enable these and other emerging healthcare practitioners to enter clinical practice. Important decision points were the determination of the scope of practice of these new professionals, appropriate levels of state board recognition (licensure, registration, and certification), and stipulations for supervision and prescribing activities (Ballenger & Estes, 1971).

BOX 2-1
Summary of Stages in the Development of the New Health Professionals

STAGE I—IDEOLOGY

- The existence of an appropriate social, medical, and political climate; medical personnel factors; and educational influences leads to a coherent rationale and expected role necessitating the creation of a new category of health personnel.
- This rationale must gain the acceptance of critical existing stakeholders in the health system (e.g., physicians and nurses, government health policymakers, educational institutions, medical regulators, state legislators, and health administrators).
- The climate in which the conceptualization of new health occupations develops helps set the stage. Stakeholders must perceive a benefit. Public policymakers must be convinced that introduction of a new health profession will benefit society by improving health services and not directly threaten existing professions.

STAGE II—IMPLEMENTATION

- Key health policy, medical education, and organizational collaboration grow to implement the conceptual framework, educational preparation, and professional regulation of the new profession.
- Critical areas must be defined: length and level of training, curriculum content, scope of practice, legal status and mechanisms of regulation, sponsorship and funding, and credentialing.
- Academic institutions begin to develop educational programs.
- Levels of state recognition (licensure, regulation, or certification) of practice activities for new practitioners entering medical practices are organized. Systems of educational sponsorship, academic recognition and accreditation, professional credentialing, occupational regulation, and definition of practice scope are established.

STAGE III—EVALUATION

- Conduct and evaluation of organized health services research and public policy analysis are designed to measure the levels of clinical performance effectiveness and practice characteristics of the new professional: measurement of levels of acceptance by patients, physicians, and other professionals; content and quality of care; cost-effectiveness; practice deployment; and role satisfaction.
- Studies begin to examine longitudinal trends of provider utilization patterns and professional demographics in the health system.

STAGE IV—INCORPORATION

- Steady growth and acceptance of the new professionals occurs.
- Utilization extends from original generalist/primary care roles to include specialty areas.
- Clinical practice settings include private solo and group medical offices; hospitals, health facilities, and organizations; academic centers; managed care systems; long-term care facilities; and public health clinics.
- Legislation is promulgated in states, authorizing medical licensing boards to regulate the new health professional.
- Regulations are adopted permitting new professionals in health workforce supply and requirements planning.
- Summary policy reports on impact and practice experiences are published.

STAGE V—MATURATION

- Acceptance and institutionalization of the profession among the health occupations occur.
- The acceptance of educational institutions is evidenced by faculty appointments for PA educators.
- Professional utilization patterns are characterized by steady, ongoing demand for practitioners' services by both patients and physicians and continuing utilization in a variety of medical care settings.

STAGE VI—GLOBALIZATION

- Growth extends to other governments; these countries modify the model of the nonphysician clinician.
- Program development changes to adapt to the nuances of each country.

To support the entry of PAs into clinical practice, in 1970, the House of Delegates of the AMA passed a resolution urging state medical licensing boards to modify health occupations statutes and regulations to permit PAs to qualify as medical practitioners. Among the first states to amend medical acts allowing PAs to practice were Colorado, North Carolina, California, and New York. On the federal level, important leadership in the early nurturing of the PA concept was provided by the government in the form of grant support for PA educational programs. Legislative initiatives included the Allied Health Professions Personnel Act of 1966 and the Health Manpower Act of 1968. PA programs quickly sprang up in medical centers, hospitals, and colleges; state legislatures and private foundations provided support for education programs as well.

State Regulation

The legal basis of PA practice is codified in state medical practice statutes granting authorization to licensed physicians to delegate a range of medical diagnostic and therapeutic tasks to individuals who meet educational standards and practice requirements. Authority for medical task delegation is based on the legal doctrine of *respondeat superior,* which holds that it is the physician who is ultimately liable for PA practice activities and mandates that physicians who employ PAs appropriately define and supervise their clinical actions. State acts exempt PAs from the unlicensed practice of medicine with the stipulation that they function with physician supervision.

Professional activities and the scope of practice of PAs are regulated by state licensing boards, which are typically boards of medicine, boards of health occupations or, in some instances, separate PA licensing boards. Laws define PA qualification requirements, practice and professional conduct standards, and the actions of the PAs. State laws commonly require physicians to delineate the practice scope and supervisory arrangements of PAs. Medical practice acts define the boundaries of PA practice activities but tend to vary considerably by state, particularly with regard to scope of practice, supervisory requirements, and prescribing authority. This variability led to barriers in practice effectiveness in a number of states. After 40 years, all of these barriers have been overcome.

As originally envisioned, the role of a PA working with a physician encompassed the full range of clinical practice areas: office, clinic, hospital, nursing home, surgical suite, and patients' homes. In many states, laws were written to give PAs a scope of practice, allowing physicians to delegate a broad range of medical tasks to PAs. This latitude allows PAs to exercise a degree of clinical judgment and autonomic decision-making within the parameters of state scope of practice regulations and the supervisory relationship. Although innovation tended to precede legislation, eventually laws and policies were considered essential for PAs to be fully effective in practice. Geographic practice isolation in rural and frontier settings may, by necessity, result in varying degrees of offsite physician supervision and require the PA to exercise some autonomy in clinical judgment, particularly when the PA is the only available onsite provider. Regulatory reluctance to support such physician–PA relationships in satellite and remote clinical settings restricts the PA in extending and providing services that might otherwise be unavailable.

Practice regulations have progressed from a delegatory model achieved by amending medical practice acts to a regulatory/authority model wherein healthcare licensing boards are explicitly authorized to govern PA practice (Davis et al., 2015). Typical state regulatory acts establish PAs as agents of their supervising physicians; PAs maintain direct liability for the services they render to patients. Supervising physicians define the standard to which PA services are held vicariously liable for services performed by the PAs under the doctrine of *respondeat superior.*

Practice Qualification

Over a number of years and by the actions of state legislatures, a standard emerged for PA practice: qualification as a PA requires that individuals be graduates of an accredited PA educational program and pass the PANCE.

Physician Assistant Education

Establishment of formal accreditation standards for PA programs marked an important milestone for the PA profession. Initially established by organizations affiliated with the AMA in 1971, the Council on Education for Allied Health developed standards for PA program accreditation, promulgated as the *Essentials of an Approved Educational Program for the Assistant to the Primary Care Physician.* Authority for PA program accreditation was set within the Commission on Accreditation of Allied Health Education Programs (CAAHEP). In 2000, the Accreditation Review Committee on Education for the Physician Assistant (ARC-PA) became an independent accrediting body for the PA profession, separate and independent of the CAAHEP. Over the years, the accreditation criteria underwent frequent revisions reflecting changes in educational preparation in a rapidly developing field. The *Essentials,* as they were called, were revised and updated in 1978, 1985, 1990, 1997, and 2000. Minor changes are made frequently. Accreditation is necessary for PA programs to receive federal Title VII grant funding and in most states for program graduates to qualify for entry to practice. The *Standards*, as they were later referred to, define the necessary core components of PA educational programs, the nature of institutional sponsorship, the curriculum content, clinical training affiliations, basic and clinical science course offerings, faculty qualifications, and admission and selection guidelines (McCarty et al., 2001). Early versions of the *Standards* were written to permit PA educational programs a wide degree of latitude to create curricular configurations based on a structure awarding several types of academic degrees.

Period 3: Evaluation and Establishment (1976–1980s)

The Comprehensive Health Manpower Act of 1973 was an important legislative milestone, marking the inclusion of PA program funding support programs. Since then, federal awards supporting PA educational programs have totaled more than $200 million. In fiscal year 2002, programs received $6.4 million, although by 2008, the amount dispensed under Title VII for PA programs declined to about $2 million.

A great deal of health services research was performed during the 1970s and 1980s examining the impact of PAs when introduced into medical practice. Both the PA and the NP concepts and related advanced practice nursing programs were novel medical education experiments, and their outcomes were the target of intense social research focus. After a decade of studies, more than 100 research publications revealed that PAs were well accepted, safe, and effective practitioners in medical care delivery. Studies also showed that patient acceptance of the PA role was high and that most PAs worked in primary care practices in medically needy areas (US Congress, Office of Technology Assessment, 1986).

PAs can lower healthcare costs while providing physician-equivalent quality of care. Even though PA cost-effectiveness has not been conclusively demonstrated in all clinical practice settings, substantial empirical and health services research supports this finding. The present increasing use of and market demand for PAs in clinical practices would be unlikely if they were not cost-effective to some degree. There is evidence that the organizational setting is closely related to the productivity and possible cost benefits of PA utilization.

Initial PA practice distribution tended to reflect the federal and medical sector intent that PAs assume primary care roles in areas of need. Early recruits to the PA profession typically were individuals with extensive levels of prior healthcare experience (e.g., military medical corpsmen, registered nurses, physical therapists, and emergency medical technicians), factors thought to contribute to their ability to function effectively with a minimal level of physician supervision. Selection of physician preceptors in rural areas was then and remains a goal of many of the programs. After graduation, many PAs selected primary care physicians located in rural or medically underserved communities.

Many of the seminal evaluations of PA use were performed in ambulatory practice and in health maintenance organization (HMO) settings. In such settings, PA clinical performance has been impressive. Their productivity (number of patient visits) has been shown to approach and sometimes exceed levels of primary care physicians. PA productivity rates in a large group model HMO show that the physician/PA substitutability ratio, a measure of overall clinical efficiency, was 76%. This assumed a practice environment in which PAs were used to their maximum capacity to perform medical services (consistent with educational competency and legal scope and/or supervision) and that they worked the same number of hours per week as physicians.

By the end of the first decade of practice for PAs, experience and empiric research indicated that US medicine's adoption of the PA had been generally positive. PAs were responsive to the public and the medical mandate to work in generalist and primary care roles in medically underserved areas. As their numbers pushed 10,000 in 1980, PAs were gaining recognition as being competent, effective, and clinically versatile healthcare providers after major health research studies revealed their clinical effectiveness (US Congress, Office of Technology Assessment, 1986).

An important element in the acceptance and use of PAs was the development of a single pathway to licensure based not only on formal education but also on a nationally standardized certification examination. Recognizing the need for a credentialing body, which would be organizationally separate from the profession, the NCCPA was formed in 1973 and formally chartered in 1975. The NCCPA administered the first PA certifying examination in 1973 and began issuing certificates shortly thereafter. Soon the PANCE became recognized as the qualifying examination for entry to PA practice by a rapidly increasing number of state medical licensing boards. The NCCPA was established with federal and private grant support and assistance from the AMA and was closely linked to the NBME in the development of the PANCE and later the recertifying examinations for PAs. During the late 1970s and early 1980s, the PANCE examination and the NCCPA certification process had become incorporated into the practice acts of most state medical practice statutes. By the 1990s, successful completion of the PANCE became a universal qualification for PA practice.

Period 4: Recognition and Incorporation (1981–1990)

By the early 1980s, PAs as well as the other non-physician health professions (such as NPs and nurse-midwives) had become widely used and accepted and their roles in specialty practice expanded. The cumulative results of the past decade of health services research and practical experience with PAs were overwhelmingly positive, with the specific measures being patient and healthcare professional acceptance, quality of care, cost-effectiveness, productivity, and clinical versatility (Schafft & Cawley, 1987; US Congress, Office of Technology Assessment, 1986).

For a time, it appeared that the sole focus of PA practice would be primary care, although not all demand for PA services was in primary care. The PA role broadened during the 1980s when utilization extended beyond primary

care into inpatient hospital settings and specialty areas. The trend toward specialization by PAs was the result, in part, of their clinical versatility and the health workforce demand. Market forces were at work and many medical and surgical specialties realized that the services of a PA could be used on inpatient hospital floors and in various settings. In 1977, the percentage of PAs working in the primary care specialties—defined as family practice, general internal medicine, and general pediatrics—was 77%. In 1981, the percentage had fallen to 62%. From 1981 to 2001, the percentage had settled at 50%. Over the same period, the percentage working in surgery and the surgical subspecialties rose from 19% to 28%, and PAs in emergency medicine rose from 1.3% to 10% (and continues to grow).

During the early 1980s, the prediction of the Graduate Medical Education National Advisory Council of a rising number of physicians in the workforce prompted questions about the future of PAs. Yet after a few years of doubt, during which utilization was sluggish and several PA educational programs closed (e.g., University of Indiana, Johns Hopkins University, and Stevens College), the PA profession continued to evolve and gain ground.

Recognition of PAs occurred during the 1980s on several levels. At the federal level, two landmark events signaled incorporation of the occupation into the healthcare workforce mainstream. Perhaps the most significant of these was the congressional passage in 1986 of an amendment to the Medicare law providing reimbursement policies for PA services under Medicare Part B (the Omnibus Budget Reconciliation Act, 1986). Recognition by Medicare, the largest health insurance program in the nation, indicated the legitimacy of PA services in medical care service delivery.

Another event that represented a major landmark for the profession on the federal level was the attainment of commissioned officer status among uniformed services in 1988. Although this milestone tends to have little impact on PAs today, it was highly significant at the time and involved efforts on many levels to obtain. Physicians, nurses, physical therapists, and administrators were commissioned. PAs had gradually moved from senior enlisted ranks to warrant officers, but full commissioning was a ceiling that was not breached until the Air Force did away with warrant officers and commissioned their PAs as full officers. Given the rich history between the military and the PA profession, this event was of particular significance and satisfaction to the profession.

A less obvious but no less important set of events that occurred during this time was the increasing number of states passing legislation to update medical practice acts recognizing PA practice. This achievement was incremental, yet the progress in the aggregate was significant. Then (as well as now), many policy changes occurred on the state level. Most of them were enactments or substantial improvements. Good Samaritan laws were enacted to protect PAs. Policies changed to allow PAs to work some distance from a physician. Reimbursement restrictions were lifted in some states, and in others, PA programs were inaugurated with tax dollars.

Research on PAs, their behaviors, and their comparisons to physicians began to appear. More than just anecdotal observations, experiments, manipulation of variables, and hypotheses began to drive the research. The research emerged as credible, and critics became fewer in number.

On an organizational level, the AAPA headquarters in Alexandria, Virginia, was erected in 1987. The building, modeled in Georgian architecture characteristic of the area, marks the establishment of the PA profession as a permanent member of the health professions on the national organizational level.

Period 5: Maturation and Establishment (1991–2001)

By the 1990s, the PA profession had achieved a remarkable degree of integration in US medicine. Over the preceding 30-year period, they gained acceptance and incorporation in healthcare delivery, federal policies endorsed their presence in society, and they reached a critical mass as a profession.

As a recent entrant, in contrast with other new professions, the PA profession was consolidated early in its representative organization and became well stabilized. Among the notable indicators of further advancement of the profession is how often it is incorporated into national health policy projections and debate. Longevity has added depth to PA roles and status. On the federal level, PAs have been considered relevant players in healthcare reform under various proposals. Significant achievements included the passage of enabling legislation in all states and prescribing in all states. For example, the Balanced Budget Act (BBA) of 1997 better clarified the Medicare policy of PA reimbursement. States have modified their practice acts to enable PAs to practice with few barriers. Together with primary care physicians and NPs, PAs are considered essential members of the US primary care workforce. During this period, healthcare reform and universal medical care access became a political instrument for politicians. President William J. Clinton was pushing for health reform, as were many legislators. First Lady Hillary Rodham Clinton was the keynote speaker at the AAPA convention in 1993. In 1992, Mrs. Clinton convened a working committee to overhaul the federal system of healthcare and extend the care to all people. To do so, she included PAs, NPs, and nurse-midwives in the mix. Subcommittees were formed to assess the role and responsibilities of PAs.

There was much speculation that, if Clinton-era healthcare reform legislation passed, the demand for primary care providers to serve the uninsured population would be strong. This demand, in turn, would result in a heightened market for PAs and other primary care providers. For the PA profession, this possibility was seen as a potential boom period during which the number of programs and graduates would markedly expand. Although the Clinton reform plan did not become law, the expansion of the PA profession indeed occurred. From 1994 to 2001, the number of PA education programs doubled, as did the number of annual program graduates. A number of papers generated from this spurt of activity assessed the role of the PA and NP in managed care organizations, which may have stimulated employment.

The power of marketing came into play in unexpected ways. The award-winning television show *ER* did much to raise awareness about the role of PAs in healthcare delivery. A bright, personable, intelligent, knowledgeable, and sympathetic figure was found practicing in various PA roles in the hospital and before the camera from one week to the next for a few years.

Period 6: Global Expansion (2001 to present)

For PAs, the new century was heralded in a number of ways. The evolution of enabling legislation was complete, with Mississippi being the last state to grant licensure for PAs. In 2007, Indiana became the last state to grant prescription rights to all PAs. More than 50 years of change have taken place: from the first graduates to the granting of enabling legislation, prescribing rights, and reimbursement nationally. What started as a noble experiment in the back room of a medical school evolved into a system of healthcare delivery across 50 states and most of the US territories. Countries such as Canada, Great Britain, Germany, Australia, India, Saudi Arabia, Liberia, Ghana, South Africa, and The Netherlands are producing their own graduates. Increasingly, the world is recognizing and allowing PAs to work. More than 115,000 people have graduated from formal PA programs, and more than 100,000 are working clinically.

By 2014, the PA profession encompassed professional practicing in primary care as well as in specialties and subspecialties. As if to add legitimacy, the federal government in the United States (the Department of Veterans Affairs and the military) and Canada (military) are the largest single employers of PAs.

In 2014, the $2.9 trillion cost for healthcare in the United States had steeled its citizens to do something in regard to efficiency, organization, and financing. PAs represented an opportunity for change for consumers, purchasers, providers, and insurers. Healthcare was no longer dominated by a fee-for-service model, and the majority of Americans had been pulled into managed care organizations that were more oriented toward health prevention and wellness than toward illness—a situation ideal for PAs with their training and emphasis on health promotion. The HMOs and preferred provider organizations (PPOs) also attempted to limit "unnecessary care" and offer networks of providers who could deliver a set of healthcare benefits for a fixed fee. Medicine became a corporate endeavor, and the PA was the ideal employee who could assume care for many routine cases of medicine and do it well with little supervision.

The worldwide expansion of the PA concept is perhaps the major landmark of this era. Globalization of PA development marks it as a stellar profession worthy of being adopted in other cultures and lands. For countries such as The Netherlands, South Africa, the United Kingdom, Australia, and Canada to embrace PAs is testimony that this occupation has merit worth emulating. The policies and practices of these countries means the concept of the PA will be redefined and modified in ways not fully anticipated by its developers. However, the PA is no longer an American product. Whereas the PA still embodies the role of assistant to the physician, this role means different things to different governments.

History has a way of repeating itself. Some of the social issues worked out between 1980 and 2000 in the United States for PA inclusion will become struggles for some other countries (and might need to be worked out again). Organized medicine in such countries may oppose the development and expansion of the PA role. What will most likely prevail is some modification of the assistant to the physician that emerges in the best interest of the people whom medicine serves. If the PA movement is found wanting, it will die. On the other hand, the current number of physicians is insufficient to meet the public's needs. With demand driving public outcry for more medical care access, the only alternative to doubling the cadre of physicians is to expand the presence of the PA.

THE MODERN PHYSICIAN ASSISTANT PROFESSION

The history of the PA profession is a remarkable one from a number of standpoints. Visionaries such as Eugene A. Stead, Jr., Richard Smith, Harvey Estes, Henry Silver, Loretta Ford, and others believed that lack of improvements in healthcare delivery demanded transformation. From what became a prime impetus for change, the PA emerged. Instead of the "one great man" theory that often precedes important social movements, a few great people with similar ideas that fit the medical and societal needs of that time founded the PA profession. Today the product has exceeded even the boldest imagination of its creators.

In modern medicine, the creation of the PA marked the occurrence of physicians voluntarily deciding to share with another healthcare provider the key intellectual and professional functions of performing medical diagnosis and treatment. These activities were legally and functionally in the sole domain of physicians until the creation of PAs.

Some assert that curriculum revisions to increase primary care experiences for medical students should consider the approaches developed and used in PA educational programs. Innovation has flourished in PA programs partly because of their multidisciplinary design and partly because they have greater latitude in making curricular adjustments. PA programs have been pioneers in incorporating topic areas increasingly recognized as important in medical education: behavioral sciences; communication sciences; the humanities; epidemiology, preventive medicine, health promotion, and disease prevention; geriatrics; and community-based practice and community-oriented primary care. Educators of PAs are also proven innovators in the development of effective strategies in deploying graduates to medically underserved areas and in primary care specialties. The cumulative experiences of PA programs, including those ensconced in academic health centers, teaching hospitals, colleges, and universities, are successful educational endeavors. There are 200 accredited PA programs in the United States and more than a dozen outside of the United States (along with others in development) that prepare competent and versatile generalist providers capable of handling most patient problems encountered in many settings.

To what degree has the PA profession succeeded in fulfilling a key objective of its creation: service in meeting the needs of medically needy populations? A traditional part of the social mission of medicine has been to provide health services that meet the needs of a nation's population. American medicine continues to be criticized as being overly specialized and unresponsive to the health needs of many citizens. Since the 1980s, the US workforce policy reform debate has centered on policy questions of the accountability of the nation's workforce to meet societal healthcare needs, in particular the needs of the uninsured, the rural citizens, and the medically underserved. Government study groups have concluded that the present system of health professions education and composition in the United States seems ill fit to meet the nation's future needs for healthcare providers. US policymakers remain frustrated with the realization that, despite the substantial expansion of physician numbers over the past 2 decades as well as the long-standing federal Medicare subsidy of graduate medical education, the number and percentage of physicians who select primary care continues to dwindle. The creation of the PA and the NP professions has helped to alleviate this shortage, but demand for services continues to outstrip supply in rural and underserved areas. America has failed to produce a balanced healthcare workforce and has fallen short of meeting the nation's need for generalist medical care services and universal access to care.

For the creation of the PA to have occurred, the critical issue of practice autonomy had to be addressed. Medical sociologists regard autonomy as the most important defining attribute of a professional within occupations, particularly the health occupations. Medicine, like law and religion, have long been regarded as the true professions: Physicians possess their own language and distinct body of knowledge, collect direct fees for their services, are autonomous in function, and are largely self-regulated. The dependent-practice role of PAs and their willingness to function within the practice of the physician and under supervision has been a critical factor in their acceptance, utilization, and success. The decision to establish the role of the PA as a dependent professional role—one characterized by a close practice relationship with a supervising physician—was a product of the collective wisdom of the profession's founders. They recognized that acceptance and use of these new providers held a direct relationship to the perceptions of physicians regarding the threat PAs might present in terms of income and professional domain. Dependent practice for PAs represented the central condition on which physician groups first accepted the PA concept. That PAs practice with supervision has always been the major factor in their acceptance and use.

There is little question that the American experience with PAs has been successful. This is due, in large part, to a close educational and practice relationship with physicians, an affiliation that stands them in good stead. Many similarities exist between the medical training approaches of PAs and primary care physicians. They are now well integrated into many medical practices, all working with physicians, nurses, and others on the healthcare team.

Conventionally defined "barriers to practice" clearly affect levels of PA clinical productivity in a broad sense, and differences in the delegatory styles of physicians are important determinants of PA practice effectiveness. Formalized barriers to practice effectiveness (e.g., restrictive regulations and payment ineligibility) represent the major limiting factors in PA use. This is manifested in clinical practice style, overlap, and in many instances, scope of practice. Professional domain ("turf") issues arise almost universally between health professionals. Yet despite this, physicians now share more of their medical diagnostic and therapeutic responsibilities with PAs than they did in 2000. That they continue to share medical functions is a result of generational shifts, social forces, changing healthcare environments, and the inevitable division of complex labor.

SUMMARY

In the turbulent 1960s, a decade of change in many areas of US society, a fundamental restructuring of the division of medical practice labor evolved. The introduction of the PA and the NP, along with the rebirth of the nurse-midwife in North America, represented a major transformation in US medical practice. The role of the PA was created to assume a scope of practice that included medical tasks previously reserved for physicians. The concept developed with a medical and societal expectation focusing on extending the capabilities of physicians in the delivery of primary care, particularly to medically underserved populations and those in rural areas. After 4 decades of existence, PAs have gained widespread recognition in nearly all aspects of medical care delivery in the United States and the concept has extended globally.

In terms of its educational systems, the PA profession has evolved successfully in preparing tens of thousands of PAs for active medical practice. The present model of PA education and certification gives graduates an opportunity to obtain employment in a primary care or generalist area or in a specialty or subspecialty area and to have clinical career-long specialty flexibility. There is strong evidence that PA educational approaches have been successful in preparing healthcare providers for employment in the healthcare system and beyond. The creators of the profession looked at models of nonphysician health personnel, such as the European *feldsher*, the Chinese barefoot doctor, and the military corpsman. This examination gave credence to the notion of developing a more rational structure of healthcare personnel, one that made more efficient use of the training and capabilities of physicians and provided the opportunity to utilize nonphysicians to maximal effectiveness.

The trend toward international utilization of PAs represents a type of coming full cycle in the natural history of these personnel. Now PAs are recognized for their clinical versatility and assist industrialized countries in addressing medical workforce shortages. PAs are particularly valuable in supplementing doctors and replacing physicians in areas of physician shortage. In some systems, reluctance to create a new category of practitioner exists—a concern sometimes raised by nurses. However, the PA concept may encourage highly qualified people into the health system who might not otherwise have been attracted to it.

The use of various health professionals has at times been championed as an attack on medical elitism and the professional establishment, as was the circumstance with the barefoot doctor. Stead believed that the medical profession has been arrogant in its stance toward entry policies and pathways leading to medical licensure. PAs have demonstrated high levels of patient acceptance and function with shorter training than that of physicians. Early critiques of PAs were that they represented a second tier of medical care. Yet PAs have been able to augment the delivery of primary care to various patient populations, including the poor, those in medically underserved areas, and other disadvantaged members of society, and they do this in proportions greater than physicians. The employment of PAs in various roles, spanning most primary care functions as well as a wide swath of technical and public health and preventive medicine duties, appears to be an appropriate niche in the systems of many countries.

References

The following citations are key to supporting this chapter's content. You can find a complete list of citations for all chapters at www.fadavis.com/davisplus, keyword *Hooker*.

Ballenger, M. D., & Estes, E. H., Jr. (1971). Licensure or responsible delegation? *New England Journal of Medicine, 284*, 330–332.

Bureau of Health Manpower Education. (1971). *Selected training programs for physician support personnel.* Washington, DC: National Institutes of Health, Department of Health, Education and Welfare.

Carter, R. (2001). From the military corpsman ranks. *Perspective on Physician Assistant Education, 12*, 130–132.

Davis, A., Radix, S., Cawley, J. F., Hooker, R. S., Walker, C. (2015). Access and innovation in a time of rapid change: Physician assistant scope of practice. *Annals of Health Law, 24*(1), 286–336.

Holt, N. (1998). "Confusion's masterpiece": The development of the physician assistant profession. *Bulletin of the History of Medicine, 72*, 246–278.

Marzucco, J., Hooker, R. S., Ballweg, R. M. (2013). A history of the Alaska physician assistant: 1970–1980. *Journal of the American Academy of Physician Assistants, 26*(12):45–51.

McCarty, J. E., Stuetzer, L. J., & Somers, J. E. (2001). Physician assistant program accreditation—history in the making. *The Journal of Physician Assistant Education, 12*(1), 24–38.

Schafft, G. E., & Cawley, J. F. (1987). Geriatric care and the physician assistant. *The physician assistant in a changing healthcare environment.* Rockville, MD: Aspen.

Schneller, E. A. (1978). *Physician assistants: Innovation in the medical division of labor.* New York: Ballinger.

Silver, H. K. (1971). The syniatrist. A suggested nomenclature and classification for allied health professionals. *Journal of the American Medical Association, 217*, 1368–1370.

Starr, P. (1982). *The social transformation of American medicine.* New York: Basic Books.

Stead, E. A., Jr. (1967). The Duke plan for physician's assistants. *Medical Times, 95*, 40–48.

US Congress, Office of Technology Assessment. (1986). *Nurse practitioners, physician assistants, and certified nurse-midwives: A policy analysis* (Health Technology Case Study 37). Washington, DC: Government Printing Office.

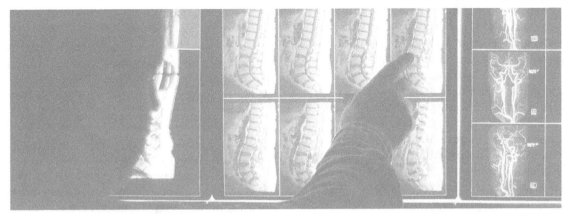

CHAPTER 3

CURRENT STATUS: A PROFILE OF THE PHYSICIAN ASSISTANT PROFESSION

RODERICK S. HOOKER ■ JAMES F. CAWLEY ■ CHRISTINE M. EVERETT

"Facts do not cease to exist because they are ignored."

—*Aldous Huxley*

The physician assistant (PA) of the new millennium does not fit any convenient stereotype. No longer just a creation of the United States, the profession is a product of various countries and has the capability to adjust to any healthcare environment. The role of the PA has been shaped over a half century to meet the needs of people around the world by adapting to various medical disciplines and health systems. The United States alone has produced more than 110,000 PA graduates and, as of 2016, at least 100,000 are actively certified (National Commission on Certification of Physician Assistants, 2016). Outside of the US there are more than 2,000 PA graduates of new and emerging educational programs—sometimes with different names, such as *physician associates* and *clinical associates*. Practice and employment settings are diverse,

ranging from family medicine in urban areas to surgery in rural locations.

The PA profession was asked by its early proponents to prove that it could provide quality care to the underserved, reduce the perceived personnel shortage in healthcare, and make the lives of physicians less harried. Many of these goals were achieved in the first few years within the confines of the limited number of personnel being trained in relatively small programs and occurring in three countries almost simultaneously. However, the criteria by which effectiveness is judged have changed, and the healthcare context has also shifted radically, raising new questions about the role of PAs.

Describing the characteristics of PAs requires drawing a profile, incorporating contemporary data regarding their practice activities, distribution, specialties, productivity, and remuneration. The composition of the profession has changed considerably since a couple of decades ago. Healthcare needs are ever changing; as a result, both the role of the PA and the characteristics of the people who fill that role are dynamic. This chapter reviews the profile of PAs in an effort to further understand the profession through the demographics and characteristics of its professionals. Drawing from rich and varied data sources, a profile of the profession can be complied, with information on distribution, demographics, education, practice characteristics, and more. Although much of the information provided in this chapter describes PAs in the United States, information on PAs in other countries is portrayed whenever possible.

DATA SOURCES ON PHYSICIAN ASSISTANTS

In the early years of the development of PAs, obtaining reliable data on their deployment was difficult. The budding American Academy of Physician Assistants (AAPA) had been able to retain information on many of the programs and graduates, but systematic and uniform data gathering was not standardized. Henry B. Perry was the first to systematically survey US PAs. A research council was formed to advise the AAPA's board of directors. The council made a series of recommendations for collecting data and determining what research questions were in need of answering. Beginning in the late 1980s, the AAPA and the associated PA programs began earnestly collecting and reporting data. This process began a generation of reports about cross-sectional information and trends. As the body of PAs grew, other agencies, such as the Medical Group Management Association, state medical boards, and federal agencies, began collecting information and making it available for analysis.

After more than 4 decades of research and careful planning, a number of important data sources for the PA profession emerged, and more have emerged globally. Using these data sources allows for analysis of trends in the PA profession and PA behavior. Some of the more usable databases are discussed in the following sections. Together, these records provide a remarkable breadth and depth of information about the profession.

American Academy of Physician Assistants

One valuable information source for Americans is the AAPA set of databases. What is known about PAs, on a cross-sectional basis, is attributable in part to the AAPA's general survey databases and master file. These periodic surveys provide detailed and timely information on socioeconomic aspects of the PA profession. The AAPA census collects this information as part of its annual membership renewal and has been collecting this information in some form for all American PA programs and their graduates. Initially, this database was used to compile information on AAPA membership, but it later expanded to contain employment trend data on a large proportion of the PA population. The AAPA membership has waxed and waned; as of 2016, it was approximately 35,000, or one-third of all PAs currently eligible to practice. Like many professional associations, membership has varied and participation rates have declined. Approximately 9,000 PAs responded to the AAPA survey in 2015.

Physician Assistant History Project

The PA History Project (PAHx) is supported by the PA History Society and maintains an international archive of history and development that is housed in the corporate headquarters of the NCCPA and is underwritten by the NCCPA. This collection of information includes documents, publications, reports, communications, memorabilia, uniforms, photographs, and ephemera. A catalog of this information is available online. The collection was started by Duke University professor Reginald Carter and continues under the guidance of the Society.

Physician Assistant Education Association

The *Annual Report on Physician Assistant Educational Programs* is a compilation of data from the annual survey of PA programs. Whereas the AAPA census database relies on individual responses from academy members, the PAEA's annual report uses data gathered from PA programs. The Physician Assistant Education Association (PAEA) membership funds the *Annual Report* and makes data available for further analysis. Data of interest include student characteristics, faculty rank and tenure, salary of faculty and staff, and trends in enrollment.

Centralized Application System for Physician Assistants

The Centralized Application System for Physician Assistants (CASPA) is operated by the PAEA. This national application service emerged in 2004 and has become an important Web-based application system for at least 90% of PA programs. This system standardizes the application process and documents the transcripts and characteristics of the PA aspirant. As a result, educators and analysts can obtain unique perspectives on trends in applicants.

Association of Postgraduate Physician Assistant Programs

The Association of Postgraduate Physician Assistant Programs (APPAP) periodically surveys and collects information about the activities of these programs and their residents. (For more information about postgraduate educational programs, see Chapter 4, "Physician Assistant Education").

National Commission on the Certification of Physician Assistants

A source of information that overlaps somewhat with the AAPA is the National Commission on Certification of Physician Assistants (NCCPA). The NCCPA registers all PA graduates who have sat for the Physician Assistant National Certification Examination (PANCE) and the Physician Assistant National Recertifying Exam (PANRE).

The NCCPA Health Foundation within the NCCPA created a new online data collection tool, the PA Professional Profile, which collects data from certified PAs as they log continuing medical education.

Accreditation Review Commission on Physician Assistant Education

The Accreditation Review Commission on Physician Assistant Education (ARC-PA) has a database on characteristics of developing and existing PA programs. Although this database is confined to US programs, its value as a source of information about new PA program trends is beginning to be explored. The ARC-PA Web site lists accredited and new programs seeking provisional accreditation. The information is supplied by the institution seeking accreditation status along with a plan for how the program will achieve its intended goals. The ARC-PA stipulates a number of requirements for accreditation; for example, the program must have at least three certified faculty PAs, and the medical director must report directly to the PA program director. A PA program can lose its accreditation status if it violates the standards set by the ARC-PA.

State Medical and Physician Assistant Boards

All 50 states, the District of Columbia, and the US territories maintain registries and databases on PAs, the locations where PAs are licensed to practice, and PA characteristics. In many states, such as Utah, Iowa, and North Carolina, annual and semiannual data on the human capital used in healthcare services are collected. These sources provide opportunities for more detailed examination on the role and behavior of PAs.

Federal Sources

Databases within the uniform services, the Department of Veterans Affairs, and other federal agencies serve as important sources on the use and activities of PAs. For example, the National Practitioner Data Bank is a depository of information on litigation and misadventure regarding PA and other practitioner activity. The Bureau of Labor Statistics collects information on employment statistics by state, county, metropolitan areas, and other variables. It also projects what the demand for occupations is likely to be in 5 and 10 years. The National Centers for Health Statistics have continuous data on ambulatory care, hospital discharge data, emergency department use, and hospital outpatients.

Proprietary Databases

A handful of agencies provide provider information for a fee. For example, Optum Provider Data Solutions, a health workforce database, is used by many insurance companies to identify legitimate and nonsanctioned providers for reimbursement. Other private for-profit sources include SK&A, Healthcare Data Solutions, MedTies, and the National Center for the Analysis of Healthcare Data.

Global Data Sources

Data on PAs who are certified and work outside of the United States is also growing. PAs in the United Kingdom have experienced rapid development since 2015. This requires more systematic surveying, a task taken on by the Faculty of Physician Associates at the Royal College of Physicians (formerly the U.K. Association of PAs) and more than 25 PA programs, underwritten by the National Health Service. Improvements in this process will contribute to the collection of more and better data. Data collected in The Netherlands on PAs is a government process. Canada periodically surveys its members.

DISTRIBUTION

PAs are distributed across the globe, not only in the United States but also in Australia, Canada, Germany, Ghana, Guyana, India, Republic of Ireland, Liberia, Netherlands, New Zealand, Saudi Arabia, South Africa, and the United Kingdom. However, the supply of PAs varies considerably from country to country. No two countries have the same type of PA and none have the same configuration of education, credentialing, accreditation, or certification. Yet all produce a health professional who works closely with physicians and appears to effectively substitute largely for the same type of labor.

United States

The United States, with 50 years of PA development, has the largest number of PAs clinically licensed to practice. At the end of 2016, approximately 100,000 PAs were in active clinical practice in the United States (Table 3–1). The distribution of PAs within the United States varies greatly by state, ranging from

TABLE 3-1
Physician Assistant Statistics

General	
Ever eligible to practice (1967–2016)	>110,000
Clinically active (of those eligible to practice in 2016)	>100,000
Female	75%
Age (mean years)	42

Industry	
Physician Offices	50,510
General Medical and Surgical Hospitals	19,380
Outpatient Care Centers (includes federally qualified health centers)	6,040
Federal (government)	2,410
Colleges, Universities, and Professional Schools	2,210
Offices of Other Health Professionals	1,190
Specialty Hospitals (except psychiatric and substance abuse)	790

Primary Specialty Of The Practice	
Primary care (family/general medicine, general internal medicine, general pediatrics)	34%
Surgery/surgery subspecialties	23%
Internal medicine subspecialties	7%

Data combined from American Academy of Physician Assistants. (2013). *AAPA Physician Assistant Survey Report.* Alexandria, VA: Author; Hooker, R. S., & Muchow, A. N. (2014). Supply of physician assistants: 2013–2026. *Journal of the American Academy of Physician Assistants, 27*(3), 39–45; Hooker, R. S., & Muchow A. N. (2014). The 2013 census of licensed physician assistants. *Journal of the American Academy of Physician Assistants, 27*(7), 35–39; and US Department of Labor, Bureau of Labor Statistics. (2014). Occupational Employment and Wages, May 2014, 29-1071 Physician Assistants. Retrieved from http://www.bls.gov/oes/current/oes291071.htm

60 licensed PAs per 100,000 populations in Alaska to 3.9 PAs per 100,000 populations in Mississippi (Figure 3–1). Approximately 14% of PAs are licensed in two states, which may explain some of the anomalies that exist between the number of PAs taken by employment settings versus individuals.

Population alone cannot account for all state variations. Mississippi, for example, is ranked 31 in population yet is tied with Guam for the lowest number of PAs and the leanest PA-to-population ratio in the country. One reason for the concentration of PAs in states such

FIGURE 3-1
PAs per 100,000 Population by State, 2015.*

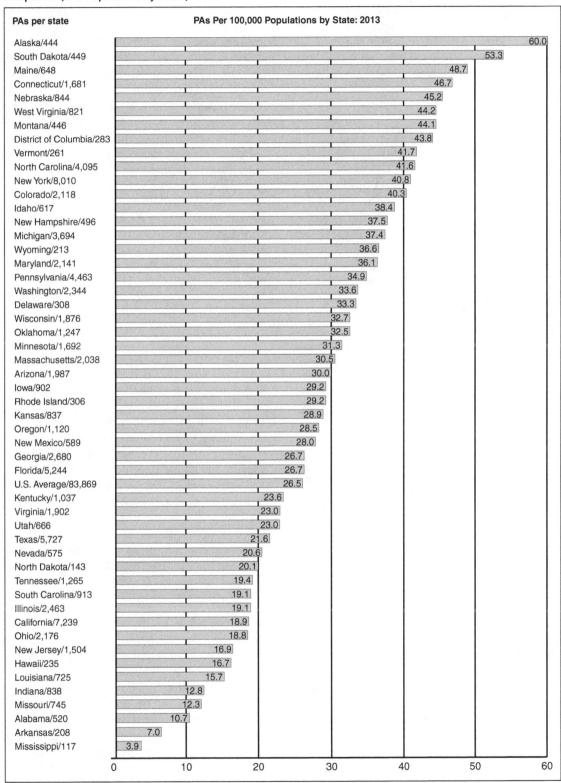

Number of PAs per 100,000 is based on state-licensed PAs in 2015 and the 2015 US Census.

as New York, Texas, and California is the high number of PA training programs in these states and the population density of the states. Locations with state-supported PA programs also see many of their graduates remain in the state. The geographic distribution of PAs in the healthcare workforce also appears to be associated with the following factors:

■ Market demand and salaries
■ Enabling state legislation (ability to practice and prescribe)
■ PA programs within the state

Although most of the US PA graduates are distributed throughout the continent, a few hundred report that they reside overseas. Some work in the US territories (e.g., Guam, the Virgin Islands, and American Samoa), whereas others work in US military settings (e.g., Iraq, Middle East, Europe, Japan, and Korea), for private agencies that have medical facilities outside the United States (e.g., in Central America, Southeast Asia, and Saudi Arabia), or for the Department of State, Central Intelligence Agency, Department of Defense, or Peace Corps.

Among those PAs who work in the United States, the communities in which they practice are diverse, ranging from the most rural communities to inner cities. The 2013 *American Academy of Physician Assistants (AAPA) Physician Assistant Survey Report* revised its classification regarding the practice location of PAs. The report shows that 87% practice in metropolitan regions; approximately 9% work in inner cities. Only 6.7% of practicing PAs work in small rural and frontier communities that are not adjacent to metropolitan areas, and another 5.4% work in nonmetropolitan areas that are adjacent to metropolitan areas (large rural) (AAPA, 2014).

Worldwide

The PA movement is active abroad in such countries as The Netherlands, Canada, Great Britain, Ghana, India, South Africa, Liberia, and Australia. As of 2016, PA development is also in some stage of development or demonstration in Germany, New Zealand, and Republic of Ireland. Figure 3–2 illustrates some of the growing information about PAs globally.

Although the aggregate number of PAs clinically active in these countries may be a bit more than 1,000, PAs are gaining greater visibility. For example, the United Kingdom has inaugurated the *Faculty of Physician Associates at the Royal College of Physicians,* which has become the professional association of U.K. PAs. Concurrently, the National Health Service is underwriting a rapid expansion of PA education development. The United Kingdom has approximately 200 physician associates, but this number is expected to grow with the development of 25-30 or so new programs. Growth in the number of PAs is also likely to occur in The Netherlands, where approximately 1,000 PAs are formally trained and distributed in many specialties. PAs are also growing in India, South Africa, and Canada, as the scarcity of doctors becomes more apparent. Canada has approximately 300 practicing PAs (including 120 in uniform) (Table 3–2).

DEMOGRAPHIC DATA

The demographics of the PA profession have changed as healthcare has changed. What began as an avenue for returning male veterans in the 1960s and 1970s is now an occupation in which females outnumber males and professionals vary in age, ethnicity, educational background, and experience. The percentage of PAs with military experience of any kind (active duty or reserves) is shrinking. Many students now enter PA programs as their first chosen careers and graduate in their late 20s, which has changed the profile of the PA profession.

Age

In the United States, the median age of PAs at graduation has declined since the 1970s. The average age of a PA at the beginning of a career is approximately 29 years. Shifts in the age of PA matriculates occur from time to time, and the proportion of recent graduates in the youngest age-group (younger than 24 years) has decreased. Conversely, the number of graduates in the middle age-group (ages 24 to 29) has increased 53% since 1994, as has the number of

FIGURE 3-2
Global Distribution of Physician Assistants, 2016

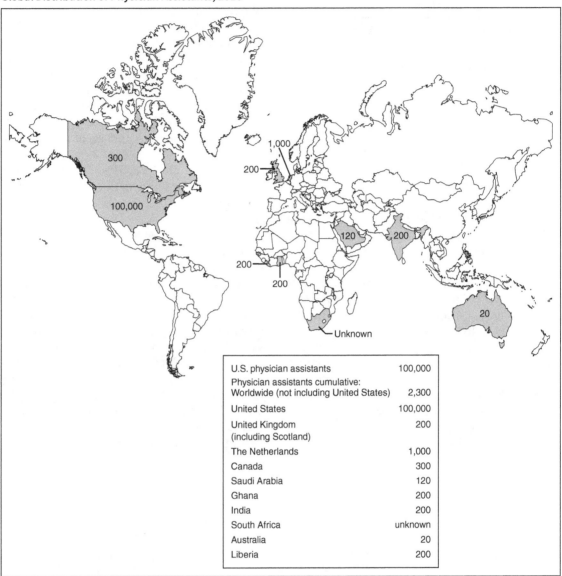

U.S. physician assistants	100,000
Physician assistants cumulative:	
Worldwide (not including United States)	2,300
United States	100,000
United Kingdom (including Scotland)	200
The Netherlands	1,000
Canada	300
Saudi Arabia	120
Ghana	200
India	200
South Africa	unknown
Australia	20
Liberia	200

graduates in the older age-group (older than 30 years), which increased 37% since 1994 (Figure 3–3). What this shift in age may indicate is a longer career duration for recent graduates because PAs commonly work well into their 60s.

According to 2015 data, the mean age of practicing PAs in the United States was 42 years (median 45; mode 32; range 22–74). On average, women PAs are 10 years younger than their male counterparts. In addition, the average age of male PAs is rising more rapidly than that of women, which might be explained by the recent influx of young women into the profession.

Gender

In 1965, the first class of PAs was all men. Women entered the third Duke University class and have been part of the PA profession

TABLE 3-2
Geographic Location of Canadian Association of Physician Assistants Members, Canada, 2015

Geographic Location	Number
Alberta	25
British Columbia	21
Manitoba	58
New Brunswick	5
Nova Scotia	27
Ontario	274
Quebec	16
Various locations (military)	110

ever since. Dr. Eugene Stead conceived of the PA profession as being composed predominantly of men because he thought they would have a greater commitment to a career and a greater willingness to meet the demands of their work. But this attitude was short lived and, by 1974, the percentage of female PAs had increased to 16% (Hooker, 2013) (Figure 3–4). Now, three-quarters of the PA workforce is female, with the class of 2015 graduating 71% women. Given these numbers, one can expect that women will remain more visible than men for decades to come.

This demographic shift is not surprising. Women have been moving into formerly male-dominated professions in large numbers since 1980. For example, the percentage of female lawyers and judges rose from 4% in 1972 to 15% in 1982. Over the same period, the percentage of female accountants rose from 22% to 38% of the total. For economists, the increase has been from 12% to 25%. These changes reflect the different educational choices made by young women since the mid-1980s. In 1968, women received only 8% of all medical degrees and 4% of law degrees. The percentages were 41% and 39%, respectively, in 2001. By 2008, 51% of medical school graduates were women. For lawyers, in 2006, the number is 25% in law practice and 44% of law school graduates.

For many women, the PA profession represents a preferred and attractive career choice over that of a physician, with its many demands and sacrifices. In fact, even women whose academic records would make them a virtual certainty to be accepted into medical school are choosing to enter the PA profession. The shorter period of formal professional training, high level of clinical responsibility, increasing practice and professional autonomy, and the career flexibility options that characterize the PA profession are important factors included in the healthcareer choices of many young women. This benefits the profession

FIGURE 3-3
Percentage Trends in the Age of PA Graduates (1984–2013)

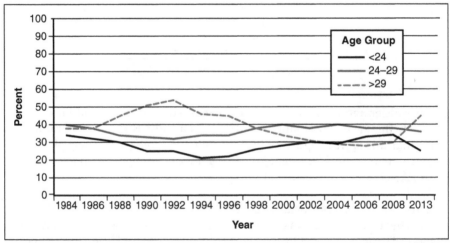

Data from AAPA, NCCPA, and unpublished data.

FIGURE 3-4
PAs by Age and Gender

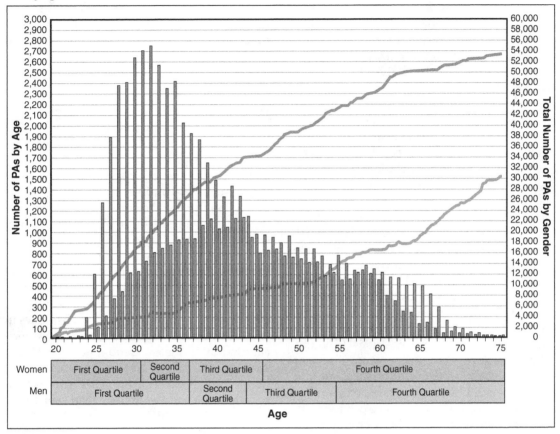

and at the same time allows women to maintain some control over their work life in a fashion that permits more lifestyle choices and family time.

Investigation of the effects of the increasing proportion of women in the PA profession in terms of productivity, wages, and career duration lies ahead. However, certain trends among practicing female PAs could lead to overall changes in the general PA profile. For example, female PAs might emulate female physicians in opting for a shorter career span and a shorter workweek as well as more cognitive roles. One observation is that female physicians are disproportionately represented in lower-paying primary care specialties, such as family practice and general pediatrics, as opposed to high-paying specialties, such as orthopedics and cardiology. Research on physicians also shows that women physicians spend

more time with patients (Hedden et al., 2014), are more likely to offer preventive services to patients, and are more likely to take different pathways of communication with patients than male physicians are. These practice patterns have also been said to be true of female PAs, although documentation on the subject is difficult to find.

Because of the shift in the gender of certain historically male-dominated occupations, modeling any healthcare workforce must consider a large set of variables. Nationally, women are 11 times more likely than men to voluntarily quit a job. Marriage also seems to affect women and men differently. Married men earn more than single men, but single women earn more than married women. This result may occur because, historically, marriage freed men of household duties and permitted more single-minded attention to jobs, but marriage has had the opposite effect for women. That too may be changing.

Women PAs earn less than male PAs even when influencing factors such as on-call hours, years as a practicing PA, years in current practice, setting, and community size are controlled (Essary & Coplan, 2014). Analysis by specialty also reveals that salary differences remain for family/general practice, pediatrics, obstetrics and gynecology (OB/GYN), emergency medicine, and orthopedics. However, no statistical differences emerge in the specialties of surgery, internal medicine, and occupational/industrial medicine. Other studies have found that female and male PAs that were hired at the same salary level did not have significant salary differences a few years later. In an analysis of PA educators, female PA educators showed statistically significant lower annual incomes than their male counterparts. The income disparity persisted when differentiated by education, rank, and position. Higher percentages of male PA faculty members were found in higher ranks and in leadership positions (Coombs & Valentin, 2014).

The reasons for salary differences are not easily explained. Shortcomings of some studies include ignoring hourly wage, productivity based on patient visits per hour or annum instead of relative value units, and total revenues generated by the PA. Other considerations to explain the differences may relate to initial starting salaries, the ability to negotiate for raises, participation in profit sharing, strengthening of a retirement fund, and the development of partnerships when private practices are examined.

Determining whether wage differences are the result of discrimination requires comparisons of groups of workers who are equally capable, experienced, and motivated. Such a comparison should be made by gender studies specialists to avoid further controversy. However, this comparison is not easy to make given the numerous factors that affect the current earnings of any worker. Economists, taking into account easily measured factors such as age, years of schooling, region, and hours of work, found that from one-half to three-fourths of the gross differences in earnings between

men and women can be explained by these factors (Lo Sasso et al., 2011). Whether the remaining differences are the result of discrimination or as-yet unquantified productivity differences will continue to be a controversial issue.

Race and Ethnicity

Racial and ethnic diversity are the cornerstones of US culture, and adequate representation of all races and ethnic groups is essential to the viability of the PA profession. Without a heterogeneous mix of the US population adequately representing the profession, the ability of the profession to meet the cross-sectional needs of the society will fall short. The proportion of survey respondents from underrepresented minorities is rising within the profession, yet the profession remains predominately white and the proportions of minorities below levels in the general population (Table 3–3). Groups showing the largest increases are Hispanics in the south-central region and African Americans in the southeast. Trend data suggest that African Americans, Native Americans, and other distinct ethnic groups are also participating in the profession more than ever before (Lelacheur et al., 2015).

Organizational efforts to improve the configuration and diversity of the PA profession are ongoing. Three PA training programs actively recruit a student body of minorities (primarily

TABLE 3-3

Number and Percent of US Physician Assistants by Race, 2013*

	Number of Respondents	Percent
Asian/Pacific Islander	588	3.8
Black, not Hispanic	454	2.9
Hispanic/Latino Origin	801	5.1
American Indian/Alaskan	77	0.5
White (not Hispanic)	14,844	94.9
Total	15,645	100

* Based on self-report from clinically practicing physician assistants.
Data from American Academy of Physician Assistants. (2013). 2013 AAPA Physician Assistant Survey Report. Alexandria, VA: Author.

African Americans). A program for Native Americans functioned for a few years in New Mexico but closed in the late 1980s. The Health Professions Educational Assistance Act and the Health Professions Scholarship Program are other endeavors designed to attract minorities to the healthcare professions. Other efforts are underway, including programs to promote the sciences to minorities, an area in which they are also underrepresented.

Education

Historically in the United States, most PAs held at least a bachelor's degree *before* enrolling in a PA program. In some cases, applicants who already have doctorate degrees are applying for PA training. Those with graduate degrees anecdotally report that their ambition to be clinically active and work with patients came late and was slow to realize.

As of 2016, all Dutch, American, and most Canadian graduates receive a master's degree upon graduation from a PA program. In the United States in 2007, 2.4% of graduates already had a doctorate degree. Doctoral preparation is also becoming an academic attainment for a career in PA education, and the number of faculty with doctoral degrees continues to grow. PA programs in other countries grant a bachelor's or a master's degree. The length of education ranges from 2 to 4 years but is generally less than 3 years.

In the United States, many PAs go on to pursue additional education after graduation from a PA program. A 2006 study identified 213 PAs who had a doctorate degree other than a medical degree (e.g., PhD, DrPH, and EdD); most of the individuals in this study acquired their doctoral degrees after graduating from a PA program. New technical degrees made available in for-profit institutions (e.g., DHSc) have made this possible with online courses and with academic requirements that are not as rigorous as those of a traditional PhD program. One case study examined the opportunity cost of such a process. A break-even rate of return for the investment had not been realized even after 10 years of employment (Makinde & Hooker, 2009).

EDUCATIONAL PROGRAMS

Global development has given rise to the number of PA programs operationally. This development is due in part to the world shortage of doctors, which is at least 4.5 million doctors. The 2,000 medical schools in 178 countries do not have the capacity to produce many more than they are already graduating. However, PA programs, which provide some of the most efficient and beneficial forms of medical education, are helping to offset this need. This observation is being realized not only in the United States but throughout the world.

United States

PA education in the United States began in 1965, with the number almost steadily rising since that time. Beginning in the 1970s, there was a foundation of 30 or so PA programs. For the first few years of PA development, the number of programs could not be determined with precision because of the difficulty with defining and counting them. In part, this was because not all were based in general medicine; there were many experiments developing specialized PAs, such as in orthopedics and surgery. Throughout the formative years of PA education, some programs merged, some folded, and some converted from specialty to primary care. This early period was followed by a decade during which the number of annual graduates remained stable or went down. However, the 1990s and the 2000s saw a boom in annual graduate outcomes, and a surge in new programs is currently underway in the United States. As of 2016, the number of US programs was 218 and growing.

The PA profession seems to be a popular career choice, perhaps as popular as allopathic medicine. The popularity of the PA profession is evidenced not only by growth in the number of programs but also by growth in the number of applicants to and graduates of those programs. That ratio (applicants per seat) is 3.5:1 for PA programs and 3.5:1 for allopathic/osteopathic schools. At the same time, more than 110,000 PAs have ever graduated from an approved US PA program. The annual supply in terms of graduates appears to be 5%, with attrition from the profession at about 3%. This growth is predicted to continue until at least 2025. By 2030, if the average of 44 graduates per program continues, the annual production of PAs will be close to 12,000 per year. Annulment (annual attrition) of PAs depends on many variables that influence the market for PAs.

California and New York account for one-sixth of PA graduates. New York, Pennsylvania, Michigan, North Carolina, and Florida are among the states with the highest numbers of annual PA graduates. At the other end of the scale, low-population states such as Arkansas and Wyoming have the fewest number of graduates from PA programs.

Worldwide

The landscape of PA programs in other countries is quite different from that in the United States. There are many reasons for this difference. The PA profession in the United States has a distribution and visibility that creates a societal awareness that might not be present in other countries. In addition, in most of these countries, a central government controls the development of most educational endeavors. This section summarizes general data about worldwide PA programs.

Canada

Canada has four PA programs with more in development. The Canadian Forces Medical Services School at Borden, Ontario, graduated the first class of formally trained Canadian PAs in 1984. The program grants a degree in collaboration with the University of Nebraska Medical Center.

In 2008, the University of Manitoba and McMaster University offered the first civilian PA training programs in Canada, which were followed by a third civilian program in 2010 launched by the PA Consortium (a University of Toronto degree delivered in collaboration with Northern Ontario School of Medicine and The Michener Institute for Applied Health Sciences) (Frechette & Shirchand, 2016).

Great Britain

As of 2016, Great Britain (England, Scotland, Northern Ireland, Wales) had 10 PA programs, with approximately 25 or more expected. At least 400 PAs have graduated since 2004. In 2013, the term *PA* was changed to "physician associate." A PA program in Scotland began in 2012 and graduated its first class in 2014. The 25-30 or so programs in development in the UK are publically funded.

The Netherlands

The Netherlands has five PA programs that produce approximately 120 graduates a year. All five of these PA programs were formed with one 10-year government budget.

Australia

As of 2016, Australia had 14 clinical PAs who were graduates of James Cook University and were employees of the State (Queensland primarily). A PA program at the University of Queensland closed after two classes graduated due to physician pressure; the program at James Cook University remains operational. Few of the graduates from the University of Queensland are working as PAs.

Taiwan

From 1990 to 2008, approximately 500 PA-like health providers were trained in large medical centers in Taiwan. Most of these were nurses who worked in large hospital settings, such as emergency departments, intensive care units, and operating theaters. However, in 2008, the Taiwan government refused to recognize these workers as PAs, both formally and informally, and so the one PA program closed and the movement ended. The nurses trained as PAs are now referred to as "practice nurses."

Liberia

Liberia has had a PA program in Monrovia since 1965, the same year the PA profession started in the United States. It is located at the Tubman National Institute of Medical Arts. A second one in Gbang, the Baptist Missionary PA program (started and run by American PA Steven Trexler), has had one graduating class so far.

Ghana started its PA movement in the mid-1960s and now has three programs. It has 3500 doctors and dentists combined, and 2500 PAs.

South Africa

Three universities in South Africa train "clinical associates" to work in locations where doctor supervision is limited. These professionals are trained to provide emergency care, conduct rounds, carry out and assist with diagnostic and therapeutic procedures, and offer holistic care to patients with a range of common acute and chronic conditions.

India

Indian PA education consists of the opportunity to earn a bachelor's degree at one of three universities and a postgraduate diploma at two universities. All five programs are in large private medical institutions and academic health centers associated with large hospitals. Most of the programs have been developed or influenced by physicians trained in the United States or the United Kingdom. To date, approximately 1,000 PAs have graduated from the programs. Unfortunately, many depart due to lack of scope of practice or regulation by the Ministry of Health (MoH), and the education pipeline has difficulty keeping up the supply of PAs. In response, the MoH has put forth a bill in Parliament to bring in a Council for Allied and Healthcare Professionals that will include physician associates. The IAPA intends to change the name to *physician associate,* as the term *physician assistant* is not protected and is commonly used to refer to a wide range of personnel, including medical assistants and others.

Germany

The first PA program in Germany began in 2005. To date, four PA programs are operational. These programs have produced approximately 100 graduates, all with a nursing background. The PA model of shifting tasks from medical doctors to PAs appears to be growing among senior physicians and hospital administrators. Although the development of a German PA movement is in its nascent stage, the training, deployment, and evolution of PA training programs appears underway.

PRACTICE CHARACTERISTICS

Medical practice is how a clinician identifies and defines himself or herself. Practice characteristics are the features of the discipline considered typical to PA practice and are reflected somewhat by the physician workforce, which has become increasingly specialty oriented. The American Medical Association annually tracks more than 125 disciplines, and the specialty orientation of PAs seems to parallel the activity of physicians, up to a point. After a decade in which PAs were largely deployed in primary care, more recent patterns reveal a trend toward PA practice in nonprimary care specialties as well as their employment in urban and rural settings, in inpatient as well as outpatient settings. These trends overlap with the type of employers who employ PAs. One large employer in the United States is the federal government. However, the 5,000 or so hospitals in the United States are also growing their utilization of PAs in myriad roles, including emergency medicine, intensive care units, and hospitalists.

Practice Setting

The practice setting is the patient care environment in which a clinician works—the primary employer of the PA. Although concise nomenclature has not emerged for identifying where PAs practice, the Bureau of Labor Statistics has created a classification system and a set of useful terms that identify where PAs are principally employed.

Practice settings are grouped into five categories: medical offices, general medical and surgical hospitals, outpatient care centers (e.g., rural community and migrant health centers), federal medical centers, and university-based medical centers.

United States

For US PAs, the patterns of practice began primarily in outpatient general practice and then began moving to hospitals and large group practices. Today, the distribution of PAs by practice setting tends to parallel that of physician distribution, in that most PAs are employed in group practice–type settings or in hospitals. Women are more likely to work in group practices than men are. A shift occurred in the early 1990s, revealing an increase in hospital-based physician practices. Another shift in the early part of this century has led more PAs to hospital-based employment. Since the year 2000, only minor shifts in the trends of practice setting have occurred. However, as solo physician practices fade and changes in resident hours worked per week affect hospital staffing, a gradual shift of employment into groups and medical centers is underway.

According to large cross-sectional studies of patient visits using National Ambulatory Medical Care Survey and National Hospital Ambulatory Medical Care Survey data, as of 2013:

- Almost one-fifth of PAs (19%) work in hospitals, which includes university and other hospital settings. The remaining work in such settings as public and private ambulatory clinics, health maintenance organizations (HMOs), geriatric facilities, occupational health settings, correctional systems, and other healthcare practices and institutions (Table 3–4).
- Almost 55% of PAs work in solo or group private practices (Table 3–5).
- Nearly one-half (44%) of PAs work in either single-specialty or multispecialty group practices. Single-specialty group practice is the largest specific category of practice setting.
- More than one-tenth of PAs work in emergency departments, and another tenth work in hospital outpatient departments.
- There is a difference in the proportion of women who are not in clinical practice (17%) versus men (5%).

The federal government is the largest employer with more than 3,000 when those in uniform are added to the civilian sector. According to the Bureau of Labor Statistics (2015), about 4% (4,400 out of 91,600) of clinically active PAs were employed by a state or federal government agency in 2014. Within the federal government, the Department of Veterans Affairs employs the most PAs—a bit more than 2,000. Uniformed services are the second largest government employer of PAs.

TABLE 3-4
Physician Assistant Principal Practice Settings, United States, 2013

Setting	Percent
Intensive care unit (ICU)/critical care unit (CCU) of hospital	2.2
Inpatient unit of hospital (not ICU/CCU)	10.3
Outpatient unit of hospital	7.4
Hospital emergency room	10.1
Hospital operating room	6.5
Other unit of hospital	1.5
Federally qualified rural health center	3.5
Other federally qualified health clinic (not rural)	1.9
Other community health center	1.9
Freestanding urgent care clinic	2.9
Freestanding surgical facility	0.4
Solo practice physician office	11.9
Single-specialty group practice	22.2
Multispecialty group practice	9.3
Health maintenance organization facility	1.3
Nursing home or long-term care facility	0.8
University/college health facility	0.6
School-based health facility	0.4
Other outpatient facility	1.9
Correctional facility	1.0
Industrial facility	0.5
Retail outlet	0.2
Mobile health unit	0.1
Patients' homes	0.1
Other	1.3
Total	100

Data from American Academy of Physician Assistants. (2013). *AAPA Physician Assistant Survey Report.* Alexandria, VA: Author.

Canada

Of the approximately 300 PAs employed in Canada, roughly one-third are in the military providing various services around the globe. At least 140 PAs are in Ontario working in emergency medicine, community health clinics, and hospitals. A growing number of PAs and "clinical assistants" are in Manitoba working in hospital-based roles. Both provinces have PA programs. Clinical associates in Manitoba are international medical graduates who have moved to Manitoba and now work in a special classified category that has considerable overlap with PAs but are not certified PAs (Jones, 2015). A

TABLE 3-5
Distribution of Physician Assistants by Primary Clinical Employer

Primary Clinical Employer	Clinically Practicing PAs		Non–Clinically Practicing PAs		Primary Care PAs	
	Number	Percent	Number	Percent	Number	Percent
Solo Physician Practice	1,394	11.7	28	11.2	699	21.4
Single-Specialty Physician Group Practice	3,858	32.4	60	23.9	1,062	32.5
Multi-Specialty Physician Group Practice	1,949	16.3	23	9.2	696	21.3
University Hospital	1,516	12.7	60	23.9	123	3.8
Other Hospital	2,307	19.3	50	19.9	286	8.8
Physician Practice Management Company	256	2.1	—	—	58	1.8
Military Branch or Government Agency (including VA)	577	4.8	21	8.4	299	9.1
Retail Clinic System (e.g., Minute Clinic)	66	0.6	—	—	45	1.4
TOTAL	11,923	100.0	251	100.0	3,268	100.0

Source: AAPA. (2013). Unpublished data.

third province, New Brunswick, introduced PAs in emergency medicine locations in 2011 (Frechette & Shrichand 2016). Enabling legislation in Alberta occurred in 2016.

Great Britain
The majority of the 400-plus PAs who have graduated in Great Britain are paid through some arrangement with the National Health Service; few work in private practices. In England, many are employed in emergency medicine settings and outpatient clinics.

The Netherlands
Most of the 1,000 or so PA graduates in The Netherlands work in a medical specialty or hospital-based role. The majority specializes in some form of medicine, and many provide services in a combination of inpatient and outpatient settings. A few PAs are employed in a general practice role. For the most part, the demand is in the medical and surgical specialties.

Australia
As of 2015, Australia had 14 clinical PAs who were graduates of James Cook University and were employees of Queensland Health.

Liberia
The vast majority of healthcare in Liberia is rendered by PAs. Before the outbreak of the Ebola virus in 2014 and 2015, the country had

4 million people and only 150 doctors. As a result of the outbreak, the vast majority of healthcare in Liberia is now rendered by its 1,000 practicing PAs, who provided much of the care during the Ebola crisis (Oliphant, 2014). Unfortunately, by the end of the crisis at least 17 PAs had died from the Ebola virus.

South Africa
The scope of practice of clinical associates in South Africa allows them to assist physicians predominantly (although not exclusively) in district-level healthcare services, with a focus on primary care. The intention is that they will work in the public healthcare service; although they are not prevented from going into the private sector, they cannot work independently and the mechanisms are not yet in place for their employment in private practices or hospitals. Clinical associates work under the continuous supervision of a "registered medical practitioner" (a doctor), who is identified by the service in which the clinical associate is working and must be known to the clinical associate.

India
Of the 1,000 or so PAs who have graduated in India, only 400 PAs appeared to be active in clinical care because of the lack of scope of practice and regulation by the MoH. Two-thirds of PAs in India work in the surgical

specialties. The majority works in cardiology and cardiac surgery. Other specialties that have seen growth include general internal medicine, nephrology, rheumatology, cardiology, and transplant surgery.

Germany

Details on Germany's PA force are difficult to fully appreciate because of the ambiguity of the term "PA." Although the number of PA graduates is estimated to be 100, little is known about their roles and employment.

Types of Practice/Specialization

Although the initial mandate for PAs, as envisioned by Smith, Estes, Silver, and their successors, was to serve as assistants to any physician, more than two-thirds have entered specialty and subspecialty practices with equal success. PA specialization began at an early stage, marked by the founding of specialty-focused educational programs in pediatrics and surgery in the late 1960s and the establishment of a surgical postgraduate program in 1972. For many years, due largely to the influence of federal funding dollars, the direction of the profession took a turn toward general medicine (later titled *primary care*). In the late 1970s, a majority of PAs worked in family medicine. But as the profession evolved and grew in the 1980s and 1990s, specialization increased as more PAs entered specialty practices. This trend led to the formation of more specialty and subspecialty societies within the AAPA and the emergence of more postgraduate educational programs. (For more information about postgraduate educational programs, see Chapter 4, "Physician Assistant Education.")

After 5 decades of PAs working in the US healthcare system, the percentage of those who work in the primary care specialties has declined, and those employed in hospital-based and specialty care practices has correspondingly increased. Most practicing PAs are in medical specialties outside of primary care. According to the latest AAPA physician assistant survey, the percentage of those working in primary care specialties has fallen to the lowest levels recorded in the past several decades. One-third of the nation's PAs in active clinical practice work in the primary care clinical practice specialties, which includes the areas of family medicine (25.9%), general internal medicine (5.2%), and general pediatrics (2.5%) (AAPA, 2013). This total is down from the 62% of PAs reported to work in primary care in 1980. It also contrasts the one-fifth (22.6%) of PAs who work in general surgery and the surgical subspecialties and the 10.5% who work in emergency medicine (Table 3–6). Women are more likely than men, by a small margin, to be in family practice. Of the PAs who do work in primary care, few work in pediatrics, geriatrics, and women's health. (For more information, see Chapter 5, "Physician Assistants in Primary Care.")

The shifting of PAs out of primary care practice parallels that of physicians, whose numbers in primary care have also trended down.

TABLE 3-6
Percentage Specialty Distribution Trends of US Physician Assistants for Selected Years

Specialty	Year (Number)									
	1974	1978	1981	1987	1994	1996	2000	2002	2008	2013
Family practice	43.6	52.0	49.1	38.7	37.2	39.8	36.5	32.1	25.9	25
General internal medicine	20.0	12.0	8.9	9.5	7.7	8.3	8.8	8.4	5.2	4
General pediatrics	6.2	3.3	3.4	4.0	2.5	2.7	2.6	2.6	2.5	2
General surgery	12.1	5.5	4.6	8.8	2.8	3.1	2.7	2.5	2.5	4.5
Surgical specialties	6.8	6.2	7.7	13.8	19.1	8.3	17.4	19.2	22.6	26
Medical specialties	3.9	6.3	2.7	7.1	7.4	5.8	8.11	9.4	9.3	10.9

Data from American Academy of Physician Assistants. (2015). *AAPA Physician Assistant Survey Report.* Alexandria, VA: Author.

Dwindling numbers in primary care run counter to the long-held traditions and priorities for PAs to serve in generalist practice and in medically underserved communities. Although general medicine remains the major practice thrust of the PA profession, trends emphasizing specialty practice in the PA profession continue. An intriguing, but unanswered, question is how much primary care is actually provided by PAs working within specialty practices? In addition, primary care figures differ depending on who is counting. In the United States, some nurse practitioner (NP) organizations include women's health (obstetrics and gynecology) as a primary care discipline and the government includes geriatrics as a primary care discipline; however, in all other countries, primary care is exclusively family or general medicine. Industrial and environmental (occupational) medicine, public health, military medicine, geriatrics, and corrections medicine are also largely primary care disciplines that are functioning under unique names. Military PAs tend to select "Internal Medicine or Family Medicine" on the AAPA census.

However one defines "primary care," the evidence that PAs are moving toward specialization is unequivocal. PAs are distributed into dozens of different medical and surgical specialties. They also remain scarce in psychiatry, anesthesiology, pathology, pediatrics, obstetrics, gynecology, geriatrics, and radiology. Genetics, one of the newest frontiers for medicine, already has a small but growing cadre of PA experts. For more information on PA specialization, see Chapter 6, "Physician Assistant Specialization: Non–Primary Care."

Types of Employers

PA employers—the organizations and individuals who provide jobs for PAs—are diverse and changing. Before the 21st century, many PA employers were solo or small group practices. Since that time, large shifts in types of employers have taken place. The *economy of scale* is the theory that best explains this shift in an entrepreneurial market more than any other reason.

Hospitals

The percentage of PAs employed by hospitals has been growing since the late 1990s. As the proportion of PAs in primary care practice has declined, the rates of PAs working in acute care settings in medical and surgical specialties and subspecialties have risen correspondingly. Hospital cutbacks in physician residency programs, curtailed availability of international medical graduates, and the cost-effectiveness of full-time inpatient jobs are all key factors in the expanding role of the PA and the number of PA positions in inpatient care. (See Chapter 7, "Physician Assistants in Hospital Settings.")

Public Service: Military, Federal, and State

The US federal government is the single largest employer of all healthcare providers. In 2015, 2,410 PAs were federally employed in the Veterans Health Administration. In the same year, about 1,150 PAs served in uniformed services branches on active duty. They are distributed among the Army, Air Force, Navy, and Coast Guard (Department of Homeland Security). A growing cadre is in the Department of Veterans Affairs health system. About 150 PAs work in the US Public Health Service (which includes the Bureau of Prisons), where the existing limitations in the available supply of PAs results in ongoing vacancies in medical staffing. For example, the Indian Health Service (IHS) employs 35 full-time equivalent (FTE) PAs, about one-third of whom are Native Americans. PAs are also employed in the Department of State, the Department of Health and Human Services, the US Customs Service, and the Department of Defense, and others serve at the White House. The distribution of PAs in the various government agencies is shown in Table 3–7.

Managed-Care Systems

PAs, NPs, and primary care physicians are highly visible in managed healthcare systems. Findings from a 1994 survey of 10 health maintenance organizations (HMOs) nationwide and data from several other HMO studies estimated that there are approximately 18 PAs or NPs per 100,000 HMO enrollees, with a range from 0 to 67 PAs and NPs. A Group Health Association of America study found the mean

TABLE 3-7
Government Employers of Physician Assistants, 2014

Employer	Number of PAs
Army (active duty)	610
Air Force (active duty)	270
Navy (active duty)	235
Coast Guard (active duty)	42
National Guard and Reserves	410
Veterans Affairs	1,680
Bureau of Prisons	60
Public Health Service	140
Other federal government	377

number of full-time physicians per 100,000 enrollees to be 142.3; the number of primary care physicians was 68.7 per 100,000 enrollees. When PAs and NPs were factored in, an inverse relationship existed (Dial et al., 1995). This observation suggests that PAs and NPs are substituting for primary care physicians in these settings in underappreciated levels, providing direct patient care to all categories of patients. NPs and certified nurse-midwives tend to provide more OB/GYN care than PAs, but PAs and advance practice nurses are used extensively in primary care.

An example of the extensive integration of PAs in HMOs exists at Kaiser Permanente in Portland, Oregon. This prepaid group practice has an enrollment of more than 450,000 members, staffed by 550 FTE physicians and 150 FTE PAs and NPs within 29 clinical departments. PAs who practice in primary care areas and specialty care roles are fully integrated as members of the health provider team. The Kaiser Permanente Center for Health Research has measured longitudinally the clinical productivity, costs, and practice characteristics of both PAs and NPs in the HMO/managed care setting.

The Southern California Kaiser Plan employs roughly 500 PAs and NPs alone. Other HMOs that employ large groups of PAs and NPs include Pilgrim/Harvard Community Health Plan in Boston; Health Insurance Plan of Greater New York; Medstar in the District of Columbia; Geisinger and University of Pittsburgh in Pennsylvania; the Mayo Clinic in Rochester, Minnesota; Group Health Cooperative of Puget Sound in Seattle; Intermountain and the Family Health Plan Systems in Utah, California, and other western states. More than two-thirds of all group-model and staff-model HMOs employ PAs and/or NPs.

Major factors receiving increased attention in managed healthcare systems relate to the clinical capabilities and cost-effectiveness of PAs in such settings. In the HMO setting, PAs and NPs have long played important roles in the clinical staffing patterns. PAs and NPs have proven themselves capable of delivering most of the healthcare services required at physician-equivalent levels of quality of care and at lower costs than physicians. When clinical productivity of PAs, as measured by the number of outpatient care visits per day, is compared with the patient visit rates of primary care physicians and NPs, PA clinical productivity is equal to and, in some settings greater than, that of other primary care providers.

COMPENSATION

Compensation refers to the money and benefits an employee receives. It is often the leading source of job interest and job satisfaction (Hooker et al., 2015). Salary and wages, benefits, and additional incentives are all components of compensation and have been topics of interest since the AAPA began collecting demographic information in the mid-1990s.

Salary and Wages

Salary is the amount of direct annual compensation in money that a wage earner receives. The salary range of experienced PAs is quite wide because PAs work in a wide variety of clinical settings, have many different arrangements with their employers, and have a large and varied skill set. Eighty-two percent of PAs report receiving their base pay in the form of a salary; 17% indicate that they receive an hourly wage. The median wage for a PA in 2013 was $44.70 per hour. The median annual salary is $92,970 (twice the median salary of the average American), with a range of $62,030 to $130,620 (Table 3–8). In 2015, according to AAPA data, the mean salary for all PAs was $102,000 annually. The

TABLE 3-8
Wage Estimates for US PAs, 2014

Percentile	10%	25%	50%	75%	90%
Hourly wage	$30.82	$39.47	$46.07	$55.18	$64.77
Annual wage	$64,100	$82,090	$95,820	$114,760	$134,720

Data from US Department of Labor, Bureau of Labor Statistics. (2014). Occupational Employment and Wages, May 2014, 29-1071 Physician Assistants. Retrieved from http://www.bls.gov/oes/current/oes291071.htm

earning for a 30-year PA career (in 2013 dollars, median figure) is estimated at $2,800,000.

Not surprisingly, PAs with more experience command higher salaries. When income distribution is viewed as a probability density, the data show a curve with the left side fatter than the right. This lopsided curve is classic for salary distributions and is predictable because income increases with experience at a fairly even pace. Eventually, some peak density is attained and then decreases exponentially at higher levels of income. The ever-diminishing tail represents the very few, who for various entrepreneurial reasons, have incomes two to four times greater than their cohorts.

The states in which PAs earn the highest wages are Rhode Island, Nevada, New Hampshire, New Jersey, and Washington. The states with the lowest wages are Louisiana, District of Columbia, and Pennsylvania (Table 3–9). Wages also vary by practice setting (Table 3–10).

Quella, Brock, and Hooker (2015) argue that because annual PA salaries have continued to exceed inflation for more than 10 years, the demand for PAs is likely to continue to exceed supply, and wages will likely rise accordingly for a few years to come.

Benefits

In addition to salary, PAs receive other perquisites, such as insurance benefits, paid leave (vacation, sick time, and maternity leave), and reimbursement for continuing medical education (CME). Table 3–11 describes the findings for insurance benefits, benefits other than insurance, and the mean number of days available for various leave categories.

TABLE 3-9
Physician Assistant Wages by Geographical Location: 2014

States With Highest Employment Physician Assistants			
State	**Number**	**Wage**	**Annual Wage**
New York	10,410	$48.22	$100,290
California	9,230	$49.43	$102,800
Texas	5,360	$51.63	$107,390
Pennsylvania	4,950	$46.98	$97,710
Florida	5,020	$41.84	$87,020

Top-Paying Wage States for Physician Assistants			
Rhode Island	250	$53.45	$111,180
Nevada	750	$54.19	$112,700
New Hampshire	530	$52.77	$109,760
Texas	5,360	$51.63	$107,390
Washington State	1,990	$51.63	$107,390

Data from US Department of Labor, Bureau of Labor Statistics. (2014). Occupational Employment and Wages, May 2014, 29-1071 Physician Assistants. Retrieved from http://www.bls.gov/oes/current/oes291071.htm

TABLE 3-10
Physician Assistant Wages by Practice Setting: 2013

Site of Employment/ Employer	Number Employed	Hourly Mean Wage	Annual Mean Wage
Office of physicians	53,280	$46.77	$97,270
General medical and surgical hospitals	19,810	$47.51	$98,830
Outpatient care centers (e.g., clinics)	6,520	$48.84	$101,600
Federal government (e.g., Department of Defense, Veteran's Health Administration)	3,290	$41.08	$85,450
Colleges and universities	2,330	$44.00	$91,53

Data from US Department of Labor, Bureau of Labor Statistics. (2014). Occupational Employment and Wages, May 2014, 29-1071 Physician Assistants. Retrieved from http://www.bls.gov/oes/current/oes291071.htm

The benefit structure for state and federal government workers tends to be more encompassing than that for those in the private sector (Table 3–12). For example, in the federal system, vacation time amounts to 4 weeks per

TABLE 3-11
Percentage of Physician Assistants Receiving Specified Fringe Benefits*

Description	Benefit Reimbursed by Employer			Benefit Not Reimbursed
	95%–100%	50%–94%	1%–49%	
Professional liability insurance (N = 16,595)	98	1	0	2
Individual health insurance (N = 15,325)	48	36	7	9
Family health insurance (N = 11,638)	25	36	11	29
Dental insurance (N = 14,625)	31	31	10	28
Disability insurance (N = 14,317)	44	18	8	31
Term life insurance (N = 13,597)	41	15	10	35
Pension/retirement fund (N = 15,079)	23	21	39	17
State license fees (N = 16,148)	73	2	1	24
DEA registration fees (N = 13,667)	78	1	1	20
NCCPA fees (N = 16,043)	65	2	1	33
AAPA dues (N = 15,793)	64	2	1	33
State PA chapter dues (N = 14,444)	57	2	1	41
Specialty organization dues (N = 11,571)	46	2	1	50
AAPA Annual Conference (N = 13,973)	57	8	4	30
Credentialing fees (N = 15,312)	75	2	1	21

AAPA = American Academy of Physician Assistants; DEA = Drug Enforcement Administration; NCCPA = National Commission on Certification of Physician Assistants.
*Percentages may not sum to 100 due to rounding.
Data from American Academy of Physician Assistants. (2007). *2007 AAPA Physician Assistant Census Report.* Alexandria, VA: Author.

TABLE 3-12
Annual Days of Paid Vacation, Sick Leave, and Medical Education for Physician Assistants by Employer

Description	Mean	Median	Standard Deviation
Annual days of paid vacation leave (N = 14,057)	18	15	6.8
Annual days of paid sick leave (N = 9,216)	10	9	6.9
Annual days of paid medical education leave (N = 11,942)	6	5	2.3

Data from American Academy of Physician Assistants. (2007). *2007 AAPA Physician Assistant Census Report.* Alexandria, VA: Author.

year, in addition to 12 holidays. Sick leave is generous, and health, dental, malpractice, and life insurances are automatically covered. The retirement benefits of federal, state, and sometimes municipal employment make this sector particularly attractive for recession-resistant employment.

Additional Incentives

As the PA–physician relationship evolves on an employer–employee level, compensation arrangements negotiated by PAs will continue to undergo change. Some PAs report receiving several forms of compensation from their primary employers. Common forms of additional compensation include overtime pay, event-call pay, and on-call pay (such as pay for wearing a beeper or being close to home for consultation). More than one-third (36%) of full-time PAs report taking call for their primary employer. The average time on call per month for those PAs who take some call but are not always on call is 104 hours.

Some forms of compensation, such as overtime, are incentive bonuses directed as payment for PAs who perform work outside of a typical workweek. Twenty percent of PAs report receiving an incentive based on productivity or performance, either the practice's performance or their personal performance (most federal and state employees do not earn bonuses). Approximately two-fifths (38%) of those who receive an incentive based on productivity and performance report that the incentive is based on revenue that the PA generates. Bonuses range from $5,000 to $13,000. Moreover, almost 15% of PAs report additional earnings, ranging from $10,000 to more than $20,000, often in the form of dual employment or reserve/National Guard roles.

CME Funding

Additional benefits to PAs include funding for CME, which averages approximately $1,400 per year. Eighty-eight percent PAs who work full time report having CME funds available to them from their primary employer.

Funds for Expenses

More than 97% of PAs report that their employers pay 100% of their professional malpractice liability insurance. Approximately two-thirds also report that their employers pay their AAPA dues (64%), state license fees (70%),

NCCPA certificate maintenance fees (63%), AAPA annual conference registration fees (59%), and US Drug Enforcement Administration registration fees (72%).

PHYSICIAN ASSISTANT CAREER CYCLE

The career cycle of a PA is gradually coming into focus. One estimate is that at almost all graduates remain in a clinical role for the first 10 years. However, after that first decade of PA employment, the trend is a downward curve, with an average of 2.9% of the workforce leaving the field due to retirement, unemployment, emigration, or death. The replacement rate is approximately 5%. Approximately 75% of PAs remain in their careers until the traditional retirement age, between 62 and 65 years (Figure 3–5).

Job Satisfaction

One relevant factor regarding retention in this workforce is that PAs tend to be highly satisfied with their careers. This observation alone may explain the low attrition rate. The job satisfaction observation also suggests some

FIGURE 3-5
PA Career Curve

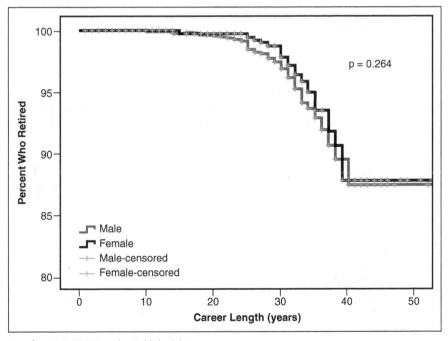

Data from AAP, NCCPA, and unpublished data

stability of the profession (Hooker, Kuilman, & Everett, 2015).

PA Role and Career Flexibility

Among many significant attributes of the generalist nature of PA education is the ability to adapt to new roles and change careers. In a study of 42 annual graduation cohorts and tracking a representative number of responses to annual AAPA surveys, the role or career focus of 49% of all PAs changed at least once. Often, the changes were significant (for example, a change from family medicine to surgery or from dermatology to emergency medicine). The mean time from one role to a substantially different one was, on average, 3.5 years. While almost half of the PAs in the study changed careers, the other half remained in their role choice throughout their careers. One interpretation of this observation is that it might help to explain why the PA profession remains high on job satisfaction reports and turnover low.

Attrition

If career retention is one side of the PA professional coin, attrition is the obverse side. Attrition (or annulment) is the gradual and natural reduction of membership or personnel from the profession. Surveys of PAs on a nationwide basis and in selected populations confirm that about 85% of all US PAs who have ever graduated remain working in the 2016 US labor force. This level of professional retention is higher than that seen in most health professions and may be as high as the level of physician retention. Only airplane pilots are thought to have a higher rate of retention. Historically, at least in the early 1980s, men, former military medical corpsmen, and graduates of military PA programs had the lowest attrition rate.

Clearly, a number of PAs drop out of the profession because of health, retirement, death, parenting responsibilities, career change, and career burnout. However, some use their PA background and experience to branch into related fields. Still others acquire additional formal education and use that as a stepping-stone to a different career. Employment experiences and education lead many PAs into more complex and advanced roles in management, health, and academia. Some have shown the ability and interest to expand their horizons in the healthcare field by creating their own new roles and opportunities. Program alumni surveys estimate that approximately 4% of all PAs have gone on to medical, osteopathic, dental, chiropractic, or podiatric school. A considerably larger number have sought graduate education (for example, a master's degree in public health, education, business administration, or public administration).

Attrition to some degree seems inevitable but does not appear to be a major problem for the PA profession. In any profession, a proportion of people are expected to explore new and expanding areas of opportunity, and the PA profession has appeared to be a reasonable springboard for these aspirations. Because a large number of PAs sought this profession after making one or more career changes, it seems only natural that they be afforded this view as well if they seek career latitude or an alternative role.

Employment Flexibility

Part-time work is an integral part of the labor force and occurs in almost all careers. In the United States, *full time* means 32 or more hours per week and *part time* is typically defined as fewer than 32 hours per week. When all occupations (not just healthcare workers) are examined, women make up the bulk of part-time workers (72%) nationally. In the aggregate, they are usually married (with the husband or partner present in the household) and are sometimes considered secondary wage earners. Although an age-participation profile is not available, most part-time PAs fall into this category as well. However, apart from the fact that only 9% of PAs practice a workweek short of full time, the distinction between full-time and part-time employment from the data presented here does not differ significantly.

Part-time PAs are more likely to work in primary care (71% full time vs. 56% part time). The type of setting, ethnicity, and number of years in current position are only marginally different between those PAs who work full time and those who work part time. The fact that so few PAs are part time is seen as remarkable when compared with other healthcare professions, including nursing and medicine.

Dual Employment

In 2014, at least one-seventh of the 102,000 certified PAs reported two or more clinical positions. Dual-employed PAs average 10 additional hours a week in their secondary position. More than 43% of PAs working two positions report that the main reason is to supplement their earnings. The average number of hours reportedly worked by *all* certified PAs is 40.6 per week, and the average number of patients they see per week is 76. With a secondary clinical position added, PAs average more than 50 hours and report seeing an average of 98 patients per week. PA role research reveals an added dimension to a national provider productivity statistic requiring refinements to annual output calculations.

FUTURE PROJECTIONS AND RESEARCH

As the national profile of PAs changes, some predictions about what the profession will look like in 2020 can be made. Females will continue to dominate the profession, accounting for as much as 75% of the workforce. This gender presence is seen across society in many different fields and professions (e.g., dentistry, medicine, veterinary sciences, military, and academics). Although some programs may be inclined to enroll their classes in roughly even numbers of men and women, they must draw upon the applicant pool presented. Since the mid-1980s, the PA profession has attracted more women than men and—with the exception of the military— this trend is likely to continue.

Second, although the average age of PAs in the workforce has slowly increased to approximately 45 years (median), data from the AAPA suggest that aging PAs are no longer remaining in the workforce into their 70s as they once did. Finally, the average age of graduates from PA programs is and will likely remain relatively stable, at around 29 years.

Future studies should address the following questions:

- Do employers of PAs have different expectations of women and men in different practice settings?
- Are employers of PAs equally satisfied with the job performance of both men and women?
- Do male PAs ask for or receive more frequent and larger raises than women do?
- Have changes occurred in the ways women and men are perceived in their roles and in how they are reimbursed?
- What experiences discourage or block female PAs from obtaining jobs with greater potential for productivity, income, and advancement? What can female PAs do to alter discriminatory practices?
- Do PAs in Canada, The Netherlands, UK, and US have similar job satisfaction scores and career expectations?
- How does family medicine PA role delineation differ amongst different countries?

SUMMARY

Data on PAs indicate that they are improving the specialty and geographic maldistribution of the medical workforce in the United States. PAs are more likely to work in primary care fields and in smaller communities and augment areas of medical need working with physicians (and are increasingly making major contributions in this area). The average age of the PA clinically employed is 42 years, and the length of employment is approximately 9 years (range 1 to 40 years). For students, the average age at graduation is 29 years (range 22 to 59). One of the problems with the work-related rewards received by PAs appears to be that they will reach an early peak in the first several years after entry into the profession and then plateau. This issue may be a concern for individuals who enter the PA profession early in age and have career aspirations to eventually work as something other than a clinician. An older individual who has been employed for some time and then makes a career move to become a PA may see this as career advancement.

Regardless, the PA profession is attracting a wide segment of society and blossoming globally. It is a career move for most entrants, and most remain in the career throughout their working lives. The presence of a PA in any population is a catalyst for change. How the PA profession will shape society remains an unanswered question.

References

The following citations are key to supporting this chapter's content. You can find a complete list of citations for all chapters at www.fadavis.com/davisplus, keyword *Hooker*.

American Academy of Physician Assistants (AAPA). (2008). *2008 AAPA Physician Assistant Census Report*. Alexandria, VA: Author.

American Academy of Physician Assistants (AAPA). (2014). *2013 AAPA Physician Assistant Census Report*. Alexandria, VA: Author.

Coombs, J., & Valentin, V. (2014). Salary differences of male and female physician assistant educators. *The Journal of Physician Assistant Education*, 25(3), 9–14.

Dial, T. H., Palsbo, S. B., Bergsten, C., Gabel, J. R., & Weiner, J. (1995). Clinical staffing in staff- and group-model HMOs. *Health Affairs*, 14(2), 168–180.

Essary, A. C., & Coplan, B. (2014). Ethics, equity, and economics: A primer on women in medicine. *Journal of the American Academy of Physician Assistants*, 27(5), 35–38.

Fréchette, D., & Shrichand, A. (2016). Insights into the physician assistant profession in Canada. *Journal of the American Academy of Physician Assistants*, 29(7), 35-39.

Hedden, L., Barer, M. L., Cardiff, K., McGrail, K. M., Law, M. R., & Bourgeault, I. L. (2014). The implications of the feminization of the primary care physician workforce on service supply: A systematic review. *Human Resources for Health*, 12, 32.

Hooker, R. S., Kuilman, L., & Everett, C. M. (2015). Physician assistant job satisfaction: A narrative review of empirical research. *Journal of Physician Assistant Education*, 26(4), 176–186.

Hooker, R. S., Robie, S. P., Coombs, J. M., & Cawley, J. F. (2013). The changing physician assistant profession: A gender shift. *Journal of the American Academy of Physician Assistants*, 26(9), 36–44.

Jones, I. W. (2015). Should international medical graduates work as physician assistants? *Journal of the American Academy of Physician Assistants*, 28(7), 8–10.

LeLacheur, S., Barnett, J., & Straker, H. (2015). Race, ethnicity, and the physician assistant profession. *Journal of the American Academy of Physician Assistants*, 28(10), 41–45.

Lo Sasso, A. T., Richards, M. R., Chou, C. F., & Gerber, S. E. (2011). The $16,819 pay gap for newly trained physicians: The unexplained trend of men earning more than women. *Health Affairs*, 30(2), 193–201.

Makinde, J. F., & Hooker, R. S. (2009). PA doctoral degree debt. *ADVANCE for Physician Assistants*, 17(3), 30–31.

National Commission on Certification of Physician Assistants. (2016). *2015 Statistical Profile of Certified Physician Assistants: An Annual Report of the National Commission on the Certification of Physician Assistants*. Retrieved from http://www.nccpa.net/research

Oliphant, J. (2014). *How you can help during the ebola crisis* [Online]. Retrieved from https://www.aapa.org/twocolumn.aspx?id=3389#sthash.vJfVJhWr.dpuf

Perry, H. B., III. (1977). Physician assistants: An overview of an emerging health profession. *Medical Care*, 15(12), 982–990.

Quella, A., Brock, D. M., & Hooker, R. S. (2015). Physician assistant wages and employment, 2000–2025. *Journal of the American Academy of Physician Assistants*, 28(6), 56–63.

Shi, L., Samuels, M. E., Ricketts, T. C., III, & Konrad, T. R. (1994). A rural-urban comparative study of nonphysician providers in community and migrant health centers. *Public Health Reports*, 109(6), 809–815.

Smith, D. T., & Jacobson, C. K. (2015). Racial and gender disparities in the physician assistant profession. *Health Services Research*, 51(3), 892–909.

US Department of Labor, Bureau of Labor Statistics. (2014). *Occupational employment and wages, May 2014, 29-1071 physician assistants*. Retrieved from http://www.bls.gov/oes/current/oes291071.htm

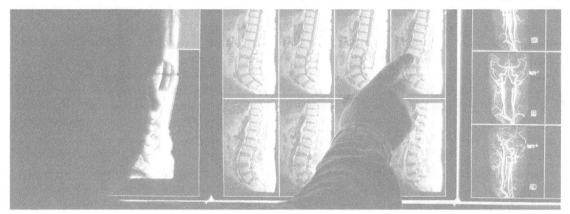

CHAPTER 4

PHYSICIAN ASSISTANT EDUCATION

RODERICK S. HOOKER ■ JAMES F. CAWLEY ■ CHRISTINE M. EVERETT

"The great difficulty in education is to get experience out of ideas."
—*George Santayana*

Physician assistant (PA) educational programs were created in academic institutions that were preparing traditional healthcare professionals, such as doctors and nurses. The PA curricula were based on new ideas and represented a hybridization of medical and nursing educational models. The first three creators of PA education—Smith, Stead, and Silver—borrowed heavily from allopathic medicine and traditional nursing theory. The intent was to prepare clinicians for roles to expand medical care services. In the intervening decades, PA educational programs have become well established in academic health centers and other institutions of higher education in the United States, The Netherlands, England, Australia, South Africa, Liberia, Ghana, and Canada. Essential to the introduction of the PA was the support of the medical profession and the federal government in all these countries. In the United States, the medical profession encouraged legal efforts in recognition of PA practice,

and the government granted financial support for the development of PA educational programs in 1971. However, government support for this burgeoning profession is hardly unique to the United States; almost all other countries with PA programs have experienced federal, state, or provincial enactment and support, including The Netherlands, United Kingdom, Canada, Australia, and South Africa. India being the exception. In their development and evolution, PA programs have helped influence concepts and trends in health professions education and have pioneered methodologies in decentralized clinical education, multidisciplinary approaches, and curriculum innovation.

EARLY DEVELOPMENT OF PHYSICIAN ASSISTANT EDUCATIONAL PROGRAMS

The first PA programs began in academic medical centers and evolved with sponsorship from a wide range of educational institutions as well as clinical organizations. The Duke University program offered one educational model for PA training, but others soon followed. The Medex

Program at the University of Washington, the 4-year program at Alderson-Broaddus College, and the Child Health Associate Program at the University of Colorado were established and fostered alternative and effective models for PA education in the US. The military programs of the Air Force and the Navy were among the first group of health center programs, beginning in 1971. By the late 1970s, PA programs had emerged in a variety of institutions, including medical schools, universities, 4-year colleges, community colleges, and technical and vocational schools as well as in teaching hospitals, correctional systems, and the federal healthcare systems.

As PA programs developed, one of their hallmarks was to be educationally efficient. Early programs were structured as short versions of medical school. Instead of partial-year education with time off, the PA education concept was to complete 24 to 36 months without significant breaks. Most programs were set in academic health centers where a rich infrastructure of clinics, educators, libraries, and other resources were at hand. This intensive education permitted a shorter process that produced educated clinicians available immediately upon graduation to be available for patient delivery services.

Another asset of PA education was diversity of setting. Diversity in sponsoring institutions was enhanced because PA education was not founded on an entry-level academic degree but instead was based on a competency model. This diversity resulted in a variety of curriculum models incorporating philosophies and approaches that were innovative and on the forefront of medical education. These models were designed for the recruitment of individuals with extensive healthcare experience and intended to meet specific national, state, and community needs.

Federal Support

For 5 decades the US federal government supported PA education through a series of small grants. PA education was included in Public Health Service (PHS) Title VII, Section 747, funding through the Bureau of Health Professions of the Health Services and Resources Administration. At times the levels of federal funding for Title VII programs waxed and waned, but federal funding has nonetheless been important to the growth and institutionalization of many PA educational programs in the United States. Spanning the years 1970 to 2010, funding has totaled more than $210 million. Congressional appropriation of PA educational programs through Title VII has promoted the expansion of enrollment within existing PA programs and has provided start-up funding for new programs.

For the 2013 fiscal year, a total of 39 programs were awarded federal grant support under the Title VII PA Grant Award Program, compared with 32 funded programs in fiscal year 2007. The investment in PA programs appears to have been a sound policy, and the rate of return has been higher than anticipated. Programs have been responsive to federal grant initiatives that target service in rural and medically underserved areas and delivery of primary care to needy populations (Physician Assistant Education Association [PAEA], 2014).

CHARACTERISTICS OF PHYSICIAN ASSISTANT PROGRAMS

As of 2016, the United States had 218 PA programs, and anticipated growth to 240 or more by 2025 (Figure 4–1). At least 41 new programs are in the accreditation pipeline. In addition, the number of programs in such countries as Australia, Canada, The Netherlands, the United Kingdom, India, South Africa, Ghana, and Saudi Arabia is growing. In fact, the United Kingdom has plans for 25-30 additional programs by the end of 2017 (Table 4–1 and Figure 4–2).

Across the board, many of these programs share similar characteristics with regard to their location, duration, curricula, faculty and student makeup, and other factors. For example:

- Almost three-quarters of US PA programs are in universities, with the remaining one-quarter in 4-year colleges, a few in community colleges, and one on a military base. Almost all of the non-US PA

FIGURE 4-1
Histogram of US Physician Assistant Programs

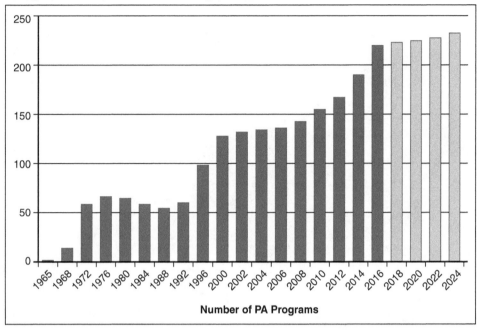

Number of PA Programs

TABLE 4-1
Summary of PA Programs Worldwide

Country	Year of First PA Graduation	Number of Clinically Active PAs (2015)	Number of PA Programs (2016)	Projected PAs (2020)
Australia	2012	20	1	40
Canada (PAs and not CAs)	2005	250	4	400
Germany	TBA	Unknown	2	TBA
Ghana	TBA	200	3	TBA
India	TBA	200	3	400
Ireland, Republic of	2017	0	1	60
Liberia	1965	200	2	
The Netherlands	2004	1,000	5	1,400
New Zealand	NA	0	0	Unknown
Saudi Arabia	2010	120	1	80
South Africa (clinical assistants)	TBA	Unknown	3	125
United Kingdom (physician associates)	TBA	75	6	425
United States	1967	99,500	200	120,000

programs are also in universities, frequently with medical schools.

- In most countries, the education process averages 26 to 36 months (average 106 weeks).
- In 2016, all US PAs were awarded a graduate degree. More than 90% of all PA programs award a master's degree. The type of master's degree offered varies; examples include Master of Science (MS), Master of Physician Assistant Studies (MPAS), Master of Science in Physician Assistant Studies (MSPAS),

FIGURE 4-2
Global Distribution of Physician Assistant Programs, 2014

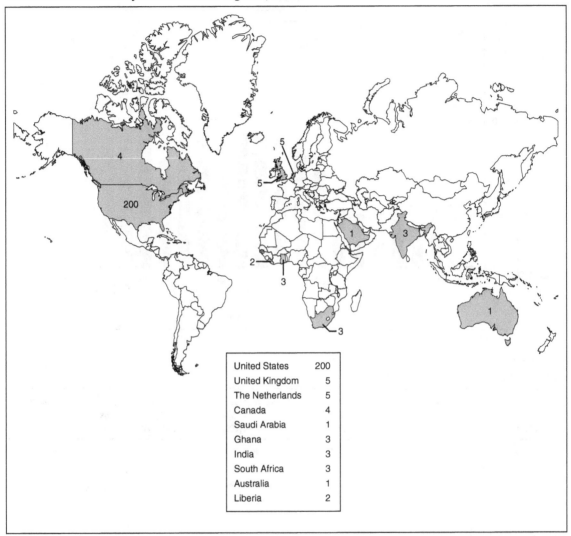

United States	200
United Kingdom	5
The Netherlands	5
Canada	4
Saudi Arabia	1
Ghana	3
India	3
South Africa	3
Australia	1
Liberia	2

Master of Physician Assistant Practice (MPAP), and the Master of Physician Assistant (MPA).

- Program enrollment and capacity have climbed steadily, with unfilled capacity under 10% (PAEA, 2014).

Costs of a PA Program

Educational institutions that sponsor PA educational programs are required to display tuition information on their websites. Table 4–2 shows data regarding PA program tuition levels, classified by public versus private institution. As might be expected, there is a significant difference in mean in-state tuition between public institutions versus private ones. The difference between public and private tuition is approximately $40,000. There is also a significant difference between the mean of public in-state and out-of-state tuitions. For PA students enrolled in a 26-month (average) professional phase of a PA program, the mean in-state resident tuition is $63,098; for nonresidents, $73,617 (2014 dollars). At present, more specific data on student choices in terms of

TABLE 4-2
Tuition by Type of US PA Program

	Public Sponsorship	Private Sponsorship
Number of schools	38	110
Resident tuition range	$8,5595–$70,319	$41,125–$137,291
Nonresident tuition range	$17,447–$117,347	$41,125–$137,291
Mean resident tuition	$33,838	$73,007
Mean nonresident range	$62,774	$73,282
Length range (months)	21–36	21–90
Average length	26.45	27.24
Class size range	18–103	18–98
Average class size	43.48	43.20
Average public program cohort tuition generated (assuming all resident rates × mean class size)	$1,558.238	N/A
Average private program cohort tuition generated (assuming all resident rates × mean class size)	N/A	$3,402.784
Total tuition per matriculant cohort (assuming resident rates in 38 programs)	$90,379.013	N/A
Total tuition per matriculant cohort (assuming nonresident rates in 110 programs)	N/A	$374,306.330

program attendance, financing resources, debt levels upon graduation, and consequent influence on practice choices are lacking. In 2014, the average total budget for a US PA program was $2,221,751.

Accreditation

Accreditation Review Commission on Education for the Physician Assistant

The Accreditation Review Commission on Education for the Physician Assistant (ARC-PA) assesses entry-level programs in the United States. Establishment of formal accreditation standards for PA programs marked an important milestone for the PA profession. The ARC-PA is the sole accrediting agency responsible for establishing the standards for US PA education and for evaluating programs to ensure their compliance with the standards. A standalone agency not embedded in any professional society, the ARC-PA is an important influence in PA education by developing a standard of curriculum. This ARC-PA influence has been instrumental in the state licensing process of PAs. The state licensure requirements in all US jurisdictions require a PA

to show that he or she is a graduate of an ARC-PA–approved program in good standing at the time of graduation. Moreover, a PA cannot sit for the Physician Assistant National Certifying Examination (PANCE) unless he or she is a graduate of an approved program. Continued certification is not a requirement for licensure in all jurisdictions.

The ARC-PA was initially established by an affiliated organization of the American Medical Association (AMA) in 1971 under another name, the Council on Accreditation of Allied Health Education Programs (CAAHEP). The AMA's Council on Medical Education first wrote the standards for PA program accreditation and was the primary overseer of many allied health standards. Thus, the Subcommittee of the Council on Medical Education became the *de facto* accreditation body and included representatives from the American Academy of Family Physicians (AAFP), American Academy of Pediatrics (AAP), American College of Physicians (ACP), American Society of Internal Medicine (ASIM), AMA, and Association of American Medical Colleges (AAMC). A document produced by the Subcommittee Council on Medical Education became the *Essentials of an Accredited Educational Program for the Assistant to the Primary Care Physician.* The AMA House of Delegates, with the endorsements noted and on recommendation of the Council on Medical Education, adopted these *Essentials,* clearing the way for the approval of educational programs that met or exceeded the requirements of the Joint Review Committee on Educational Programs for PAs (the predecessor of the ARC-PA).

As the quality of accreditation and the sophistication of assessing PA programs improved, the evolution of the accreditation process dictated that it become its own regulatory agency. The ARC-PA became an independent accrediting body in 2001.

ARC-PA Standards

The *Standards* document has undergone a number of revisions, with the latest changes to the fourth edition occurring in 2014. Prior versions of the *Standards* have set the tone for all aspects of PA program operation, including curriculum design and content. All key aspects of program operation are addressed in the *Standards.* These areas include administration and sponsorship, personnel, financial resources, operation, curriculum, evaluation, fair practices, laboratory and library facilities, clinical affiliations, faculty qualifications, admissions processes, publications to include on websites, and record-keeping. One underappreciated influence of the *Standards* has been the promotion of PA program curriculum creativity and innovation, particularly in institutions that have relied on traditional modes of medical education.

Although the ARC-PA does not prescribe curriculum length, preclinical and clinical content must include supervised clinical practice experiences, instruction in interpersonal and communication skills, and a number of patient-assessment and patient-management topics. Clinical education is required in a variety of settings to reflect breadth and depth of content and must include outpatient and inpatient settings as well as emergency departments. This clinical experience is, for the most part, undertaken in academic teaching facility settings, and inpatient clinical rotations are usually conducted in an experiential team format consisting of PA students,

medical students, and residents, led by a staff attending physician on a clinical rotation assignment basis. The required content areas of the preclinical curriculum are anatomy, physiology, pathophysiology, pharmacology and pharmacotherapeutics, and genetic and molecular mechanisms of health and disease. In the clinical curriculum, the required areas are emergency medicine, family medicine, internal medicine, surgery (including operative experiences), and medical care across the life span (e.g., pediatrics, prenatal care, geriatrics, and women's health).

Accreditation Process

ARC-PA accreditation is a voluntary determination and nearly all US PA programs participate in the accreditation process. Programs lacking ARC-PA accreditation are ineligible for federal grants, and their graduates are unable to apply for national certification or state licensure, thereby leaving them unable to practice.

ARC-PA considers applications for provisional and continuing accreditation. Institutions considering accreditation for a proposed or existing program must follow specific guidelines for conducting a comprehensive self-analysis to assess their performance in educating students. Programs must comprehensively document their operations and undergo several onsite evaluations before the request for accreditation is approved.

The ARC-PA *Standards* stipulate that the program must have:

- A full-time, 12-month faculty program director who is a National Commission on Certification of Physician Assistants (NCCPA)-certified PA or a physician
- A medical director who reports to the program director (the program director and medical director must be separate)
- At least three full-time equivalent (FTE) principal faculty positions (one of which may be the medical director if the position is equal to or greater than 0.6 FTE)
- Three faculty who are currently certified as PAs or licensed in the state as PAs

Accredited PA programs are subject to periodic reviews and onsite evaluations, a requirement for maintenance or retention of accreditation status.

Faculty

A mixture of healthcare professionals and professional educators are used within PA education programs. These educators include physicians and PAs (both master's- and doctoral-level instructors) with backgrounds in the basic medical sciences, the behavioral and social sciences, and various other disciplines. In 2015, approximately 1,600 PAs and 500 non-PAs were employed in US PA programs nationwide.

Data on Faculty in US PA Education Programs

The professional faculty of a PA program typically consists of a full-time program director (usually a PA who holds a master's or doctorate degree), a medical director (usually a physician serving part time), and an average of 4.3 FTE personnel serving in various PA faculty instructional roles. The total number of employees per program ranges from 3 to 13, with an average of 1 FTE for every 7.7 students enrolled.

In 2013, the average annual salary for PA academicians was $85,785 (compared with the average annual salary of $86,204 for practicing PAs). Whereas females fill the majority of PA program faculty positions, males hold the majority (60%) of program leadership positions,

such as the role of program director. In addition, male PA faculty members earn more on average per than female faculty members (e.g., at the associate professor level, the differences is $10,000) when all things are considered.

Advancement and Tenure

Most PA faculty are nontenured or not on tenure tracks (75%). Only 6% are at the rank of professor. Traditional criteria for promotion and tenure have presented some difficulties for PA faculty because faculty members are responsible for the academic administration of programs. Typically, administrative accomplishment is a minimal consideration in promotion and tenure decisions that usually reflect a "publish or perish" academic attitude. On the other hand, PA program faculty, given a finite time frame and limited faculty resources, tend to believe that the successful implementation of academic programs and production of competent graduates takes precedence over research and publications. Alternative definitions of scholarship have been developed by many institutions and are used to broaden their criteria for consideration in faculty promotion and tenure decisions.

Trends of PA program faculty in tenure-track positions or holding tenure over the past 5 years are shown in Figure 4–3. Despite a growth in the number of PA educational programs and

FIGURE 4-3
Trends of PA Faculty by Academic Rank, 2003–2012

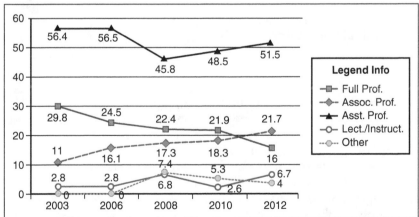

Data compiled from Physician Assistant Education Association's Annual Reports of PA Educational Programs in the United States, 2003–2012.

students during this time frame, the percentages of faculty either in tenure-accruing positions or tenured positions have declined. Nationally, about one-third of all college and university faculty members are tenured; in PA education, the percentage of PA faculty holding tenure rose slightly from approximately 5% in the 1990s to 8% in 2014.

Only a small percentage (7%) of US PA faculty members has earned the rank of professor. Around 10% have earned the rank of "associate professor," whereas 87% are classified as either "assistant professors" or "instructors." The composition of PA faculty remains largely at the junior level in most sponsoring institutions. Due to the attention this disparity has raised, the rise of PA educators in the university ranks is beginning to change.

Attrition

Attrition is the reduction of a workforce due to members leaving an agency or institution. According to annual surveys conducted by the PAEA, faculty attrition rates in PA programs have averaged roughly 11% to 12% per program per year. Over the 20-year period examined by the PAEA, respondents reported that 1,387 personnel left their positions. The overall 20-year mean is 69.3 personnel departing per year—an average of 0.9 persons departing per program per annum.

The reasons for departing PA teaching are not well known, but one finding suggests that salary is *not* among those reasons. One item that does seem to stand out a dissatisfaction among PA faculty is the lack of promotion as academics instead of administrators (Graeff, et al. 2014).

Program Directors

Program directors administer academic units with an annual budget averaging near $1.8 million or more, teach and evaluate an average of 44 students per program per year, and supervise an average of 10.1 faculty and 2.5 administrative staff. For institutions with ARC-PA accreditation, PA program directors should be certified PAs or physicians; others may assume the role, but institutions must provide the ARC-PA with justification for such appointments.

The role of a PA program director has evolved and become more complex. Directors are essentially academic unit administrators (i.e., department chairs) who are responsible for setting and maintaining the mission and goals of the program, supervising and evaluating the faculty, selecting qualified students, supervising administrative staff, attaining and maintaining compliance with accreditation criteria, managing the budget, relating to senior institutional administration, and promoting the program and the PA profession within and external to the institution.

Medical Directors

The role of a PA program medical director has consolidated over the years. Once a central member of the program faculty, medical directors now often serve on a part-time basis (0.2–1.0 FTE). One survey found that 50% of medical directors have a time commitment of less than 15% and one-sixth have a time commitment of more than 50%; 100% participated in curriculum planning and committee function, most notably the admissions committee; and 100% participate in direct student instruction. Rarely do medical directors mentor students or faculty or participate in or guide research projects.

Applicants

Almost all applicants to US PA educational programs do so through the Central Application Service for Physician Assistants (CASPA). Established in 2001, CASPA has centralized the application process and improved the ability to understand the PA applicant pool by allowing applicants to complete one online application and designate multiple programs to receive it. CASPA first verifies the materials for authenticity. This process of centralization enhances student choices and decreases falsified applications.

Number of Applicants

In response to forces in the healthcare professions marketplace, PA educational programs have seen steady increases in the number of program applicants, with annual increases ranging from 11% in 2007 to more than 20% in

2014. Applicants in 2014 designated an average of six schools on their CASPA applications. The rise in the number of applicants is thought to be due to such factors as:

- Improved visibility of the PA profession over half a century
- Opportunity to pursue a graduate degree
- Attractive income of PAs
- Ability to enter medicine without prolonged education

Application to US PA programs is competitive, and the applicant pool yields well-qualified candidates. In 2015, each available seat in existing PA programs listed with CASPA (approximately 200 programs) yielded 3.5 applicants per available seat. These proportions are similar to figures reported for US medical school applicants.

Applicant Demographics

The PA pipeline is determined by the general interest in the profession (applicant pool) as constrained by the capacity of educational programs. The PA profession appears to be popular among young adults, and a declining trend in the age of applicants continues, decreasing to 26 years in 2014, compared with 27.5 years in 2005 and 28 years in 2002. Most (73%) applicants are female. The average first-year student has an overall undergraduate grade point average (GPA) of 3.49 and science GPA of 3.43. For comparison, the typical first-year US medical school student is 23 years old, with an overall GPA of 3.67 and science GPA of 3.61; of the students entering medical schools in 2010, 53% were male.

The top undergraduate majors of applicants to PAs programs are biology, psychology, health science, exercise, nursing, medical technology, premedical, and sciences. The mean number of years of prior healthcare experience is 3.6 years, with 55% of self-reported healthcare experience being direct patient care. Applicants commonly identify this health-related work experience as the leading influence in choosing to learn about the PA profession and apply to a PA program. Most applicants take the Graduate Record Examination (53.9%); only 4.2% take the Medical College Admissions Test.

A review of data compiled by the PAEA provides useful insights into the types of students entering PA programs and the projected outcomes for those students:

- As of fall 2013, total first-year enrollment in entry-level programs was 7,887.
- Of the total number of students enrolled as first-year students for 2013, 71% were women; in addition, 28% were nonwhite students, and 7.3% were Hispanic.

Factors Influencing the Decision to Become a Physician Assistant

Data examining the reasons aspirants seek to become PAs are sparse. Using anecdotal sources, a list of motivators that are thought to influence individuals who apply to PA school was compiled. No one single motivating factor has emerged to explain why people choose a career as a PA. Some faculty members believe the prime factor for young women to select a PA education over medical school is that the shortened time to achieve a professional career allows more options for family planning. However, some factors that influence an individual's decision to become a PA have been identified. Although typical students plan a career in healthcare during high school, the decision to become a PA generally occurs later in life. A significant proportion selects the PA profession as their first health career. Other students decide to become PAs after first ruling out medical school and researching the PA profession. Dissatisfaction with a previous healthcare career is a moderate motivator for some. However, after potential students learn about the profession, they may take 3 to 4 years before they begin the enrollment process. The lag time from learning about the PA profession to starting the enrollment process typically results from time spent meeting application requirements, applying, being accepted, and finally enrolling.

A number of other factors can influence a person's choice to become a PA. Interestingly enough, PAs and other professionals continue to be the dominant force influencing students to consider a PA career. Personal contact with practicing PAs is probably the most effective recruitment tool for the profession. However, the factor of "following in a parent's footsteps" has also started to emerge as an influence. Since 1985, dozens of adult children have followed their PA parents' careers to become PAs (a few enrolling at the same time). Having a family member who is a PA or a physician or having a PA as a primary care provider is a strong influence on the decision to become a PA.

Selection Criteria

PA programs use a variety of criteria to select qualified students. Selection measures for predicting successful completion of PA training may include scores from the Scholastic Aptitude Test (SAT), Minnesota Multiphasic Personality Inventory (MMPI) scores, ACT, or GRE; transcript GPAs; and records of length of previous healthcare experience (depending on the program). Other criteria often include a personal essay, letters of recommendation, and an interview. The way in which these elements are weighted in a given program depends on the mission of the PA program and factors relating to institutional preference. Many educators believe that test results of intellectual ability and achievement are the reliable predictors of success in training programs. Specifically, SAT scores alone predicted excellent or poor student performance in the program. The MMPI test scores and previous healthcare experience appear to have little or no significance in predicting success or failure in the program or on the PANCE.

Selection criteria can change based on institutional funding, reputation, and state resident preferences (especially if the program is publicly funded). Some programs have well-defined goals—such as Christian service (e.g., Trevecca Nazarene University, Christian Brothers College, and Union College), a commitment for graduates to practice in a medically underserved area, or fluency in Spanish—that factor into their applicant decisions.

Course Prerequisites

Because PA program curricula vary considerably in content and structure, the sponsoring institution determines which courses are required for entry to PA education. The most commonly required courses were the following:

- Chemistry (86%)
- Physiology (83%)
- Anatomy (72%)
- Psychology (69%)
- Microbiology (66%)
- Biology (60%)
- English (51%)

Some research has identified a wide breadth of courses required for entry into PA programs. However, requirements vary by program. Some programs have minimal standards, whereas others have stringent course requirements that exceed those of some medical schools. A standardized set of prerequisite courses for applicants might be useful for applicants.

Prior Healthcare Experience

Although most PA programs emphasize prior health-related experience as a requirement for admission, the literature demonstrating the utility of this prerequisite does not support this requirement. There is no indication that students need prior healthcare experience to succeed in PA school and practice. In fact, one examination found no association between prior healthcare experience on the academic performance, graduate skill preparation, and employer perceptions of PA graduates. However, anecdotally, students with extensive healthcare experience are perceived as "easier" to teach by some faculty. This preference on the part of PA programs is a reflection of the early models of PA education, which tended to be based on students possessing extensive prior healthcare experience. (Recall that throughout the 1960s and 1970s, former military corpsmen and medics were viewed as some of the more suitable PA students.)

The requirements and acceptable definitions of "experience" vary by program. CASPA categorizes experience into "direct patient care" and "health-related" experience. Some programs require a definitive number of hours of direct patient care experience. A few schools do not recognize volunteer hours as sufficient, whereas other schools "strongly recommend" or simply do not require any healthcare experience at all.

Because there remains a great diversity in the type and duration of prior healthcare experience required by schools and recommended by practicing PAs, prospective students often are forced to ask themselves (and admissions committees): "Does experience really matter?" As admissions committees try to look at the "total package" for each applicant, it becomes difficult to justify how much prior healthcare experience is necessary to enter a PA program. Furthermore, because schools vary on what they consider appropriate experience, a prospective student may find himself or herself eligible for some programs but not others.

A survey of PAEA programs reported that three-quarters of new students worked in a healthcare field, regardless of patient contact, with 11% having worked in healthcare for more than 9 years (PAEA, 2014). According to an American Academy of Physician Assistants student survey, 31% of new student respondents had never worked in a healthcare field with direct patient-contact experience. When that number is compared with the percentage of students who reported any healthcare experience in 2007, a growing number of students start PA school with little or no direct patient contact experience.

Despite the lack of evidence correlating previous healthcare experience with success in PA education and the profession, some still feel it is important to mandate healthcare experience in new applicants. It is not unreasonable to assume that some experience in healthcare would help a student learn more in the limited amount of time they have as a PA student. Students with a background in healthcare know some of the language and culture of medicine and may have less difficulty deciphering jargon and acronyms in classes and lectures. Others believe it represents a proxy for maturity or life skill experience. Another strong argument for the experience requirement is that it brings with it a degree of exposure to the "real world," which usually involves holding a job and possessing the sense of responsibility that comes with it (Dehn, 2002). Finally, some believe that students who enter a PA program with significant clinical experience may find it easier to get through the clinical phase of the program.

However, prerequisites that are too diverse from program to program and prerequisites that are difficult to fulfill (e.g., 3–4 years of hands-on healthcare experience) may be detrimental to the profession because such restrictions limit potentially successful individuals from pursuing the career (Higgins et al., 2010). Ultimately, as the profession grows, more work is needed to determine the influence and effects of previous healthcare experience on matriculating and graduating students because many inexperienced but compassionate and motivated first-career individuals make good PAs.

On average, new PA students reported 32 months' experience, down from an average of 56 months in 1992. However, these statistics do not differentiate between direct patient contact experience and "other" experience. Therefore, the average 32 months' experience reported by new students may be in healthcare positions requiring fairly different skill sets and experiences than those required for PAs.

Many applicants come from decidedly clinical settings, such as emergency medical services, nursing, medical assisting, and medical laboratories. In fact, nurses, including NPs and licensed practical nurses, made up almost one-fifth of the 2002 student body, although that percentage has changed considerably. Paramedics account for approximately 20% of students. Some applicants come from other branches of the medical field, such as psychology, pharmacy, and allied health disciplines. Unfortunately, the historical healthcare experience of applicants and matriculates is not consistently collected and no newer data are available.

Students

The number of PA graduates has steadily climbed; approximately 7,000 PAs entered the workforce in 2015. One study predicts a 72% increase in the PA supply by 2025 (Hooker & Muchow, 2014). Estimates may underestimate the rapid expansion of PA programs expected over the same time. Moreover, retention rates are extremely high; only 2% had withdrawn from the cohorts who started in 2011 and graduated in 2013 (PAEA, 2014).

As the number and capacity of PA programs has steadily grown, concerns have emerged regarding whether growth is sustainable in the face of shortages of faculty and clinical training sites. Increasing numbers of students across the health professions have pushed demand and competition for a limited number of existing clinical slots. Some PA programs have begun paying for clinical rotations, often disrupting long-standing institutional relationships.

Student Demographics

Demographic patterns observed among PA students for the first decade of the profession showed clear male predominance. As a result of a steady increase in the proportion of women in the PA profession since 1985, women now comprise approximately 75% of all practicing PAs and an even larger percentage of PA students (Hooker et al., 2013). More than 8,000 first-year students enrolled in 190 programs in 2014; approximately 75% were female.

Factors Influencing the Decision to Enroll in a Program

Among those students accepted into a PA program, the most common factors that influenced the decision to become a PA were primarily the desire for "health-related work" and the encouragement of a "PA acquaintance" or "other health professional." These factors account for one-half of all reasons for choosing a PA career and have important implications for recruiting additional PAs.

Once a PA program has selected an applicant, the decision is in the applicant's hands. This decision is primarily influenced by two factors: PA program location and program reputation. The reputation factor is interesting because there is no consensus among applicants regarding which programs have superior reputations. Once a student has selected a program or has graduated from that program, there is an inherent belief among individuals that he or she made the correct educational institution decision.

International Medical Graduates

International medical graduates (IMGs) are doctors who have been to medical school outside of the United States. Some IMGs are US citizens who were not educated in the United States, whereas others are not US citizens. Historically, the process of IMGs attempting to become PAs has had its share of controversy. Specifically, concern arose over IMGs attempting to obtain advanced placement in PA programs and shortcut their way through the codified steps to PA licensure (Jones, 2015). Additional controversy resulted when some states funded "fast-track" to recruit IMGs into PA programs. In fact, IMGs constitute between 23% and 28% of physicians in the United States, the United Kingdom, Canada, and Australia. Low-income countries, such as India, China, and Pakistan, supply between 40% and 75% of these IMGs.

Despite such controversy, IMGs have a presence in PA education, including in programs outside of the United States. Medex Northwest, the University of Washington's PA Program, has trained more than 30 IMGs as PAs since 1980. The success of this venture is in contrast to other PA programs, some of which do not accept IMGs. The academic performance of Medex IMGs created few issues during the didactic phase of the Medex program. These students tended to be "average" students academically. Some IMGs had communication difficulties or role socialization and transition concerns; some had issues regarding a lack of assertiveness and discomfort dealing with crisis. The Medex clinical training model, however, includes close monitoring of student performance and frequent clinical site visits. This ongoing evaluation allowed faculty observation of the IMGs and their adaptation as PA students. The IMGs—many of whom had worked as translators or lower level healthcare workers in the United States—generally had an easy transition to the clinical phase of training. Most expressed gratitude to be back in significant clinical roles. All graduated "on time," and none were required to repeat any clinical rotations. All 39 Medex IMG PAs passed the national PANCE on the first try (Wick, 2015). The notion of IMGs transitioning into PAs remains controversial. Whether they are good fits or take up space that could be filled by younger first-career applicants is a topic that requires further discussion and data.

Predicting Success as a Physician Assistant Graduate

Without a definition regarding what constitutes an "effective PA," educators have turned to the only quantifiable indicator: the PANCE. Researchers have studied predictors of success in education programs to validate and improve admission requirements and course curricula. One study examined the predictive value of the PANCE among a small sample of 88 PA students and found little to predict in terms of demographics (Asprey et al., 2004). Another examined PANCE scores of 38 programs in the early 1990s and found master's-prepared PAs had higher average percent pass rates on the PANCE and higher average core scores than bachelor's-level program graduates. Programs with long accreditation status were found to perform significantly better on the clinical skills portion of the PANCE than those with less-established accreditation. Later, it was found that master's-prepared PA graduates performed better on the PANCE examination than non–master's-prepared graduates.

A study involving a large sample of 18,000 test takers found that master's-prepared graduates did slightly better on the PANCE than bachelor's-level graduates. Program characteristics, such as tuition, length of program, public versus private, medical school affiliation, and region of the country made no difference in PANCE scores. Neither did class size or the age or gender of the student. The authors concluded that, in this sample, little quantitative difference existed to predict who will pass and who will fail the PANCE in relation to an academic degree (Hooker et al., 2002) (Figure 4–4).

Program Organizational Role

The hierarchy of a program within a sponsoring institution varies (Figure 4–5). A program may be a division (subdepartment) of a medical school department (e.g., Duke University School of Medicine, Department of Family Medicine, Division of Physician Assistant Studies), or it may be a department in a School of Health Professions (e.g., School of Health Professions, University of Texas, Southwestern, Department of Physician Assistant Studies). An increasing number are becoming departments

FIGURE 4-4
PA Graduates Projection

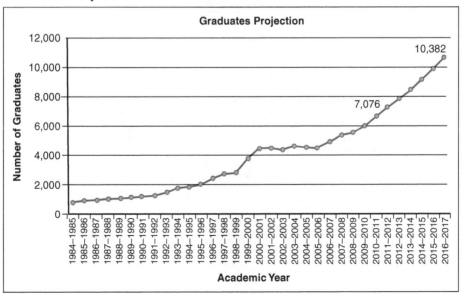

FIGURE 4-5
PA Faculty by Highest Degree, 2003–2012

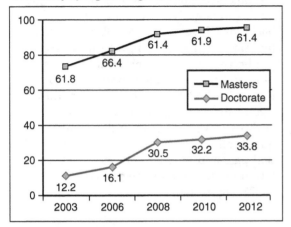

Data compiled from Physician Assistant Education Association's Annual Reports of PA Educational Programs in the United States, 2003–2012.

in schools of medicine within health sciences divisions (e.g., The George Washington School of Medicine and Health Sciences, Health Sciences Programs Division). Some programs are schools within themselves (e.g., Pacific University School of Physician Assistant Studies).

It appears that PA programs are increasingly set in academic units such as departments or divisions.

In a survey of 91 PA programs, 65% were within departments and 29% were standalone departments (Wright et al., 2009). Three-fifths (59%) resided in private institutions; of these institutions, two-thirds (67%) were sections within departments and 26% were, themselves, departments. Approximately one-half of all programs surveyed (46%) were located in academic health centers. The majority were embedded within a department (64%); 26% were at the departmental level. One-fifth (18%) of all PA programs reside in medical schools (Figure 4–6).

One-half of PA program directors (52%) report directly to a dean, 9% to an associate dean, 21% to a department chair, 6% to a provost (or equivalent), and 12% to "other" staff members. Between 2000 and 2008, one-quarter (26%) of all programs moved up in their hierarchical arrangement within the institution and 14% anticipated change by 2010 (e.g., shifting from a section in a Department of Family Medicine to a Department of PA

FIGURE 4-6
Physician Assistant Organization Chart

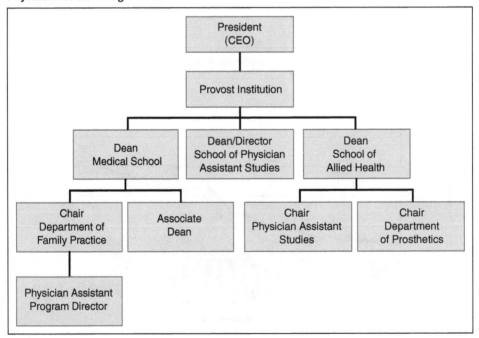

Studies). This substantial variation among institutions sponsoring PA programs likely reflects evolutionary development more than organizational rationale. How programs function and effect change within institutions remains to be explored.

Spread over 141 accredited programs in 2013, the average number of students in a PA program at any time (first, second, and third years combined) was 108. The mean number of students enrolled in first-year classes is 42 (range 40 to 173). The highest number in capacity is in the Interservice Physician Assistant Program (IPAP), capable of enrolling more than 200 students annually (three classes each year), which is substantially larger than the second largest program. Almost all students in US programs are full time.

First-year enrollment in PA programs increased from 24 students in 1984 to 47 in 2013. This increasing trend continues and may be due to a number of factors, such as efficiency in teaching large classes, demand for employment, application demand, quality of applicants, and institutional pressure to enroll more and/or maximize tuition. The irregularity of the trend is due to new programs entering with smaller classes, pulling the mean down until they ramp up to their desired size.

PHYSICIAN ASSISTANT PROGRAM CURRICULA

The philosophy of PA programs is one of a broad-based approach to primary care health professions education. This focus has resulted in curricula that provide PA students with a strong foundation in primary care and general medicine while preparing them to enter a wide range of specialized clinical areas.

The traditional philosophy of PA education has been based on demonstrating a standard level of clinical competency. Unlike most other health professions, PA education initially avoided assignment of a specific academic degree for entry-level preparation. In describing this philosophy, the PAEA Graduate Education Council stated that "proficiency in the clinical skills identified as being necessary for future competence in primary care/generalist practice would be the 'gold standard' of PA educational preparation, rather than necessitating adherence to institutional requirements for a specific academic degree."

Curriculum Overview

The format of the typical PA program is an intensive 26-month (range, 24 to 36 months), medically oriented curriculum that educates the student in medicine. Approximately one-half of that time (12 months) involves didactic instruction in the basic and clinical sciences, followed by a similar period of rotating clerkships and preceptorships in all major clinical disciplines (although this format is increasingly blended, with clinical experience included in the first year and additional theoretical lectures in the second year).

The basic science curriculum is usually structured to provide an in-depth understanding of structural features characterizing body tissues and organ systems, biochemical mechanisms regulating body metabolism, and nutrition. It also reviews the physiological controls that govern body system functions, which form a foundation on which to build an understanding of the pathophysiology and behavioral alterations that cause clinical manifestations of illness. These topics form the basis for understanding the management of illnesses and injuries.

In most US PA programs, the curriculum is based on the medical school model. A typical PA program is about 50 weeks shorter than a typical medical school program, but the primary educational objectives are similar. Both physician and PA education provide students with the theoretical knowledge and technical skills needed to perform therapeutic and diagnostic procedures accurately. Like medical schools, PA programs use a format of didactic and clinical training. However, the average PA program spans 27 months with minimal breaks, whereas the average medical school spans 48 months of instruction and breaks between school years 1 and 2.

Curriculum Topics

A few studies have dealt with the subject of what should be learned in PA programs. One found that most PA programs were teaching what medical school educators had already been teaching—that the core of medicine is history taking and physical examination. In addition to teaching the proper approach to the patient and certain clinical skills, programs included technical skills such as urinalysis, blood analysis, electrocardiogram (ECG) interpretation, hearing and vision screening, Papanicolaou scrapings, application and removal of casts, tuberculosis skin testing, interpretation of radiographs, parenteral injections, bacteriology testing, suturing, and pulmonary function testing.

Primary Care Education

Curricular innovations in health professions education that have focused on the clinical preparation of providers for primary care roles originated within now-prominent PA programs. PA programs using decentralized training approaches—such as those seen at the University of Washington Medex Northwest PA Program; the Stanford University Primary Care Associate Program; the University of California, Davis; Lock Haven University; and the University of Utah PA Program—have paved the way for other programs in their efforts to develop effective methods in placing PA graduates in medically underserved areas.

PA educators remain sensitive to changes in the healthcare environment, and program curricula undergo regular review and modification. Experience indicates that this flexibility results in newly employed PAs who adapt easily to many practice settings. For example, the University of Texas-Pan American and Lock Haven University are innovative curricula that prepare primary healthcare providers for practices in areas with underserved populations.

To address areas essential to the preparation of competent primary care providers, PA programs commonly include instruction on preventive medicine, substance abuse prevention and treatment, healthcare for the homeless, women's healthcare, geriatric medicine, environmental and occupational medicine, mental health, and a practical orientation to developing skills in the delivery of clinical preventive services. Other examples of innovations of PA programs in focusing on primary care have been

the long-standing inclusion of such topics as health education, epidemiology, communication skills, and biomedical ethics. These subjects have only relatively recently been regarded as important in undergraduate medical education.

Skills and Procedures

Each PA program seeks to develop within each student a strong foundation in the basic and clinical sciences of medicine. The education process may reflect a traditional medical school curriculum and even share classes with medical students, or it might introduce multidimensional assessment and decision analysis techniques that are unique to the particular PA program.

A comprehensive survey of Colorado PAs found that almost all of them learned 39 common procedures (Box 4–1). Eight procedures (including reading chest and long-bone x-ray films, suturing, splinting, interpreting ECGs, and performing pelvic examinations, Papanicolaou smears, and urinalysis) were performed more than once per month by at least 50% of PAs in their practices. Three procedures (performing cardiopulmonary resuscitation, lumbar puncture, and suprapubic aspirations) were used less than once per year by more than 90% of PAs. The leading skills needed for any PA practice were history taking, physical diagnosis, and patient management.

In examining the content of PA clinical activities, a study of Arizona family medicine practices found differences between providers by types of procedures. Fetal monitoring and respiratory procedures occur across all three clinician types, suggesting overlap in skills and ability (although at different rates). Dermatological procedures appear to be unique to PAs and physicians, but PAs were more likely to perform wound suturing than the other two providers. In this study, only joint injection seemed to be more likely performed by physicians.

Clinical Rotation

PA education is built on the apprentice concept—that a student learns best by doing. The clinical rotation is when the student sees

Skills Most Frequently Performed by PA Students

PROCEDURES
- Cardiopulmonary resuscitation
- Electrocardiogram (perform, interpret)
- Fingerstick and heelstick
- Fluorescein Wood's lamp examination
- Parenteral injection (intradermal, subcutaneous, intramuscular)
- Lumbar puncture
- Suprapubic aspiration
- Urethral catheterization
- Venipuncture

LABORATORY TECHNIQUES
- Agglutination test for mononucleosis (read)
- Blood smear (perform, read)
- Culture (perform, read)
- Gram stain (perform, read)
- Sensitivity plate (read)
- Stool examination for occult blood
- Urinalysis (dipstick, microscopic)

PATIENT CARE
- Chest radiograph (read)
- Intravenous line (set up, start, monitor)
- Long-bone x-ray film (read)
- Papanicolaou stain (perform)
- Pelvic examination
- Suturing
- Wound care (burns, casts, splints)

SCREENING TESTS
- Articulation screening
- Denver Developmental Screening Test
- Hearing screen
- Vision screen

pediatrics, prenatal care and women's health, general surgery, emergency medicine, and psychiatry/behavioral medicine (Fig. 4–7).

Such clinical experiences can vary in length from a few weeks to a few months. Many programs also add components on rural health, public health, care in nursing homes, addiction medicine, and certain specialties, such as orthopedics, pulmonology, forensic medicine, radiology, intensive care, urology, gastroenterology, corrections medicine, and sports medicine.

Supervised Clinical Practice Experiences

Traditionally, the clinical rotation phase (i.e., preceptorship) of training for PA students is the final step in the professional socialization process (however, when this stage occurs varies among institutions). During the preceptorship stage, PAs must learn the proper attitudes and techniques for managing patients with professionalism and appropriate clinical judgment—the essence of appropriate medical practice. With the science of medicine learned primarily from lectures, books, and laboratory work, the art of relating to patients is acquired through imitative role modeling, intuition, and trial and error. Views about patients tend to change the most during this time, as students gain clinical experience and expertise.

The preceptorship is an experience shared by a physician mentor and a student. This experience is not trivial because the physician may become a lasting role model in the memory of the student and shapes the PA's career. During preceptorship, the physician guides the PA through the cardinal learning experiences of medicine—exploring, examining, and cutting into the human body; dealing with the fears, anger, sense of helplessness, and despair of patients; meeting urgent situations; accepting the limitations of medical science; and being confronted with death—for the PA to achieve professional self-actualization.

Preceptorships do not come easily, and good preceptors are even harder to find. A PA student may have to compete with medical students from the host institution or students

patients, either in conjunction with an experienced clinician or on his or her own with an experienced clinician assessing the student's evaluation of a patient. The clinical settings in which these encounters occur vary and can be outpatient or inpatient, including primary care offices, tertiary care centers, birthing centers, and nursing homes. Although specific clinical rotations are not required for each clinical discipline, a PA program is obligated to give every student clinical experiences in family medicine, general internal medicine,

FIGURE 4-7
Procedures in Family Medicine by Type of Provider

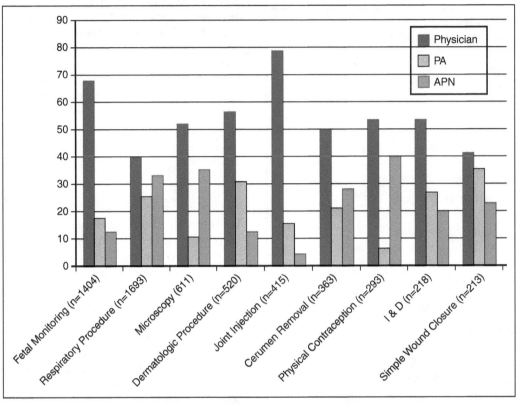

Tabor, J., Jennings, N., Kohler, L., Degnan, B., Eng, H., Campos-Outcalt, D., & Derksen, D. (2016). AzCRH 2015 Supply and Demand Study of Arizona Health Practitioners and Professionals. University of Arizona Center for Rural Health.

from other PA or NP programs for clinical slots with a preceptor. One critical issue for many PA programs is the availability of clinical training sites. With the expansion of medical student and PA student educational programs, the number of educational slots for clinical students in practices and teaching hospitals are at a premium, particularly in certain disciplines such as pediatrics and women's health. This shortage has led some programs to begin paying to precept students; in 2008, 8% (nine programs) responding to the PAEA Annual Survey reported payment to sites and/or preceptors. Additional concerns that can affect preceptorships include using one site too often (preceptor fatigue) or overusing a facility that already has clinicians with too many students. Higher tuition and debt burden are the reasons most often cited for not purchasing preceptorships. Outside of the United States, PA programs tend to value this human capital as valuable and as a standard pay preceptors for their time to work with students.

Many preceptors enjoy the intellectual and social stimulation of training students. Some see mentoring as an effective tool for recruiting new employees or the opportunity to be challenged by bright students. Others dismiss the notion of a professional obligation to train those who follow them into medicine. However, the pressures placed on clinicians to meet performance expectations have often been cited as a reason that some clinicians elect to discontinue preceptorship due to the conviction that it "slows them down," thus decreasing productivity.

A survey asked 115 clinical preceptors of the University of New Mexico PA Program to assess their experience as clinical teachers, interest in teaching topics, preferred delivery modes, and rewards of teaching. Their responses showed that preceptors' interests and needs varied. More importantly, it allowed the faculty opportunities to address preceptor needs and make better matches of students to preceptors at their sites (O'Callaghan, 2007).

Graduate Level Education

Educators and researchers in many health profession disciplines have long wrestled with the "degree debate" regarding the appropriate entry-level credential. This process represents a natural progression in the maturation of many professions. Debates are often discomforting and require many years to achieve general consensus within the representative educational programs. For example, as early as 1958, the field of occupational therapy began deliberations as to what educational level was best suited for the profession. Nearly 30 years later, the American Occupational Therapy Association (AOTA) endorsed a gradual shift to the master's degree as the entry-level degree for its profession. Similarly, the physical therapy profession began a transition to an entry-level master's degree over a 10-year period back in 1979, which met with continued debate. Their guidelines for educational programs, as revised in 1997, standardized the physical therapy entry-level degree at the master's level. Now US PT and OT programs award a technical doctorate. NPs determined that the NP education award was the Master of Science in Nursing (MSN) degree. The doctorate of nursing practice (DNP) is an institutional option, and the trend is to award this degree to all advance practice nurses upon graduation.

A similar pattern of evolution is being observed in the PA profession. When the first educational program was founded, the mandate for programs was to produce safe and competent clinicians and to get them into the field as soon as possible. PA education was a competency-based model, consisting of 2 or 3 years of college work with certain prescribed courses plus vocational training. Often, a certificate of completion was the only credential awarded upon completion of the educational program. As time passed and PA educational programs

evolved, sponsoring institutions, such as Alderson-Broaddus College in 1970, began to award academic degrees along with the certificate of program completion.

The first PA program to award a master's degree for entry-level training was the Child Health Associate Program at the University of Colorado in 1975. As PA education evolved, individuals argued that a master's degree is consistent with the quantity and quality of intellectual work to which PA students are subjected and that the level of academic rigor in PA programs was well beyond bachelor's-level work. PA students develop the power of critical reasoning, the capacity to generalize, and the ability to find and evaluate clinical information so they can practice evidence-based medicine. Using this line of reasoning, one can conclude that PA education is at a higher level than undergraduate and that a master's degree is the appropriate credential for the profession.

In 1990, only three programs in the United States (6% of all programs) awarded a master's degree; by 2008, 76% did. Now, a master's degree is universal in the United States. It is also the favored degree in three of the four PA programs in Canada and the five programs in The Netherlands. By 2020, PAs programs throughout the United Kingdom will also award graduate degrees. Typically, programs award the Master of Science (MS), Master of Physician Assistant Studies (MPAS), or Master of Health Science (MHS) degree. The average program length has increased from 24 months in 1987 to 26 months in 2007 (range 12 to 31 months). Didactic curriculum has increased from 1,004.5 hours in 1991 to 1,594 hours in 2007. The increases in didactic curriculum and consequent increase in total program length are likely related to the higher degrees granted by contemporary programs. Table 4–3 shows the various degrees awarded by PA educational programs. Two US programs have signaled they will award a doctorate to PA graduates with some additional work.

Until recently, the ARC-PA *Standards* did not address the educational level at which PA education should be provided. In the second edition of the *Standards*, the operative language was: "This version of the *Standards* reflects the realization that a commonality in the core

TABLE 4-3
Credentials Awarded by Physician Assistant Programs, 2011 (N = 164)*

Credential	Number
Certificate	27
Associate	4
Baccalaureate	23
Bachelor of Science (BS)	8
Bachelor of Science in Physician Assistant (BSPA)/Bachelor of Science in Physician Assistant Studies (BSPAS)/Bachelor of Physician Assistant Studies (BPAS)/Bachelor of Physician Assistant (BPA)	7
Bachelor of Medical Science (BMS)	1
Bachelor of Clinical Health Services (BCHS)	1
Bachelor of Health Science (BHS)/Bachelor of Science in Health Science (BSHS)	4
Other Baccalaureate Degree	2
Master's	154
Master of Science (MS)	29
Master of Physician Assistant Studies (MPAS)/Master of Science in Physician Assistant Studies (MSPAS)/Master of Physician Assistant Practice (MPAP)/Master of Physician Assistant (MPA)	81
Master of Health Science (MHS)/Master of Science in Health Science (MSHS)	12
Master of Medical Science or Master of Science in Medicine (MMS/MSM/MMSc)	24
Master of Public Health (MPH)	4
Other master's degree	6

*Note: Some programs award more than one credential. Data from Physician Assistant Education Association (PAEA). (2012). Twenty-Eighth Annual Report on Physician Assistant Educational Programs in the United States, 2011–2012. Alexandria, VA: PAEA.

curriculum of programs has become not only desirable, but also necessary in order to offer curricula of sufficient depth and breadth to prepare PA graduates for practice in a dynamic and competitive healthcare arena." Additionally, the *Standards* are intended to "reflect a graduate level of curricular intensity." In 2014, the ARC-PA modified the fourth edition of the *Standards* to indicate that the establishment of new PA programs may occur only at institutions that can award a bachelor's degree or higher. Yet the *Standards* do not specify any delineation of curricular content relative to the credential awarded upon successful completion of the educational program.

Unlike other health professions, there is not a single type of master's degree awarded for PA education, but instead there has emerged a wide variety of master's degrees granted by sponsoring institutions. The Council on Graduate Medical Education endorsed educational content that includes "principles of statistics and epidemiology, learning how to search efficiently for 'current best evidence,' knowing the relative value of different types of evidence, and knowing when and how to apply evidence to the care of an individual or patient group." Achieving this degree of knowledge and clinical expertise requires a greater breadth and depth of graduate professional education than competency-based undergraduate models are typically able to accommodate.

In some instances, institutional requirements dictate the form the master's degree is to take. In other institutions, the award of a master's degree means that such a degree comprises a set number of graduate credits and contains specific quantitatively oriented courses. Finally, the configuration of the master's degree should take a distinctly academic identity as opposed to a professional degree in which traditional institutional academic requirements may not be present.

As programs converted to the master's degree, most adjusted their curricula to include additional courses in research-related subjects such as biostatistics, research methodology, and data analysis. Almost all US programs have made this change. Converting programs were surveyed as to which course(s) were added to the curricula. Common responses were research methods in epidemiology (20%), research methods in statistics (11%), and a long list of research/quantitative courses. When converting, PA programs were asked if the conversion necessitated a change in their mission and goals; 34% indicated that it did, and 21% indicated that it did not. In terms of whether changing to the master's degree caused them to lengthen the program, 32.6% indicated that it did, and 22.5% indicated that it did not.

In the early 1990s, new models of PA education developed. One of these programs combined PA education with a related graduate degree program: the PA/master of public health (e.g., program at The George Washington University). In 2017 there were eight PA/MPH programs. Others offer distance education master's degree programs aimed at practicing PAs (Table 4–4).

POSTGRADUATE PHYSICIAN ASSISTANT EDUCATION PROGRAMS

PAs have educational requirements that begin immediately upon graduation from an entry-level program. Such education ranges from formal education courses to on-the-job training. For most, it is a lifelong learning process. Postgraduate education, commonly referred to as a *PA residency program* or *fellowship,* is an advanced training process available to some PAs and has steadily grown since the new millennium. It is an additional period of training in a formal setting with a concentration in a medical or surgical discipline. Postgraduate training programs allow newly graduated PAs to acquire hands-on training to improve their clinical skills and didactic knowledge in specialized areas. Trainees of postgraduate programs, sometimes referred to as fellows, perform medical tasks at a level comparable to a physician resident and may provide some economic benefit to the healthcare system. However, postgraduate residency training programs face substantial challenges. These include lack of documented value, standardized curricula, and chronicled outcomes through research.

Traditionally, residency programs were developed for medical school graduates to provide the clinical experience needed in their chosen specialty. In the past, these residencies were notorious for having extremely long and arduous workweeks. However, in 2003, the Accreditation Council for Graduate Medical Education's mandate involving the amount of hours a resident could work became policy. As a result, a new approach of using PAs and NPs emerged to help fill the gaps left by shorter resident weeks. Subsequently, 1-year formal postgraduate training programs, which followed the graduate medical education model, became more popular as a method to train new PAs in specialty fields. The Association of Postgraduate PA Programs (APPAP) helps to oversee and organize the educational curricular for the 44 programs of this nature. Programs exist that offer training in a variety of subspecialties, but most common are surgery and emergency medicine. Programs vary in length, with some as short as 6 months and others as long as 24. As of 2014, the amount of PAs with postgraduate training only accounted for "1% of the entry level program graduates per year." If the need for specialty trained PAs continues to grow, then the PA field may see an increase in the number of postgraduate programs, a greater diversity in subspecialty program types, and thus an overall higher number of PAs with specialty training.

Although PA residency programs have been in existence for more than 3 decades, they have

TABLE 4-4
Examples of Master's of Public Health/Physician Assistant Dual-Degree Programs, 2016

Program	Year Founded	Applicants/ Enrollees	Admissions Criteria	Cost	Length	Curriculum Integration
Emory University	2006	21/2	Academics and experience	$46,000	38 months	10 credits
Arcadia University	2001	N/A		N/A	3 years	6 credits
Touro College	2003	500/25	Diversity	$30,000	32 months	Total program
The George Washington University	1987	150/12	Narrative	$90,000	3 years	8 credits
University of Washington	2004	551/81	Diversity/ academics	$37,000	37 months	None

yet to establish themselves as an essential component of the profession. Some argue that increased autonomy and specialization have resulted in a need for practical, postgraduate specialty education. In addition, the numbers of PAs seeking formal postgraduate training before entering the specialty of their choice, or transferring from one specialty to another, is slowly increasing. If the PA profession follows the pattern of physicians and several other healthcare professions, postgraduate residency education may become an expectation for practitioners. Currently, the NCCPA has no residency requirements for PA certification. PAs can chose to participate in a residency or not. Each individual student must weigh the pros and cons and decide for him or herself (Will et al., 2016).

A benefit of participating in a residency program is the hands-on training that PAs receive within a specific field of interest. Generally, PA residents report substantial gains in their knowledge and skills during their training, including improvements in their abilities to establish a diagnosis; to recognize disease and pathology; to think critically; and to develop a differential diagnosis. The APPAP suggests that it would take years to attain the level of confidence and skill that can be acquired during a 1-year residency. This training can be particularly helpful in fields that are fast-paced; advanced training gives the PAs the opportunity to gain experience in their chosen specialty, which they may have not been exposed to during their clinical rotations as a PA graduate student. For example, Will and colleagues (2016) discuss the hiring and training process for a hospitalist PA, citing that hiring a PA with prior work experience still requires 6 to 12 months of on the job training, and a newly graduated hire will require even more instruction. Additionally, one study among PAs currently working in a hospitalist position found that 91% of participants would have been interested in a formal postgraduate training program, even if it meant lower pay for the first year. This finding suggests that many PAs, once having experienced what it is like to learn on the job, may actually prefer some specialized training. A residency in hospital medicine

could allow a PA to begin working as a hospitalist immediately, eliminating the need for on-the-job training.

One view is that the PA curriculum is too short to learn all of the intricacies of modern medicine (Hooker, 2009). Concentrated experience in a specialized setting is apprenticeship at its best because it combines scholarly activity and tertiary medicine. Another advantage is the complete readiness of postgraduate-trained PAs; having had the opportunity to learn from role models, they become efficient and competent in their skills and gain overall confidence. Additionally, residencies can provide practicing PAs with the opportunity to either change their specialty with confidence or simply increase their skill level within their current clinical practice.

Another added benefit of a residency is that it allows PAs to augment the care of residents who have restricted work hours due to the passing of the ACGME mandate. The mandate stipulates that residents "work no more than 24 hours of continuous patient care (with an added 6-hour transition and education period), 1 day in 7 free of patient care responsibilities, and a minimum of 10 rest hours between duty periods." PAs have been shown to be an effective way to alleviate the added pressures the mandate placed on the hospital system. A 30-year survey of the use of PAs in an Emory intensive care unit found that PAs allowed for the "expansion of services" without the addition of more medical residents. Many of these positions require a high level of specialization (Carpenter et al., 2012).

One argument against the PA residency is the idea that it promotes the movement away from the PA as a generalist, a person who has a great commodity in the healthcare field: flexibility. PAs can switch specialties without having to seek further training, allowing them to adapt to the continually evolving medical environment and play a vital role that is adaptable. Another argument is that PAs appear to be quick to learn and have a reputation for high performance. The evidence for PA residencies' producing something more than a cadre of house officers is limited at best (Hooker, 2009). This adaptability may contribute to the high rates of PA job satisfaction. Thus it follows that moving toward a more comprehensive postgraduate training system may decrease job satisfaction and move the PA toward a more inflexible physician model of specialty choice. This too may result in the profession becoming less desirable to potential students, as one of the most attractive qualities for many prospective students is the opportunity for mobility.

One other consideration is whether a PA postgraduate training program is useful or not. Dehn (2013) contends that a PA residency is redundant, arguing that because PAs practice under supervision throughout their careers, completing a residency is superfluous and not valuable. "Residencies essentially duplicate what PAs find in their typical work environments" (Dehn, 2013).

A major setback toward furthering PA residencies lies in motivating newly graduated PA students to forgo a higher salary for a much lower residency stipend. As of 2015, the median annual wage for a PA in the United States was $98,180 ($47.20 per hour × 2080 hours per year), according to the US Bureau of Labor Statistics in 2015. Contrast this with the income offered by John Hopkins University for its emergency medicine residency program, which pays a stipend of $46,000 per year for the 18-month program. Proponents of postgraduate training may argue that higher starting salaries offset this temporary deficit. However, this difference may be negated after several years of practicing, at which point postgraduate training has no correlation to salary.

Further, Dehn (2013) conducted a survey aimed at collecting information regarding job satisfaction, hours worked per week, and salary for three different PA residency program graduates comparatively. The survey showed that although PAs with postgraduate training make on average 15.1% more, they also work 15.5% more hours, thus suggesting that their higher salary is simply indicative of workload.

Postgraduate training programs may continue to develop popularity as PAs select more specialized roles. Whether this is a positive development in the PA profession will be debated, with both positions holding pertinent views. Each individual must conduct his or her own cost-benefit analysis to decide whether a specialty postgraduate training program is personally worthwhile. Educators, policymakers, employers, and members of the profession have relatively little systematic information on which to formulate opinions and make judgments about the value of PA postgraduate education programs, but these programs are established and expected to grow. A few postgraduate PA programs award a doctorate degree in science such as DSc.

FURTHER RESEARCH ON PHYSICIAN ASSISTANT EDUCATION

Despite 50 years of experience, the literature about the education of PAs and PA educational programs is limited. Following is a list of research areas in need of attention:

- **Case reports:** Writing about the development of a program from its initial conception and development to the first class can provide insight into policy development and educational start-up costs. Case reports can show how a program is structured in an institution and the organizational roles for each educator.
- **Role delineation:** What is the role of the educator in a PA educational setting? What percent of PA educators work clinically? Do lines of demarcation exist between the academic coordinator and the clinical coordinator? Does program size matter in the educational load of a PA academic? Why are increasing numbers of PA faculty attaining doctoral degrees? What does a graduate from a postgraduate PA program do? Is there some way to distinguish a postgraduate-trained PA and a PA trained on the job in the same specialty?
- **Organizational arrangements:** What are the lines of influence and organization for a PA program in a host institution? What is the optimal academic unit (e.g., school, department, division, program) for a PA program within an educational institution? Does the degree of separation from the president of a university to

the PA director have any influence on how a program functions?

- **Breadth of knowledge:** How many diagnoses should a PA know by the time of graduation? What measures do PA programs apply to ensure that graduates are attaining minimal levels of competence?
- **Quality of care:** How do programs know that the students they are graduating are prepared to deliver adequate quality of care? Does the quantity or quality of tests in PA education preparation matter on the PANCE?
- **Retention:** What are the social and economic factors that contribute retention or attrition of PA faculty? Is the turnover of PA program directors excessive?
- **Global comparisons:** How does PA education differ by country?
- **Economics:** What are the opportunity costs of a formally trained surgical PA versus a postgraduate-trained PA versus an on-the-job trained PA? Do these differences in cost of education have any predictive value on the role the PA selects?

SUMMARY

PA programs have evolved and expanded in institutional sponsorship and organizational structure. The typical program enrolls 45 students per year on average, with six faculty, a ratio of 7:1, and an increasing on-campus prominence. The education of PAs has moved from being marginal, isolated, experimental, externally funded educational operations to well-established, widely accepted, complex graduate level academic departments with a substantial applicant pool and a robust internal financial base.

What has also changed is that PA programs are no longer producing graduates that channel into primary care. The trend of more PAs choosing specialty practice positions over primary care, where now at least two-thirds of all PAs are in specialty practice, could be linked to factors such as debt level, higher salaries, and greater availability in specialty positions, but thus far findings conclusively defining such an association are lacking. Such choices could also relate to the disproportionate debt burden associated with attending privately sponsored programs, where the mean public-to-private tuition comparison is more marked. It should be noted however that, among newly graduating medical students, debt is not the leading factor associated with specialty choice. The process of specialty choice among PA graduates may or may not be similar to that of medical students. Yet another factor to consider is the ability of PAs to change specialties over the course of their careers. More than half of all clinically practicing PA have changed specialties at least once in their career, and 12% have changed specialties more than four times.

Two of the most dominant trends in PA education are the marked expansion of the numbers of programs since the 1990s, as well as graduates' resolution of the issue of the academic credential awarded on completion of PA studies.

References

The following citations are key to supporting this chapter's content. You can find a complete list of citations for all chapters at www.fadavis.com/davisplus, keyword *Hooker*.

Asprey, D., Dehn, R., & Kreiter, C. (2004). The impact of age and gender on the Physician Assistant National Certifying Examination Scores and pass rates. *Journal of Physician Assistant Education*, 15(1), 38–41.

Carpenter, D. L., Gregg, S. R., Owens, D. S., Buchman, T. G., & Coopersmith, C. M. (2012). Patient-care time allocation by nurse practitioners and physician assistants in the intensive care unit. *Critical Care*, 16(1), R27.

Dehn, R. W. (2002). Does experience count? *Clinical Advisor*, 5(1), 98.

Dehn R. (2013). PA-Is PA residency training worth it? *Clinical Advisor*. Retrieved from http://www.clinicaladvisor.com/pa-is-pa-residency-training-worth-it/article/116919

Graeff, E. C., Leafman, J. S., Wallace, L., & Stewart, G. (2014). Job satisfaction levels of physician assistant faculty in the United States. *Journal of Physician Assistant Education, 25*(2), 15–20.

Higgins, R., Moser, S., Dereczyk, A., Canales, R., Stewart, G., Schierholtz, C., et al. (2010). Admission variables as predictors of PANCE scores in physician assistant programs: A comparison study across universities. *Journal of Physician Assistant Education, 21*(1), 10–17.

Hooker, R. S. (2009). Assessing the value of physician assistant postgraduate education. *Journal of the American Academy of Physician Assistants, 22*(5), 13.

Hooker, R. S., Hess, B., & Cipher, D. (2002). A comparison of physician assistant programs by national certification examination scores. *Perspective on Physician Assistant Education, 13*(2), 81–86.

Hooker, R. S., & Muchow, A. N. (2014). Supply of physician assistants: 2013–2026. *Journal of the American Academy of Physician Assistants, 27*(3), 39–45.

Hooker, R. S., Robie, S. P., Coombs, J. M., & Cawley, J. F. (2013). The changing physician assistant profession: A gender shift. *Journal of the American Academy of Physician Assistants, 26*(9), 36–44.

Jones, I. W. (2015). Should international medical graduates work as physician assistants? *Journal of the American Academy of Physician Assistants, 28*(7), 8–10.

O'Callaghan, N. (2007). Addressing clinical preceptorship teaching development. *Journal of Physician Assistant Education, 18*(4), 37–39.

Physician Assistant Education Association (PAEA). (2014). *Twenty-Ninth Annual Report on Physician Assistant Educational Programs in the United States, 2012–2013.* Alexandria, VA: PAEA. Retrieved from http://www.paeaonline.org/index.php?ht=d/sp/i/243/pid/243

Wick, K. H. (2015). International medical graduates as physician assistants. *Journal of the American Academy of Physician Assistants, 28*(7), 43–46.

Will, K. K., Williams, J., Hilton, G., Wilson, L., & Geyer, H. (2016). Perceived efficacy and utility of postgraduate physician assistant training programs. *Journal of the American Academy of Physician Assistants, 27*(3).

Wright, K. A., Cawley, J. F., Hooker, R. S., & Ahuja, M. (2009). Organizational infrastructure of American physician assistant education programs. *Journal of Physician Assistant Education, 20*(3), 15–21.

CHAPTER 5

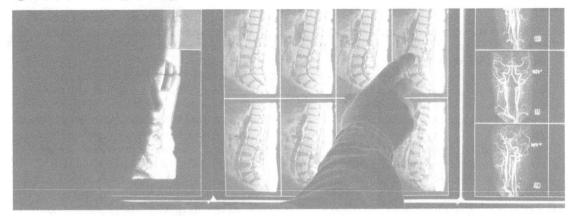

PHYSICIAN ASSISTANTS IN PRIMARY CARE

CHRISTINE M. EVERETT ■ JAMES F. CAWLEY ■ RODERICK S. HOOKER

"A half doctor near is better than a whole one far away."
—*German Proverb*

"The good physician treats the disease; the great physician treats the patient who has the disease."
—*Sir William Osler*

Primary care provides an entrance into the health system for new needs and problems and provides person-focused care over time. It delivers services for health promotion and treatment of common conditions and coordinates care delivered by specialists within a patient's family and community. The physician assistant's (PA's) central role in primary care is not surprising given the functions of primary care and the profession's historical development. This chapter discusses the functions of primary care, the roles performed by PAs within primary care, primary care specialties, and relevant federal policies. Because primary care is experiencing worldwide growth and transformation, special focus is placed on novel primary care delivery systems such as the patient-centered medical home.

THE ROLE OF PHYSICIAN ASSISTANTS IN PRIMARY CARE

The entry point for most people into the healthcare system is primary care. Not surprisingly, primary care–oriented disorders make up the vast majority of all medical conditions seen by healthcare providers. One researcher pointed out that countries with health systems that focus on primary care achieve better health levels, higher satisfaction with health services among their populations, and lower expenditures in the overall delivery of healthcare.

A fair amount of research documents that PAs contribute to the successful attainment of primary care outcomes. They are trained to diagnose and treat most conditions in primary care.

In terms of medical specialties, primary care in the US is defined as family medicine, general internal medicine, geriatrics and general pediatrics. Countries with well-established primary care systems have physicans serving as "gatekeepers," meaning that patients may not visit specialists and may not electively be admitted to hospitals without being referred by primary care doctors. To some, "gatekeeping" represents a negative element of healthcare delivery systems because patients may be denied needed care. The practice developed, however, to avoid unnecessary procedures and overtreatment, thus facilitating the appropriate distribution and use of limited resources. In the United States, people may access specialists directly, which many believe leads to increased costs and fragmentation of services.

The major focus of medical education for PA, doctor, and most nurse practitioner (NP) programs is primary care. The student entering medicine learns the principles and practice of general medical care which form the foundation on which other areas of medicine rest. Curricula for the would-be primary care clinician are organized so that the graduate can manage most medical conditions in a typical community with a normal population distribution. In many instances, primary care forms the foundation on which other areas of medicine rest. To understand the crucial role of PAs within the primary care system, we must first define *primary care.*

PRIMARY CARE DEFINED

Primary care is the provision of integrated, accessible healthcare services by clinicians who are accountable for meeting most personal healthcare needs, developing sustained partnerships with patients, and practicing in the context of family and community.

Primary care serves several key functions, including the provision of:

- Comprehensive care
- Continuous care
- Coordinated care
- Accessible care
- Patient-centered care

To meet the definition of primary care, a provider or clinic must meet all of the preceding functions. Therefore, primary care is often thought of in relation to the type or level of health services provided, such as preventive, diagnostic, and therapeutic sevices; health education and counseling; minor surgery;

and coordination of services provided by other specialty providers within the system.

Primary care is distinguished from two other classifications of healthcare delivery: secondary and teritary care. *Secondary care* is usually thought of as short-term service delivery, infrequent consultation from a specialist, or surgical or other advanced interventions that primary care clinicians are not equipped to provide. This type of care includes hospitalization, routine surgery, specialty consultation, and rehabilitation. It is possible for specialists to provide services typically considered primary care. For example, a cardiologist who offers advanced specialized care for cardiac conditions may also provide health education and disease preventive counseling. However, cardiologists would not be considered primary care clinicians because they typically do not provide the full range of primary care servcies (comprehensive care). Additionally, they typically are not the first point of contact (accessible care) and do not coordinate all providers caring for their patients. *Tertiary care* is regarded as the provision of care for complex conditions and usually involves an institution with advanced technology and specialty and subspecialty services. Examples include organ transplant units, burn centers, cardiothoracic surgery centers, and advanced trauma centers.

Unfortunately, limitations of the current primary care system, as well as the traditional structure and processes of primary care practices, do not facilitate its role. As a result, individual primary care physicians have difficulty successfully implementing and organizing the delivery of quality care. Visits to primary care clinicians account for approximately 58% of all office visits in the United States. Primary care practitioners manage an average of 4.6 clinical problems per encounter, and they are seeing an increase in the proportion of visits exceeding 20 minutes in duration. For a single physician with a typical panel of patients, it would take 10.6 hours a day to implement the recommendations for care related to chronic conditions and 7.4 hours a day to provide all recommended preventive care. This work overload, as well as limited reimbursement, has led to decreasing numbers of medical students choosing careers in primary care, resulting in shortages of primary care providers. To address these issues, one suggested strategy is to increase the presence of PAs or nurse practitioners (NPs) in primary care.

Federal Policy and Primary Care

In 1978, the Institute of Medicine (IOM) issued a major report on primary care recommending that PAs and NPs be given an important role in delivering primary care. The IOM report was inclusive and its findings were endorsed by the American College of Physicians (ACP). The report made recommendations on a number of important issues, such as PA prescriptive practices, third-party reimbursement, and enabling legislation. Both the IOM report and the ACP endorsement continue to be reiterated in many healthcare policy reports.

In addition to the IOM initiative, for more than 4 decades, federal government policies and state legislation have encouraged the use of PAs and encouraged their employment in primary care. When the Patient Protection and Affordable Care Act was enacted, PAs were recognized as qualified primary care providers. Due to the federal grant award program for PA educational programs, many PA training programs strongly emphasized primary care as the centerpiece of their curriculum. Distinct incentives were offered to programs that graduated large numbers of primary care PAs or placed graduates in practices with primary care physicians. This trend continues today with the Affordable Care Act, which set aside additional dollars to expand PA programs with stated objectives to graduate primary care PAs. Evidence to date shows that this policy is accomplishing its goal. PAs are helping to ease the maldistribution of physicians by delivering primary care to many areas in which access is difficult and physicians are not likely to practice.

The Distribution of Physician Assistants in Primary Care

All of the US states, four US territories, and four Canadian provinces enable PAs to practice; however, the ratio of PA to population is irregular and the distribution uneven in these areas. Generally speaking, those states/provinces that

have a higher concentration of universities hosting PA programs have higher ratios of PAs, with the Northeastern states having the highest density of PAs, PA education programs, and population in the United States. Five universities in The Netherlands, four in Canada, three in the United Kingdom, one each in Australia and Saudi Arabia, along with programs in Ghana, Liberia, and the US have PA programs.

The distribution of PAs also varies by metropolitan status. PAs are more likely to work in urban settings than rural ones; usually, the larger the metropolitan area, the greater the concentration of PAs. In some geographic regions, such as the far west of the United States, the ratio of PAs to population is greater than that of doctors to population. When nonmetropolitan practices are examined, however, the proportion of PAs to physicians in rural practice is 9%. The vast majority of rural practice PAs works in primary care. Geographic distribution of PAs in other countries is not known.

Despite the close link between primary care and the creation of the PA profession, the proportion of PAs in primary care has declined between 1996 and the early 2000s (Figure 5–1).

FIGURE 5-1
Physician Assistant Specialties

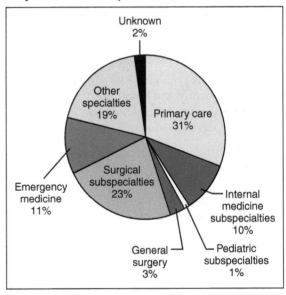

Source: American Academy of Physician Assistants (AAPA). (2011). Physician assistant census report: Results from the 2010 AAPA census. Alexandria, VA: Author.

When primary care opportunities are available, graduates willingly choose primary care over specialized practices (Figure 5–2).

APPROACHES TO PRIMARY CARE

Community-Oriented Primary Care

Community-oriented primary care (COPC) is an advanced approach to primary care practice—one designed to better meet the health needs of populations. Since PA educational philosophy is related to primary care, it is useful to understand the concept of COPC's relevance to the PA profession.

Population health tends to improve when a community approach assumes the responsibility of care beyond the individual level. A COPC approach meets the demand for curative care and at the same time considers the total population and its health needs:

> [The COPC model] is a way of practicing medicine and nursing or of providing primary care, which is focused on care of the individual who is well or sick, or at risk for illness or diseases, while also focusing on promoting the health of the community as a whole, or any of its subgroups (Kark & Kark, 1983).

Furthermore, the COPC model has been defined as "a continuous process by which primary care is provided to a defined population on the basis of its health needs by the planned integration of public health with primary care practice" (Gofin & Cawley, 2004). This COPC approach in health services delivery is one in which providers take responsibility for the health of all members of the community, whether or not they seek care. COPC is considered a practical approach to rationalize, organize, and systematize the existing resources through health interventions directed to prioritize health problems. The impact of COPC in different countries and health systems is considered relevant in the practice and teaching of family medicine as well as in healthcare reform movements addressing the future of general practice in the United Kingdom.

The COPC Approach

The main elements in the development and application of the COPC model are:

- Determination of a defined population—Assessment of the population served, which may be a community, a neighborhood, a school, a working place, a clinic, or the people registered with a practitioner. In all of these cases, essential demographic information of all members of the population is critical. This information enables access to the total population for critical intervention.
- Assessment—Assessment of the health needs of the community. The findings are used for priority setting and intervention planning.
- Community health programs—Integration of health interventions that address all stages of the natural history of disease (incorporating promotion, prevention, treatment, and rehabilitation functions) and a comprehensive focus addressing all the physical, mental, and social determinants of health.
- Accessibility—Availability of the services, taking into consideration economic, fiscal, and cultural barriers.
- Multidisciplinary health team—A team composed of different disciplines according

FIGURE 5-2
Trend in the Percentage of Primary Care PAs by Year of Graduation (1975–2008)

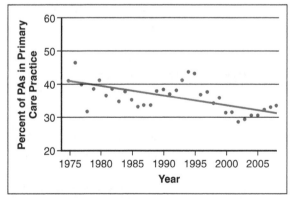

Source: Coplan, B., Cawley, J., & Stoehr, J. (2013). Physician assistants in primary care: Trends and characteristics. Annals of Family Medicine, 11(1), 75–79.

to the specific health needs of the community and the available human resources. Together with the clinical skills needed to provide high-quality healthcare, epidemiological and sociobehavioral skills are needed to respond to the community health needs while performing the activities required by the COPC approach.

- Outreach approach—"Working outside the clinical walls" to enable the team to assess directly the physical and social determinants of health at the microenvironment level.
- Community involvement—Requiring, promoting, and facilitating community participation in healthcare activities as a means for active involvement (individually and collectively) in the improvement of health. Important determinants of health, such as behavior, attitudes, and beliefs, are closely related to individual decisions in their social environment. Therefore, the involvement of members of the community can enhance the positive effects of the community-oriented health interventions. If health services are not able to meet all the needs of the population, then a COPC program should include an intersector coordination with other services serving the population (Gofin & Cawley, 2004).
- COPCs have been largely replaced by Community Health Centers.

At least three educational programs provide orientation in COPC to PA students: the University of Utah, the University of Texas Southwestern, and The George Washington University.

The Patient-Centered Medical Home

Although evidence suggests that primary care benefits the people it serves, there is little question that the healthcare system in the United States is in need of redesign. The system structure is heavily focused on secondary and tertiary specialty care, and the payment policies encourage expensive, episodic care. Despite the fact that approximately one-half of the US population has a chronic illness that requires longitudinal, coordinated care, care coordination and preventive care are often not, or are poorly, reimbursed. This approach to health-system delivery is not congruent with the needs of aging patients with chronic illnesses and is not fiscally sustainable. Successful treatment of patients with chronic illness is complex and requires care from multiple providers with a range of clinical expertise over an extended period of time. Although many patients with chronic illensses have the opportunity to benefit from the increased services that are available from multiple specialties, few will realize a benefit if the result is excessively fragmented care. A recommended solution to the mismatch between the design of the current health system and the needs of patients with chronic disease is to expand the role of primary care in chronic disease management. The recommended strategy to accomplish this is by redesigning primary care practices into patient-centered medical homes (PCMHs).

The PCMH Approach

The PCMH is an approach to providing comprehensive primary care that is supported by many physician groups. Seven principles characterize the PCMH:

1. Personal physician: Every patient has a relationship with a primary care physician.
2. Team-based care: A team of individuals at the practice level collectively take responsibility for the ongoing care of patients.
3. Whole person orientation: The full range of patient needs are met within primary care or arranged for with other qualified individuals.
4. Integrated and coordinated care: Care is integrated and coordinated across all sectors of the healthcare system and community.
5. Quality and safety: Quality and safety are hallmarks of the PCMH and include a focus on evidence-based medicine, information technology, quality improvement, and patient involvement.
6. Accessibilty: Enhanced access is available through expanded hours, open access, and new methods of communication with providers such as e-mail.

7. Affordability: Payment reform that addresses value of care coordination and other services provided in the primary care setting.

This focus on team-based care has been interpreted by some as increasing the inclusion of PAs and other professions in primary care. In fact, the Affordable Care Act specifically encourages the establishment of health teams, which "may include" PAs, to improve the quality and efficiency of primary care (Congress, 2010, Title III, Subtitle F, Sect. 3502). What remains unclear is how this new approach to primary care practice design will affect the roles of PAs.

PERFORMANCE OF PHYSICIAN ASSISTANTS AS PRIMARY CARE PROVIDERS

PAs have established themselves as a vital part of the US, Ghana, and Liberia primary care workforce and will be central for other countries as their numbers expand. Identifying the professional capacities of PAs is a critical first step to understanding their contributions.

In the beginning, the role of the PA was conceived to be one in which the PA would initially see the patient and then present the major findings to the physician. Together they would complete the patient visit. Usually, the doctor would be the one to decide on the final diagnosis and treatment and then delegate aspects of a further diagnostic or treatment plan. The PA performed the diagnostic or treatment plan based on his or her level of experience and skill, as well as the degree of trust between the PA and the physician. Something of a "hand-off" from doctor to PA would occur. A further evolution of the PA role, now commonplace, is that the PA sees the patient often without having the physician present for any part of the visit. With experience and trust, particularly in which the patient's problems are routine and typically straightforward, the physician–PA relationship develops. This is the point at which the physician may delegate a good portion of diagnostic and treatment responsibilities without the physician seeing or reviewing each patient. This process is referred to as "negotiated performance autonomy" and is the cornerstone of the PA movement (Schneller, 1978).

In some instances, patients will preferentially request the PA. In a study that presented patients with a theoretical scenario wherein they needed to find a new primary care provider, approximately 20% of patients stated that they would prefer to see a PA or an NP. With time, as the supervising doctor's confidence becomes reinforced by the skill and performance of the PA, he or she may be delegated more advanced work tasks. As the PA assumes more responsibility for the management of patients, he or she begins to work longitudinally with chronic diseases such as hypertension and diabetes. Evolution is not static and the desire to learn well or even excel tends to move the PA into more challenging roles without jeopardizing patient safety.

PA Skills

A national US practice analysis was undertaken in 2004 to assess the knowledge and clinical performance of PAs in practice. Such practice analysis is important to identify the range of skills and the set of beliefs about the domains of knowledge needed by PAs to be considered competent in their field. A total of 5,282 completed surveys and were considered representative of the PA population in years of experience, geographic distribution, and practice specialty. According to the surveys, the three skills required for most medical encounters were formulating the most likely diagnosis, basic science concepts, and pharmaceutical therapeutics. The survey also revealed eight content domains. Overall, survey responses showed few differences in the tasks performed by PAs based on the length of time worked in the profession.

Another study described the characteristics of providers and patients and the types of prescriptions written by PAs and NPs and compared these activities in metropolitan and nonmetropolitan settings. A PA or an NP was the provider of record for 3% of the primary care visits. All providers wrote prescriptions for 60% of all visits, and the number of prescriptions was 1.3 per visit. PAs were more likely to prescribe controlled substances than were physicians and NPs. In rural areas, NPs wrote more prescriptions than did physicians and PAs, but both appeared to prescribe in a manner similar to physicians in the type of medications used in their patient management. The majority of PAs in clinical practice appeared to be providing similar care and care that was similar to the care provided by ambulatory care doctors.

Productivity

In the US healthcare system, approximately 1 billion outpatient visits occurred in 2010; a PA was seen in approximately 5% of these visits. Approximately 56% were broadly defined as "primary care" (internal medicine, family practice, pediatrics, and obstetrics and women's health).

Analysis of productivity data from a national representative sample showed that, on average over 1 year, PAs performed 61.4 outpatient visits per week compared with 74.2 visits performed by physicians, for an overall physician full-time equivalent (FTE) estimate of 0.83. However, productivity of PAs varied across practice specialty and location, with generalist PAs providing more visits than their specialist counterparts. Rural productivity was higher than urban productivity, largely due to the concentration of generalist PAs in rural settings. Additionally, a policy analysis compared the productivity of solo practice physicians who employed PAs with those who did not, demonstrating that solo practice physicians who do employ PAs see an increase in the number of patient visits per week (127.2 vs. 116.4), a decrease in the number of weeks worked per year (47.7 vs. 48.6), and an increase in net income ($220,000 vs. $186,900), despite lower office visit fees ($90 vs. $96.50 for a new patient).

Additional productivity documentation may be found in a state-level analysis in Utah. Even though PAs make up only 6.3% of the state's combined clinician (physician, PA, and NP) workforce, they contribute approximately 7.2% of the patient care FTEs in the state. The

majority (73%) of Utah PAs works at least 36 hours per week and, compared with physicians, spends a greater percentage of total hours working in patient care. The rural PA workforce reported working a greater number of total hours, as well as a greater number of patient care hours, compared with the overall statewide PA workforce.

In a Dutch study of a family practice doctor (general practitioner—GP) and an American-trained PA, the productivity, based on contacts per 1000 patients, increased by 17% over 1 year after the PA was added to a solo practice office. Measured per FTE of a GP, the number of GP contacts decreased slightly (2.3%). Types of contacts, diagnoses, drug prescriptions, and new referrals to the primary care practice changed significantly. The number of PA contacts per 1 FTE PA was about 60% of that of the GPs, with clinical activities overlapping substantially. In the aggregate, the PA saw more women, children, and patients ages 25 to 44 years; performed more practice consultations; made more women's health–related diagnoses; and prescribed more drugs for dermatological and respiratory problems.

PHYSICIAN ASSISTANT ROLES IN PRIMARY CARE

The initial purpose of the creation of PAs was not specifically to become primary care providers, but to support and augment the general services of the physician, regardless of specialty. The fundamental role of the PA as a clinician was initially described as one designed to examine and gather clinical information on the patient. Over time, the role of the PA transformed from merely assisting the primary care physician to one of close interdependence with the physician employer. This evolution was not strategically planned, yet this outcome was the inevitable product of delegation and expansion of duties that occurs in almost any apprenticeship and assistantship.

One study analyzed primary care physician office encounter data from the National Ambulatory Medical Care Surveys and found remarkably few differences in the types of patients, diagnoses made, and treatment rendered by the three providers, with the exception that the mean age of patients seen by physicians was slightly greater than that for PAs and NPs. On the other hand, NPs provided counseling and education during a higher proportion of visits than did PAs and physicians. These factors aside, the study findings suggest that PAs and NPs provide primary care in a manner that is similar to physician care.

Because of the similarities between physicians and PAs, the role of PAs can now be defined based on the distribution of care between the physician and the PA. The roles that PAs can perform within the PA–physician dyad have previously been divided into the two categories of "substitute" and "supplement" (Scheffler et al., 1996). When PAs perform all functions of primary care for a subset of patients in a manner similar to physicians, they perform substitute roles. According to the philosophical ideal for primary care, this translates into assuming the tangible (the provision of the full complement of primary care services) as well as intangible attributes (patient–provider relationship) of a physician's professional role for a subset of the patients (i.e., serves as the usual provider of care). This results in distribution of care within the dyad *by patient*. This approach may be implemented for a variety of reasons, such as relieving demand for physicians and physician shortages.

PAs perform supplemental roles when they substitute for physicians *for particular primary care services or tasks* but are not providing the full scope and breadth of primary care. For example, they may be responsible for providing acute care on a walk-in basis; chronic disease management; or preventive care. This results in the distribution of care within the dyad *by task*. This approach may be taken to improve quality of care without increasing demands on physicians or reducing service costs. These role categories are important starting points for defining PA roles. They are an oversimplification, however, as significant heterogeneity still exists within each category.

Precise primary care PA role definition requires recognition of three important domains that influence how patient care is distributed within the physician–PA dyad:

1. The level of PA involvement
2. The complexity of the patients
3. The primary care services provided

These domains reflect the three key questions asked when defining the role of a PA working in collaboration with physicians: How much of the patient care should be performed by the PA for a given patient population over time? What groups of patients should receive care from PAs? What primary care services will be performed by PAs?

Level of Involvement

It is clear that PAs have the capacity to perform the majority of primary care services; however, it is unclear how the amount of care provided to a patient population by PAs affects patient outcomes. The amount of care provided by a primary care provider to a patient reflects the potential impact of that provider on quality of care and patient outcomes. The amount of care provided by primary care PAs can fall into two major categories: usual provider or supplement. PAs act as the usual provider of care by providing the majority of primary care. Alternatively, PAs can act as a supplement by providing a limited number of episodes of primary care.

Current research does not clarify if, and under what conditions, PAs acting as usual or supplemental providers are achieving optimal patient outcomes. Limited studies have evaluated the quality of care provided by PAs as usual providers of care. Studies that have explicitly evaluated the impact of supplemental PA care on patient outcomes have been limited to implementation of chronic disease–specific programs.

Complexity of Patients

A paucity of evidence is available to guide organizations and practitioners in determining the level of involvement and type of care that can be effectively delivered by PAs to patients presenting with varying levels of complexity.

Historically, the perceived role of PAs was to provide care to well and noncomplex patients for preventive care, acute issues, and treatment of stable chronic conditions. The belief that patients with complex problems and multiple diagnoses are best served by physicians working with a team of healthcare professionals still predominates today. However, the evidence supporting this traditional view is inconclusive. Many of the studies that compare the complexity of patients treated by the provider types evaluate effectiveness on the level of the episode, with most relying on provider self-report. Some observational studies found that patients seen by PAs were similar in complexity to patients seen by physicians. However, other observational studies and one experimental trial have reported that patients treated by PAs were less complex. These studies do not address the amount of care or the services provided to patients, however.

Primary Care Services Delivered

Many studies have evaluated the type of care or services that could be provided by PAs within an episode of care in a variety of settings. These studies have concluded that 85% to 90% of primary care services could effectively be provided by PAs without the direct input of a physician. Studies conducted on national datasets confirm that when the main reason for an outpatient visit is evaluated by provider type, the average scope of services provided by PAs is similar to that of doctors, but the proportion of each care type delivered may vary by provider type. For example, in a study that evaluated the care delivered in 1,200 US community health centers, a higher percentage of PA visits were for acute primary diagnoses compared with those of physicians and NPs (48% vs. 34% vs. 33%, respectively; Hing et al., 2010).

When these three domains are combined, PA roles in primary care can be defined. A study conducted in one large, multispecialty physician group confirms that primary care PAs and NPs do perform the full range of roles, even within one organization (Figure 5–3). In fact, the study suggests that PAs in primary care often perform

FIGURE 5-3

PA/NP Roles on Panels of Medicare Patients with Diabetes

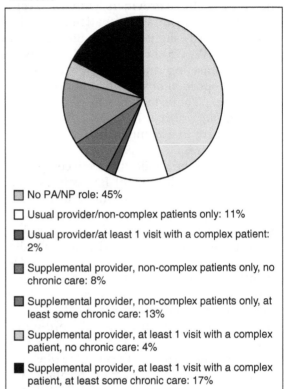

☐ No PA/NP role: 45%

☐ Usual provider/non-complex patients only: 11%

■ Usual provider/at least 1 visit with a complex patient: 2%

■ Supplemental provider, non-complex patients only, no chronic care: 8%

■ Supplemental provider, non-complex patients only, at least some chronic care: 13%

☐ Supplemental provider, at least 1 visit with a complex patient, no chronic care: 4%

■ Supplemental provider, at least 1 visit with a complex patient, at least some chronic care: 17%

Source: Everett, C. M., Thorpe, C. T., Palta, M., Carayon, P., Gilchrist, V. J., & Smith, M.A. (2014). The roles of primary care PAs and NPs caring for older adults with diabetes. Journal of the American Academy of Physician Assistants, 27(4), 45–49.

multiple roles simultaneously (average = 4). Although this finding is likely a function of working with multiple physicians and speaks to the flexibility of the profession, it is unclear if multiple-role performance is an overall benefit. Performing multiple roles simultaneously could lead to role confusion or role conflict, which could ultimately reduce PA, physician, and/or patient satisfaction.

CONTRIBUTION OF PHYSICIAN ASSISTANTS AS PRIMARY CARE SPECIALISTS

The contribution of PAs to primary care is best understood by examining the evidence in relation to each function of primary care.

Comprehensive Care

Commonly used measures of comprehensiveness include patient populations seen, scope of services provided, and rate of referral. Multiple studies have compared the scope of patients services provided by PAs and physicians in primary care settings and have concluded that PAs can perform 85% to 90% of services traditionally provided by primary care physicians. Ongoing national surveys of ambulatory medical care delivery systems demonstrate that PAs perform similarly to doctors within visits when types of patients are compared by primary diagnoses. The characteristics of patients, the reasons for medical office visits, the most frequently reported principal diagnoses, and the medications prescribed in primary care are summarized in Tables 5–1 through 5–4. These data are drawn from a national study on the content of ambulatory visits undertaken in 2007.

In a study of 1,200 US Community Health Centers, a higher percentage of PA visits were due to an acute condition (48%) compared with physician (34%) and NP visits (33%). The acute conditions were typically injury and illness. Patients with multiple chronic conditions made up nearly half of all visits. The most frequent chronic conditions reported were hypertension, hyperlipidemia, diabetes, depression, obesity, arthritis, asthma, and

TABLE 5-2
Distribution of Medical Office Visits by the 20 Most Common Principal Reasons for Visit, United States, 2007*

Rank	Most Common Principal Reason for Visit	Percentage
1	General medical examination	7.5
2	Progress visit, not otherwise specified	6.1
3	Postoperative visit	2.8
4	Cough	2.8
5	Medication, other and unspecified kinds	2.2
6	Knee symptoms	1.9
7	For other and unspecified test results	1.8
8	Routine prenatal examination	1.8
9	Symptoms referable to throat	1.7
10	Back symptoms	1.5
11	Hypertension	1.5
12	Well-baby examinations	1.5
13	Vision dysfunctions	1.4
14	Stomach pain, cramps, and spasms	1.3
15	Nasal congestion	1.3
16	Gynecological examination	1.3
17	Skin rash	1.3
18	Fever	1.2
19	Earache or ear infection	1.2
20	Diabetes mellitus	1.1
	All other reasons	56.8

*Based on a reason for visit classification for ambulatory care.
Data modified from: Hsiao, C. J., Cherry, D. K., Beatty, P. C., & Rechtsteiner, E. A. (2010). *National ambulatory medical care survey: 2007 summary.* Hyattsville, MD: National Center for Health Statistics.

TABLE 5-1
Number and Percentage of US Office Visits by Patient Age and Sex (2007)*

Age-group (years)	Females (%)	Males (%)	Total (%)	Total Number of Visits (in Thousands)
<15	7.9	8.9	16.2	147,910
15–24	5.2	23.0	7.8	70,593
25–44	13.8	6.6	21.2	194,261
45–64	16.7	11.8	19.0	264,103
65–74	7.0	5.8	12.4	113,426
≥75	7.7	5.4	13.2	120,565

*Based on a reason for visit classification for ambulatory care.
Source: Hsiao, C. J., Cherry, D. K., Beatty, P. C., & Rechtsteiner, E. A. (2010). *National ambulatory medical care survey: 2007 summary.* Hyattsville, MD: National Center for Health Statistics.

chronic obstructive pulmonary disease. The percent of visits made by patients with any of these specific conditions did not vary by type of clinician, nor were there differences in percentages of established patients seen by each type of clinician (87%–89%). In these federally funded community health centers, which almost exclusively provide primary care, the staffing ratio of PA/NP to doctor averages 30% (range: 0%–40%; Hing et al., 2010).

Results from a study in Iowa suggest that comprehensiveness of primary care services varies by geographic location. Findings

TABLE 5-3
Number and Distribution of Office Visits by the 20 Most Common Principal Diagnosis Groups, United States, 2007

Rank	Most Common Diagnosis	Percentage
1	Essential hypertension	4.2
2	Routine infant or child health check	4.0
3	Acute upper respiratory infections, excluding pharyngitis	3.4
4	Arthropathies and related disorders	3.3
5	Spinal disorders	2.7
6	Malignant neoplasms	2.5
7	Diabetes mellitus	2.4
8	Rheumatism, excluding back	2.0
9	Specific procedures and aftercare	1.9
10	General medical examination	1.9
11	Follow-up examination	1.9
12	Normal pregnancy	1.7
13	Otitis media and eustachian tube disorders	1.5
14	Asthma	1.4
15	Gynecological examination	1.4
16	Heart disease, excluding ischemic	1.3
17	Allergic rhinitis	1.3
18	Ischemic heart disease	1.2
19	Glaucoma	1.2
20	Benign neoplasms	1.1
	All other diagnoses	57.6

Source: Hsiao, C. J., Cherry, D. K., Beatty, P. C., & Rechtsteiner, E. A. (2010). *National ambulatory medical care survey: 2007 summary.* Hyattsville, MD: National Center for Health Statistics.

TABLE 5-4
Number and Percentage Distribution of Drug Mentions by Therapeutic Drug Category, United States, 2007

Therapeutic Class	Number of Mentions (in thousands)	Percentage Distribution
All drug mentions	2,250,489	100.0
Analgesics or antiplatelet agents	247,055	11.0
Antihyperlipidemic agents	123,994	5.5
Antidepressants	109,001	4.8
Anxiolytics, sedatives, and hypnotics	85,659	3.8
Antidiabetic agents	82,140	3.6
Beta-adrenergic blocking agents	77,776	3.5
Antiplatelet agents	71,193	3.2
Bronchodilators	68,049	3.0
Anticonvulsants	67,436	3.0
Dermatological agents	65,678	2.9
Proton pump inhibitors	65,092	2.9
Diuretics	63,571	2.8
Angiotensin-converting enzyme inhibitors	60,847	2.7
Antihistamines	59,620	2.6
Viral vaccines	54,691	2.4
Opthalmic preparations	47,056	2.4
Adrenal corticosteroids	44,343	2.0
Sex hormones	40,652	1.8
Nasal preparations	39,813	1.8
Antiemetic, antivertigo agents	37,241	1.7

Source: Hsiao, C. J., Cherry, D. K., Beatty, P. C., & Rechtsteiner, E. A. (2010). *National ambulatory medical care survey: 2007 summary.* Hyattsville, MD: National Center for Health Statistics.

indicated that rural primary care providers performed more procedures than their metropolitan counterparts. Among 55 responding PAs, all reported providing patient education, prescribing, interpreting radiographs, referring patients, and providing a wide range of services similar to their physician counterparts. Few differences emerged when comparing family medicine doctors to PAs in rural areas, suggesting that both clinicians provide a broad array of medical services. Evidence from five studies on referral rates and patterns by PAs in primary care indicates that referring is an activity that does not substantially differ between PAs and doctors.

Coordinated Care

Care is coordinated when patients receive appropriate care in a cost-effective manner. Many conceptualizations of care coordination exist, but all agree that communication between primary care practitioners, other healthcare professionals, and patients is a key component of coordination. Coordination of care is generally viewed by primary care PAs as a function that falls within their clinical role. Specialist physicians report willingness to accept patient referrals from primary care PAs and general satisfaction with the appropriateness and timeliness of the referrals.

Continuous Care

Continuity of care can refer to the transfer of information between episodes of care (informational continuity) or to the provision of care over time by consistent providers (longitudinal and/or relational continuity). A patient–clinician relationship is a central feature of primary care; the potential for decreased relationship exists when a provider team approach is implemented. Two studies have evaluated the relationship between continuity and quality of care. One evaluated the effects of visit continuity for patients ($N = 14,835$) of a large multispecialty practice served by primary care provider teams with PAs and NPs on patient perceptions of the quality of primary care. Patients who only saw their primary care physician reported significantly higher physician–patient relationship quality and better assessments of organizational features of care (such as access and integration of care) than those who had visits with providers other than their primary care physician. However, patients who had visits only with providers on their primary care team had significantly higher assessments of the clinical team but lower assessments of their physician's knowledge of them as a person than did those who had visits with providers off the team. The subgroup of patients who had visits with their primary care PA/NP team members reported better primary care experiences (Rodriguez et al., 2007).

Another survey of attendees of primary care clinics at five Department of Veterans Affairs medical centers ($N = 21,689$) evaluated the extent to which self-reported continuity of care related to patient satisfaction after adjusting for patient, provider, and clinic characteristics. The mean adjusted humanistic score for patients who reported always seeing the same provider was 17.3 points higher than for those who rarely saw the same provider. Similarly, the mean adjusted organizational score was 16.3 points higher for patients who always saw the same provider compared with those who rarely saw the same provider. Demographic factors, socioeconomic status, health status, clinic site, and patient utilization of services were all associated with both the adjusted humanistic and organizational scores of the scale. When continuity of care was held constant, the results revealed no differences in satisfaction between provider types (PAs/NPs and doctors; Fan et al., 2005).

Accessible Care

Accessible care is care that is easy for patients to obtain in a timely fashion. Empirical evidence suggests that PAs can improve access to care to underserved patients and open access practices. The primary care patients of PAs are slightly more likely to be female, rural, and uninsured or publicly insured than those of physicians. One study utilized administrative data and surveyed primary care clinicians, including doctors, NPs, PAs, and midwives, in California and Washington to determine whether practice in underserved areas varied by provider type. PAs demonstrated a greater proclivity for providing care to the underserved, as they ranked first or second in both states as the providers with the highest proportion of members practicing in rural areas, health professional shortage areas, and vulnerable population areas. The finding that PAs practice in greater proportion than do physicians and nurses in areas of low population density (i.e., rural areas) has also been identified in studies in Iowa and Utah.

Compared with patients reporting primary care doctors as a usual source of care, patients of PAs were more likely to live in rural areas, lack insurance or have public insurance other than Medicare, report lower perceived access to care, and/or have decreased likelihood of having some preventive care, such as comprehensive health examinations or mammograms. Despite these differences in characteristics and utilization, no differences existed in patient complexity or in self-rated health between primary care patients of physicians and PAs, suggesting that PAs can provide access to a usual source of care for a broad range of patients.

Appointment delays impede access to primary healthcare, and open access (OA) scheduling may improve the quality of primary healthcare. One study assessed whether implementing OA during a 12-month period affected practice or patient outcomes and whether the results differed by provider type. Providers (doctors, PAs, and NPs) in four practices successfully implemented OA. On average, providers reduced their delay to the next available preventive care appointment from 36 to 4 days; no-show rates declined, overall patient satisfaction improved, and continuity of care improved. However, these findings did not differ by provider type, suggesting that PAs and doctors are similar in their adaptability to complex organizational changes aimed at improving access.

Patient-Centered Care

Patient-centered care is recognized as a critical function of primary care, but agreement on a definition of this function is evolving. Most studies that have evaluated patient-centered care include patient satisfaction as an outcome. Satisfying care, in this context, means the patient completes the visit feeling that his or her needs were met. No amount of quality care by a PA will overcome the labeling of "unsatisfactory" if a patient has established a negative impression.

To assess the extent to which the experiences of patients vary according to type of primary care provider (PA, NP, or doctor), a national survey of elderly patients receiving US government health insurance (Medicare) was undertaken. The beneficiaries completing the survey identified a primary care provider and recorded satisfaction data, patient sociodemographic characteristics, healthcare experience, types of care, and types of supplemental insurance. Although a small number (3,770, or 2.8%) of respondents identified a PA or an NP as their usual primary care provider, for questions on satisfaction with their personal care clinician, results were similar across provider type. The conclusion was that Medicare beneficiaries are generally satisfied with their medical care and do not distinguish preferences based on type of provider.

Efficiency: Cost Beneficial Use of PAs in Primary Care

Another issue is whether PAs are cost-beneficial to employers. One multivariate analysis identified significant cost differences. In every condition managed by PAs, the total cost of a visit was less than that of a physician in the same department. In some instances PAs ordered fewer laboratory tests than did physicians for the same episode of care. These findings suggest that PAs are not only cost-effective from a labor standpoint but are also cost-beneficial to employers. In most cases, PAs order resources for diagnoses and treatment in a manner similar to physicians for an episode of care, but the cost of an episode of an illness is more economical overall when the PA delivers the care, which can be explained in part by the PA's lower salary.

To estimate the savings in labor costs that might be realized per primary care visit from increased use of PAs and NPs in primary care, one study examined the practices of an HMO; 26 primary care practices and data on approximately two million visits delivered by 206 practitioners were extracted from computerized visit records. On average, PAs and NPs provided one in three adult medicine visits and one in five pediatric medicine visits. The likelihood of a PA or NP visit was significantly higher than average among patients presenting with minor acute illnesses (e.g., acute pharyngitis). In adult medicine, the likelihood of a PA or NP visit was lower than average among older patients. Practitioner labor costs per visit (and total labor costs per visit) were lower among practice arrangements with greater use of PAs and NPs, standardized for case mix. The authors concluded that primary care practices that used more PAs and NPs in care delivery realized lower practitioner costs per visit than practices that used fewer PAs and NPs (Roblin et al., 2004).

Effective Care

To be effective, a PA needs to provide quality care that meets or exceeds a predefined standard, such as specified quality measures. Unfortunately, most of the quality metrics available are disease-specific measures, which are not ideal for measuring the quality of primary care. In the absence of quality metrics, care must result in outcomes comparable to those of a doctor. Several studies have compared the care provided by PAs and doctors on quality measures such as processes of care and/or patient outcomes for specific diagnoses.

HIV

In some clinics, PAs and NPs are primary care providers for patients with human immunodeficiency virus (HIV), but little is known about the quality of care they provide. One study compared eight quality-of-care measures assessed by medical record review. The quality of care provided by PAs and NPs was compared with that provided by physicians in 68 HIV care sites. The authors surveyed 243 clinicians (177 physicians and 66 NPs/PAs) and reviewed the medical records of 6,651 persons with HIV or AIDS. After adjustments for patient characteristics, most of the quality measures did not differ between NPs and PAs (and did not differ compared with those of infectious disease specialists and generalist HIV experts). PAs and NPs had higher performance scores than generalist non-HIV experts on six of the eight quality measures. The authors concluded that, for the measures examined, the quality of HIV care provided by PAs and NPs was similar to that of physician HIV experts and generally better than that of physicians who were not HIV experts. Preconditions for this level of performance included high levels of experience, focus on a single condition, participation in teams, and easy access to clinicians with HIV expertise (Wilson et al., 2005).

Common Geriatric Conditions

The treatment of common geriatric conditions by PAs is another areas that requires further study. One randomized trial found that geriatric patients who were provided with a PA case manager were more likely to have their target conditions identified (e.g., depression, cognitive and functional impairment, falls, and urinary incontinence) than were those patients who received standard care. These findings suggest that incorporating PAs in supplemental roles for target populations can increase case finding, assessment, and referral for previously underdiagnosed and under-treated or untreated conditions.

Metabolic Diseases

Multiple studies have evaluated the relationship between the type of provider and the attainment of treatment goals for diabetes, dyslipidemia, and hypertension. One analysis of 19,660 patients with diabetes, coronary artery disease, or hypertension was conducted in the VA Connecticut Healthcare System. Although significant differences were seen in the type of patients cared for by PAs/NPs and resident physicians, attainment of goals for each condition was similar, with one exception: PAs and NPs were more likely than resident physicians to attain an hemoglobin A1c (Hgb_{A1C}) goal of less than 7.5. Similarly, a study conducted on 88,682 primary care patients in 198 Veterans Administration clinics demonstrated that clinics that included NPs were associated with lower Hgb_{A1C} levels (approximately 0.31 percentage points), and clinics with PAs did not show a statistically significant difference in Hgb_{A1C} levels compared with clinics without PAs or NPs.

Another study of 46 family medicine practices measured adherence to American Diabetes Association guidelines via chart audits of 846 patients with diabetes. Compared with practices employing PAs, practices employing NPs were more likely to measure Hgb_{A1C} levels (66% vs. 33%), lipid levels (80% vs. 58%), and urinary microalbumin levels (32% vs. 6%) and to provide treatment for high lipid levels (77% vs. 56%). Practices with NPs were more likely than physician-only practices to assess HgbA1c levels (66% vs. 49%) and lipid levels (80% vs. 68%). However, these process improvements did not translate into improved outcomes, with the exception of better attainment of lipid targets in practices employing NPs. With regard to diabetes process measures in this study, family practices employing NPs performed better than those with physicians only and better than those employing PAs (Ohman-Strickland et al., 2008).

Despite these examples, most studies evaluating the effectiveness of PAs in primary care have not identified the role of the PA in the care of the patient. Because PAs can perform a variety of roles, this distinction is important to understanding how to build teams that deliver accessible, efficient, and effective primary care. Only one study to date has compared the effectiveness of different PA and NP roles in primary care. Diabetes outcomes, hospitalizations, and emergency department visits were compared for Medicare patients with diabetes who were cared for at a large, multispecialty physician group and who experienced primary care PAs and NPs in different roles. Specific PA/NP roles were associated with different quality of diabetes care and health service utilization patterns, and no single role was best for all patients or all outcomes (Table 5–5). These findings suggest that implementation of PA and NP roles may require prioritization of outcome goals and consideration of the population served.

PRIMARY CARE SPECIALTIES

This section identifies the core primary care disciplines and profiles the utilization of primary care PAs. It also evaluates how much more there is to discover about this discipline.

Family Medicine

Family medicine (historically referred to as *general medicine*) is the trunk from which all of the branches of medicine grow. It is the discipline that deals with the general medical needs of an individual and his or her family, from pregnancy and children through adolescents to adults, and on into geriatics. The family medicine doctor provides preventive care and health education for all ages and both sexes in addition to treating acute and chronic illnesses. She or he has spent 2 to 3 years in postgraduate training learning all aspects of general medicine as it affects the individual, the family, and the community as a whole. Trained in health, fitness, and all aspects of medicine, including obstetrics, gynecology, and pediatrics, the family practitioner is the source of continuity of care for the community. The rural doctor is more likely to be a family doctor than any other discipline in medicine.

The titles *family practitioner* and *family physician* have become widespread in Canada, the United States, and many other countries. The term *general practitioner* (GP) is common in the United Kingdom as well as in most other Commonwealth countries where the word *physician* is largely reserved for certain types of medical specialties, especially internal medicine. Many GPs do minor procedures, such as removing skin lesions, in their offices. Historically, they also perform major surgeries, such as tonsillectomies, hernia repairs, and appendectomies. In more rural parts of many countries, this style of medical practice continues. In the United Kingdom, the development of a formal family medicine doctor to replace the GP occurred at almost the same time as the development of the PA profession in the United States. Outside of the United States, the view

TABLE 5-5
PA/NP Roles Predicting Diabetes-Specific Outcomes and Healthcare Utilization

Primary Care PA/NP Role			Outcome Measure			
PA/NP Level of Involvement	Complex Patients	Chronic Care	≥ 2 A1c Tests	Glycemic Control	No. of ED Visits	No. of Hospital Visits
Supplemental	No	Yes	+	=	=	=
Supplemental	No	No	=	+	+	=
Supplemental	Yes	Yes	=	+	=	–
Supplemental	Yes	No	=	–	=	–
Usual Provider	Yes/No	NA	=	=	–	–

Finding reflects $p \leq .05$. Adjusted for patient sociodemographic variables (age, race, Medicaid dual-eligible, disability entitlement), clinical characteristics (ACG risk score, 16 medical conditions, and three diabetes complications), healthcare utilization, and panel characteristics (specialty of usual provider, number of patients on panel, and percent of women on panel). +, Better outcome than physician-only care; –, worse outcome than physician-only care.
Source: Everett, C. M., Thorpe, C., Palta, M., Carayon, P., Bartels, C., & Smith, M.A. (2013). Physician assistants and nurse practitioners perform effective roles on teams caring for Medicare patients with diabetes. *Health Affairs, 32*(11), 1942–1948.

of the family practitioner or GP differs depending on the country.

Generally, throughout much of the world in the past few decades, the number and type of medical specialists has increased, whereas the number of family medicine doctors and GPs has decreased. These changes may have many causes, including long working hours, the isolated nature of a solo general practice, and lower pay compared with that of most specialists.

Profile

Less than one-quarter of PAs identify their practice specialty as primary care. In 2015, approximately 19% of PAs who responded to the American Academy of Physician Assistants (AAPA) Survey census identified family medicine or general practice as the specialty they practiced for their primary employer. No studies have been done to identify all of the specific activities of PAs in family medicine; however, a list of primary care clinican tasks has been published. Additionally, the work detailing the daily activities of family medicine PAs in rural Iowa is profiled in Chapter 8, "Physician Assistants in Rural Health."

PAs enjoy strong support from family physicians, as evidenced by statements by the American Academy of Family Practice (AAFP) affirming PAs' capabilities in delivering primary care services. Several postgraduate training programs are available for PAs in family practice, providing an additional year of clinical education in this specialty.

The 2015 PA Profile in the NCCPA identified 17,090 PAs in family medicine and found that the median age of the PA was 41. Females comprised 66% of the cohort; 56% worked in an office-based private practice; 11.5% in a community health center. Most (90%) worked in an urban setting. The majority (82%) worked full time (≥32 hours per week). The median salary in 2015 was $95,000.

Internal Medicine

Internal medicine is another component of the main trunk of medicine that deals with the general medical needs of the individual adult, from adolescence through geriatrics. The term *internal medicine* is a direct translation from the German term *innere medizin*, signifying a discipline popularized in Germany in the late 1800s in which physicians combined the science of the laboratory with the care of patients. Specialists of internal medicine are referred to as *internists* and spend at least 3 years of postgraduate training learning how to prevent, diagnose, and treat diseases of the internal organs that affect adults. Internists are more likely to be basic scientists than are practitioners in the other primary care disciplines. Internal medicine includes the 13 subspecialities of medicine, including rheumatology, endocrinology, nephrology, cardiology, infectious disease, and gastroenterology.

In the United States, general internists practice medicine from a primary care perspective, but they can treat and manage many ailments and are usually the most adept at treating a broad range of diseases affecting adults. In other countries, an internist is a specialist who accepts referrals for consultation but may not follow patients longitudinally. Outside of the United States, the internist is not a primary care provider but a consultant.

Profile

In 2015, approximately 5% of all PAs in clinical practice in the United States identified general internal medicine as the specialty they work in for their primary employer. Internal medicine physician groups, as expressed in published statements of the ACP, support the role of PAs working in general internal medicine. As with physician-internists, PAs in internal medicine have practices skewed toward geriatrics. Among internists, the hospitalist movement has become increasingly popular driven, in part, by a desire by physicians to better control the circumstances of their work. It would be a mistake to believe that physicians are going to fade from the healthcare delivery scene, yet it is clear that their roles in the division of medical labor are changing.

The 2015 PA Profile in the NCCPA identified 4,290 PAs in general internal medicine. The average age was 42, females represented 72% of the cohort, and 60% worked in a office-based private practice. Almost all (84%) worked in an urban setting. The majority (83%) worked full time (≥32 hours per week), and 84% were salary-based. The median salary in 2015 was $95,000.

Pediatrics

Pediatrics is the branch of medicine that deals with the medical care of infants, children, and adolescents and is included as primary care only in the US. The upper age limit ranges from age 14 to 18, depending on the country, although adolescent medicine is an emerging area of pediatric specialization and can include youths up to age 21. The pediatrician may be more holistic than the internist as a result of having a depth of knowledge about premature birth, family dynamics, death and dying, growth milestones, mental health disorders, genetics, behavioral disorders, preventive medicine, reproduction, and injury.

Profile

PAs who specialize in pediatrics are approximately 1.5% (1,631 in 2015). One entry-level PA program specializes in pediatrics and two postgraduate programs have specializations in neonatology. The number of PAs who practice general pediatrics or a pediatric subspecialty has been steadily increasing from approximately 1,300 PAs in 1997 to 3,028 PAs in 2010 (1,683 in general pediatrics) to 2000 in 2015. The range of pediatric PA practices mirrors that of pediatricians. Most work in general pediatric settings, whereas a smaller number choose subspecialties of pediatric care. Of all pediatric PAs, two-thirds practice with general pediatricians and one-third work with pediatric subspecialists.

PAs working in the pediatric inpatient setting typically fit one of two models. Either they are employed outside the hospital and have privileges to provide inpatient care, or they are employed as medical staff on the pediatric or neonatal unit. Because pediatric PAs draw on the generalist and the specialist aspects of their medical training, they can effectively handle routine pediatric issues and can address a wide range of acute problems.

In 2015 the median age was 37. Females were 83% of the cohort, and 78% worked in a office-based practice. Almost all (83%) worked in an urban setting. The majority (74%) worked full time (≥32 hours per week), and 82% were salary-based. The median salary in 2015 was $85,000.

FURTHER RESEARCH ON PHYSICIAN ASSISTANTS IN PRIMARY CARE

The literature about PAs in primary care is limited. This section offers a brief review of areas in need of attention:

- **Regulatory environments:** Scope of practice laws vary by state within the United States and by country. What is the impact of regulatory environment on team structure and role design?
- **Organizational contexts:** Primary care is now delivered in a range of organizational settings. How do large multispecialty groups use PAs in the care of a defined population? What are the trade-offs organizations make in employing PAs and NPs? What are the overlaps in care by doctors, PAs, and NPs in the same setting?
- **Primary care team structures:** A wide variety of approaches to implementation of primary care teams exists. Teams may include additional professionals, such as social workers, pharmacists, diabetic educators, and public health professionals. What is the optimal team design to maximize outcomes? Is there an ideal ratio of primary care PAs to doctors for a given size population? What is the substitution ratio of PAs to doctors?
- **Role definition:** Although one definition of primary care PA role has been studied, this definition is limited to the delivery of outpatient care to a small subgroup of patients. Definitions that include additional primary care tasks relating to a full complement of primary care patients should be created and studied. Possible topic areas are home visits, nursing home, emergency department, and hospital coverage.
- **Organizational outcomes:** What are the costs associated with different primary care team structures and PA roles? Do the levels of physician and PA satisfaction differ with different team structures and role definitions?
- **Patient outcomes:** What is the impact of team structure and the PA role on a range of disease-specific outcomes? On general health outcomes such as functional status?

On patient healthcare utilization of resources, including specialist care, emergency department, and urgent care and hospitalizations?

- **Career selection:** Do PAs in primary care have different expectations and aspirations than those in specialty practices?
- **Retention:** What factors contribute to retention or attrition of PAs in primary care?
- **Education:** What are the links between training in primary care and patient outcomes?

SUMMARY

PAs have displayed an impressive track record in primary care since the 1960s, when the profession first emerged. Where there were once clear barriers to their full practice effectiveness, there is now recognition by national initiatives, state boards, insurance carriers, and physician groups of the vital roles that PAs play in the delivery of primary care health services. PAs have shown themselves to be safe and capable providers of primary care services. Contemporary studies suggest that PAs can and do contribute to the delivery of primary care functions, particularly the provision of comprehensive care and accessibility. Yet despite the success of PAs, rural practices and other needy sectors continue to be challenged to attract significant numbers of PA providers.

The healthcare system is currently focused on redesigning primary care into team-based, PCMHs. If PCMHs are to accomplish the goal of delivering patient-centered care with improved access, quality, and cost, an increased reliance on PAs and other healthcare professionals will result. Understanding PA roles in primary care will be a necessary first step to identifying team structures that maximize organizational, provider, and patient goals.

References

The following citations are key to supporting this chapter's content. You can find a complete list of citations for all chapters at www.fadavis.com/davisplus, keyword *Hooker*.

American Academy of Physician Assistants. (2014). *2013 AAPA Annual Survey Report*. Alexandria, VA: American Academy of Physician Assistants.

Fan, V. S., Burman, M., McDonell, M. B., & Fihn, S. D. (2005). Continuity of care and other determinants of patient satisfaction with primary care. *Journal of General Internal Medicine, 20*(3), 226–233.

Gofin, J., & Cawley, J. F. (2004). The physician assistant and community-oriented primary care. *Perspective on Physician Assistant Education, 15*(2), 126–128.

Hing, E., Hooker, R. S., & Ashman, J. (2010). Primary healthcare in community health centers and comparisons with office-based practice. *Journal of Community Health, 36*(3), 406–413.

Kark, S. L., & Kark, E. (1983). An alternative strategy in community healthcare: Community-oriented primary healthcare. *Israel Journal of Medical Sciences, 19*(8), 707–713.

Ohman-Strickland, P. A., Orzano, A. J., Hudson, S. V., Solberg, L. I., DiCiccio-Bloom, B., O'Malley, D., et al. (2008). Quality of diabetes care in family medicine practices: Influence of nurse-practitioners and physician's assistants. *Annals of Family Medicine, 6*(1), 14–22.

Roblin, D. W., Howard, D. H., Becker, E. R., Adams, K. E., & Roberts, M. H. (2004). Use of midlevel practitioners to achieve labor cost savings in the primary care practice of an MCO. *Health Services Research, 39*(3), 607–626.

Rodriguez, H. P., Rogers, W. H., Marshall, R. E., & Safran, D. (2007). Multidisciplinary primary care teams: Effects on the quality of clinician-patient interactions and organizational features of care. *Medical Care, 45*(1), 19–27.

Scheffler, R. M., Waitzman, N. J., & Hillman, J. M. (1996). The productivity of physician assistants and nurse practitioners and health work force policy in the era of managed healthcare. *Journal of Allied Health, 25*(3), 207–217.

Schneller, E. S. (1978). *The physician's assistant: Innovation in the medical division of labor.* Lexington, MA: Lexington Books.

Wilson, I. B., Landon, B. E., Hirschhorn, L. R., McInnes, K., Ding, L., Marsden, P. V., & Cleary, P. D. (2005). Quality of HIV care provided by nurse practitioners, physician assistants, and physicians. *Annals of Internal Medicine, 143*(10), 729–736.

CHAPTER 6

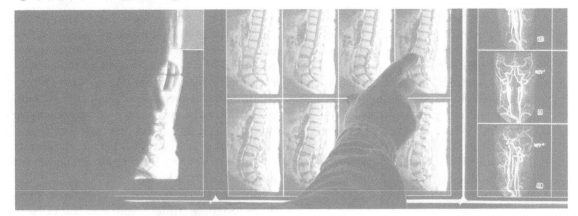

PHYSICIAN ASSISTANT SPECIALIZATION: NON–PRIMARY CARE

CHRISTINE M. EVERETT ■ RODERICK S. HOOKER ■ JAMES F. CAWLEY

"Specialization is a feature of every complex organization, be it social or natural, a school system, garden, book, or mammalian body."
—*Catharine R. Stimpson, US scholar and educator, 1992*

From the earliest days of the development of the physician assistant (PA) concept, the medical profession recognized the value of PAs and employed them in diverse settings. Now less than one-third of all US PAs work in primary care (family medicine, general pediatrics, geriatrics, and general internal medicine), and more than a quarter of PAs work in a surgical practice (e.g., general surgery, orthopedics, cardiovascular surgery, or some other surgical activity). Another quarter have roles in medical disciplines such as cardiology, nephrology, oncology, rheumatology, hematology, pulmonology, and gastroenterology. Smaller branches produce the disciplines of radiology (diagnostic and interventional), dermatology, and psychiatry. Postgraduate programs have sprung up to accommodate PAs

who wish to have additional training in various areas of medical care.

Demand for and use of PAs in specialized roles tends to fluctuate as the result of many factors (supply and demand being the leading one). However, the presence of PAs in medical subspecialty areas has expanded considerably since 1980. The wave of specialization that has swept over the medical profession has exerted widespread effects on the PA profession. Specialization has influenced the practice of medicine in profound ways, from the demise of the American general practitioner to the rise of a Byzantine world of specialty and subspecialty societies, examination processes, certification systems, and credentialing arrangements.

HISTORY OF PHYSICIAN ASSISTANT SPECIALIZATION

In an historic sense, specialization in medicine appears to be an inexorable phenomenon. Medical specialization emerged in the 19th century as a result of expanding medical knowledge and the notion that patients could be best managed through grouping patients, providers, and diseases into specific categories. Specialization was influenced by factors such as disease prevalence, advances in medical knowledge, and the use of technology, and it became well established throughout the 20th century as more and more groups of physicians formed specialty societies and formal certification processes. Today, the Accreditation Council for Graduate Medical Education recognizes at least 26 physician specialties and 126 subspecialties. Specialization is a compelling force in medicine and medical practice, and it is not at all surprising that this movement has influenced the PA profession.

Early observers of the PA noted that it was only a matter of time before specialization would transform the PA profession just as it has that of physicians. In 1972, Ann A. Bliss wrote:

> Immediately upon graduation, the physician's assistant [sic] is in considerable danger of being swallowed whole by the whale that is our present entrepreneurial subspecialty medical practice system. The likely co-option of the newly minted physician's assistant (sic) by subspecialty medicine is one of the most serious issues confronting the PA. (Sadler, Sadler, & Bliss, 1972)

Although Bliss believed that this "danger" would occur much sooner than it has, it appears that the time of reckoning with specialization has finally arrived.

The *raison d'être* of the PA profession was to work with physicians and provide medical services to populations that were underserved or that did not receive any care. While this is recounted in the history of the profession (see Chapter 2), the original intention of Eugene Stead, Richard Smith, and Harvey Estes in creating the profession has not been fully appreciated. These leaders envisioned these new practitioners as assistants to doctors in a very general and literal sense; they did not confine the activities of PAs to working only with general practice physicians. Estes intended that PAs would provide a wide number of services

for physicians in all types of medical practice areas (Estes, 1993). The original Duke curriculum was a generalist one, preparing PAs for roles in general medicine but also in specialties and subspecialties. Thus, the original design of the Medex and Duke programs was that the PA would perform medical tasks—some involving diagnosis and therapeutic management and some involving technical and routine procedures. This training relieved the busy doctor and allowed him or her more time for continuing professional education, dealing with complex patient illnesses, and seeing more patients. Both models trained PAs as all-purpose generalist assistants to doctors. This concept became markedly altered as the PA movement gained momentum in the early 1970s. The main influence was Title VII §747 and the emphasis on producing PAs and nurse practitioners (NPs) for primary care as well as promoting their employment in rural and underserved areas of care. The curricula of most PA programs receiving federal support during this time were designed with the intent that program graduates would become primary care practitioners.

Within the PA profession, specialty mix began at an early stage. For many years, largely due to the influence of federal funding for primary care education, the direction of the profession took a marked turn toward primary care and, in the late 1970s, a majority of PAs worked in general/family medicine. But as the profession evolved and grew in the 1980s and 1990s, specialization increased as increasing numbers of PAs entered specialty practices. This, in turn, led to the formation of an increasing number of specific specialty and subspecialty societies within the American Academy of Physician Assistants (AAPA) and increasing numbers of postgraduate educational programs.

These trends have continued, and as the number of PAs in specialties has increased, the number in primary care has consequently declined. The majority of clinically active PAs are in specialties. The proportion of the PA workforce practicing in general primary care decreased from 43% in 1997 to 24% in

2015. Over the same period, the percent of PAs reporting practice in adult medical specialties increased from 17% in 1997 to 26% in 2015. Ten percent of PAs practiced in urgent care in 2014, a practice area not previously included as a specialty option. The percentage of PAs working in primary care specialties fell to the lowest levels recorded in the past several decades (AAPA, 2014). About 31% of the nation's 100,000-plus PAs in active clinical practice in 2015 were employed in primary care specialties; less than one-third of all new PA graduates now enter primary care fields. This trend is in contrast to the fact that one-quarter of PAs work in surgery and the surgical subspecialties and 11% work in emergency medicine (National Commission on Certification of Physician Assistants, 2015) (Figure 6–1).

FIGURE 6-1
PA Specialty Trends, 2002 to 2014

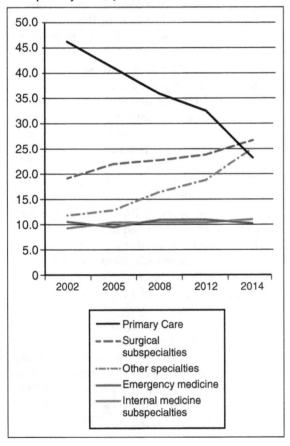

FACTORS INFLUENCING PHYSICIAN ASSISTANT SPECIALIZATION

Organizationally, specialization within the PA profession has spurred the founding of a number of specialty and subspecialty organizations. In the United States, the challenge is to retain these groups under the big tent of the AAPA because many of these specialty groups hold their own meetings with relevant continuing medical education programs. Some professional associations of specialized physicians have developed their own PA and NP certification structure. Globally, cardiovascular PAs in India take a specialized examination for certification in this surgical specialty.

Although the number of PAs has increased, the growth rate has been higher in specialties than in primary care. Because PAs are employed by physicians, are often legally required to work with physicians, and emulate physician behavior in many ways, it is not surprising that they would move into specialty practices. Most of the trends observed among physicians are also seen in PA specialization, including the trend to work in a "nonprimary" care role and the increase in wages that specialization brings (Table 6–1).

What factors influence or lead PAs to choose a particular specialty or practice? PAs probably respond to the same forces that shape physician specialty choices: the training process, the specialty that fits the lifestyle and geographic preferences of the physician, and market forces (Figure 6–2). The level of debt of newly graduating PAs may also be a determinant of specialty choice, just as it is for graduating medical students. Beyond these factors, the reasons PAs choose a particular specialty is only partially known. For PAs, the most influential factors determining specialty choice are technical orientation, income, and lack of primary care employment availability. PAs identify prevention, academic environment, intellectual content, patient–provider relationship, and peer influence as influencing factors for being in primary care.

Market forces play a significant role in specialty choice. One study showed that the specialty distribution of new graduates closely

TABLE 6-1
Physician Assistants, Specialty Groups: Trends, by Percent, 1984 to 2013

Specialty	1984	1989	1990	1992	1994	1996	2000	2002	2009	2013
Family/general medicine	54.5	37.9	33.0	31.4	33.7	39.8	36.5	32.1	24.9	23
General internal medicine	9.2	7.8	9.0	8.9	9.2	8.3	8.8	8.4	6.9	–
Emergency medicine	6.4	6.2	7.0	8.0	8.7	7.0	9.7	10.2	8.7	10.6
General pediatrics	4.1	3.6	3.0	2.5	2.3	2.7	2.6	2.6	2.4	2.0
General surgery	9.2	7.9	8.0	8.0	7.7	3.1	2.7	2.5	2.5	2
Internal medicine subspecialties	4.8	3.8	6.0	7.1	6.3	5.8	8.1	9.4	11.3	11
Pediatric subspecialties	0.0	1.0	2.0	1.2	1.2	2.1	1.5	1.5	1.6	–
Surgical subspecialties	9.0	7.5	9.0	9.8	10.5	8.8	10.4	10.0	19.5	24
Obstetrics and gynecology	3.1	4.6	4.0	3.3	2.9	3.0	2.7	2.7	2.4	3
Occupational medicine	4.1	5.8	5.0	3.9	3.4	3.0	3.4	3.0	2.1	–
Orthopedics	4.1	5.6	6.0	7.6	7.8	6.9	7.3	9.2	9.5	–
Other	7.9	6.6	6.4	6.5	7.4	8.4	9.3	10.2	10.5	11.6

Data from American Academy of Physician Assistants, AAPA Census Reports 1984–2013.

resembles that of the entire profession, and the market has the same influence on new graduates as it does on experienced PAs. Employment opportunities also likely play a role. The projected use of PAs on teams, or the trend of using PAs as replacements for residents, raises several policy issues in healthcare workforce planning. When the resident workweek was restricted to 80 hours, a significant effect on the use of PAs in hospital settings was observed with the number of PAs being employed. The most immediate effect was between the years 2000 and 2006, when the number of hospital-based PAs increased by nearly one-third.

PHYSICIAN ASSISTANTS IN MEDICAL SPECIALTIES AND SUBSPECIALTIES

In approaching the issue of specialization, this chapter focuses on medical specialties and subspecialties. As previously noted, PAs who participate in surgery or work in the surgical specialties represent a significant component of PA practice. However, this practice predominantly occurs in inpatient settings; therefore, these specialties are addressed separately in Chapter 7, "Physician Assistants in Hospital Settings." Chapter 7 also provides a review of PAs who work in intensive/acute care.

Medical specialties are generally the nonprimary care disciplines that physicians and PAs pursue. Many originate from internal medicine. Some of the medical specialties listed are surgically based, but when working in these specialties, PAs tend to function outside the operating theater.

Box 6–1 lists some of the clinical practice specialties and subspecialties in which PAs are used. The list is far from complete.

Allergy and Immunology Medicine

Immunology is the study of the immune system, including allergies. This discipline deals with the physiological functioning of the

FIGURE 6-2
The Effect of the Education Process on Physician Assistant Specialty and Location

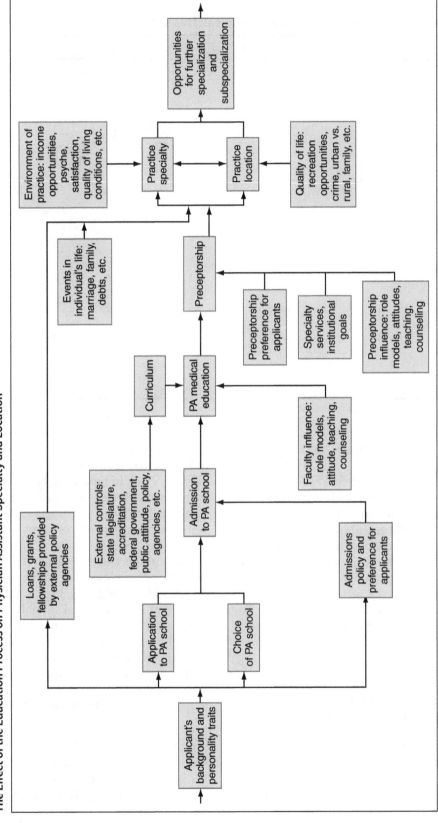

Data from Hooker, R. S. (1992). Employment specialization in the PA profession. *Journal of the American Academy of Physician Assistants, 5*(8), 695–704.

BOX 6-1
Partial Listing of Nonprimary Care Areas That Employ Physician Assistants

Allergy	Neonatology
Anesthesiology	Neurosurgery
Cardiothoracic surgery	Obstetrics and gynecology
Clinical research	Occupational health
Critical care units	Oncology (including pediatric oncology)
Dermatology	Ophthalmology
Emergency medicine	Organ procurement and transplantation
Forensic medicine and pathology	Orthopedics and sports medicine
Gastroenterology and endoscopy	Otorhinolaryngology (head and neck surgery)
Gerontology	Physical medicine and rehabilitation
Hematology	Plastic surgery and burn care
Infectious disease and immune deficiency	Public health
Interventional radiology	Rheumatology
Invasive cardiology	Substance abuse
Mental health and psychiatry	Urology
Preventive medicine	

immune system in states of health and disease; malfunctions of the immune system in immunological disorders (autoimmune diseases, hypersensitivities, immune deficiency, allograft rejection); and the physical, chemical, and physiological characteristics of the components of the immune system in vitro, in situ, and in vivo. Allergy medicine is applied immunology research used to diagnose the allergic responses to environmental stimuli and determine their treatments. Allergists tend to be internists or pediatricians, although many family medicine physicians perform allergy testing and treatment. Allergy and immunology are combined because a large overlap exists between the two disciplines and many doctors are trained in both areas of medicine. Some doctors are trained in allergy, immunology, and rheumatology.

Tasks and Procedures
Historically, allergy and immunology have not been areas widely occupied by PAs. Based on the patient's history and accompanying physical examination findings, PAs in this specialty typically orders a range of tests for allergens and lung functions via bronchodilators and spirometry and develop a preliminary diagnosis and treatment plan. On a typical day, allergy and immunology PAs see acute and chronic conditions. Sinus conditions tend to make up a large part of the patient load. In some settings, they may administer allergy desensitization injections, manage atopic dermatitis and chronic coughs, and treat acute asthma attacks. Patients may be children or adults with allergies or immunological disorders such as immunoglobulin G subclass deficiency.

Safety and Effectiveness
One study surveyed allergy and immunology practices to determine the impact of PAs on satisfaction and quality of care. This telephone survey queried 23 PAs, 21 doctors, and 54 patients from asthma practices employing PAs and 21 physicians and 55 patients from practices who did not employ PAs. The survey found patient satisfaction was higher in terms of level of care provided, responsiveness to questions, phone calls, patient education, and time spent waiting to see a provider in practices that employed a PA compared with those who did not employ a PA. Less than 1% of PAs work in allergy or immunology.

Increases in patient satisfaction and patient volume were mentioned as the top two benefits a PA provides to an allergy clinic. In addition, an increase in patient education, a reduction in appointment wait time, and the ability to spend more time with the physician or PA were mentioned by respondents as the top benefits provided to the patients by a PA (Figures 6–3 and 6–4).

FIGURE 6-3
Benefits of a Physician Assistant to the Allergy Clinic as Perceived by Each Provider (7-Point Likert Scale)

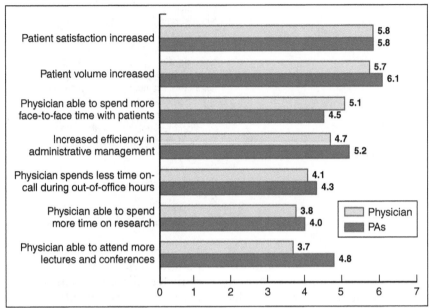

Data from Thomas, G. P., McNellis, R. J., & Ortiz, G. R. (2003). Physician assistants enhance quality of care in asthma patients. *Journal of Allergy and Clinical Immunology, 111*(Abstract Suppl.), S71–S440.

Cardiology

Cardiology is the study and management of patients with myocardial, circulatory, and valve diseases. Interventional cardiology deals specifically with the catheter-based treatment of structural heart diseases. A large number of procedures can be performed on the heart by catheterization, which most commonly involves inserting a sheath into the femoral artery (or another large peripheral vessel) and cannulating the heart under fluoroscopy.

According to estimates from the National Commission on Certification of Physician Assistants, nearly 2,500 certified PAs work in cardiology, and another 3,000 certified PAs work in cardiac and thoracic surgery. That number is expected to rise, as provider availability might keep pace with an aging population.

Results of a 2012 survey by the American College of Cardiology indicated that most cardiology PAs work in a group-practice setting (48%) or a hospital-based practice (33%). Most

respondents provided both inpatient and outpatient care (77%).

Tasks and Procedures

Practice in cardiology commonly demands range and versatility. Therefore, cardiology PAs can perform many tasks and procedures, which range from hospital admission and discharge evaluations to conducting key tests, including treadmill and stress tests, nuclear stress tests, and tilt table tests.

Cardiology PA inpatient responsibilities may include non–intensive care unit patients, writing orders and progress notes, conducting patient consults, and dictating consultations. They explain cardiology procedures to patients, monitor placement of catheters and pacemakers, and monitor chest pains that do not require evaluation by the emergency department (ED). PAs in cardiology also commonly perform such procedures as aortic balloon pump removal, elective cardioversion, central line placement, Swan-Ganz placement, sternal/thoracotomy closure, endoscopic

FIGURE 6-4
The Patient's Views: Benefits of a Physician Assistant to the Allergy Clinic as Perceived by the Patient (7-Point Likert Scale)

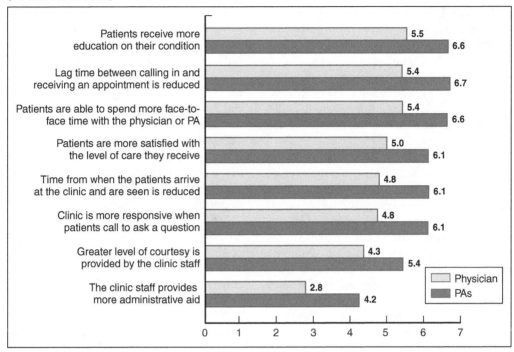

Data from Thomas, G. P., McNellis, R. J., & Ortiz, G. R. (2003). Physician assistants enhance quality of care in asthma patients. *Journal of Allergy and Clinical Immunology, 111*(Abstract Suppl.), S71–S440.

saphenous vein harvesting, and conduit vessel harvesting. Procedures that are increasingly being performed by PAs include coronary arteriography and cardiac catheterization. By performing these tasks and dealing with laboratory results and imaging studies in advance, cardiology PAs enhance continuity of care by providing cardiologists more time and easing case management.

In cardiology offices, PAs perform history taking and physical examinations of new patients, including in-depth details of cardiovascular health and general habits. They also see patients for follow-up visits, perform post-procedure site checks, titrate blood pressure, coordinate medications, and promote recovery through discussion of diet, exercise, and lifestyle issues.

PAs are also taking on disease-specific roles in cardiology. Heart failure is a condition of increasing public health and policy importance. As such, some practices employ PAs specifically to treat patients with heart failure in outpatient settings.

Safety and Effectiveness

Limited evidence is also available regarding the effectiveness of PAs in cardiology. One study evaluated the relationship between inclusion of PAs and advanced practice nurses (APRNs) in cardiology practices and adherence to seven guideline-recommended therapies for patients with heart failure. Practices that employed PAs or APRNs had similar outcomes for five of the outcomes. However, clinics that employed two or more PAs or APRNs had greater conformity to guidelines for two of the outcomes (implantable cardioverter-defibrillator therapy and delivery of heart failure education; Albert et al., 2010).

Two studies have evaluated PA performance of specific procedures generally performed by cardiologists. DeMots, Coombs, Murphy, and Palac (1987) evaluated the feasibility of PAs performing coronary arteriography. The complication rate and facility in performing the procedure were compared with those of cardiology fellows. The procedure and fluoroscopy times were similar and, more importantly, the mortality rate was zero. The rate of complications was very low compared with published standards. Additional experience with this same model and two additional PAs included an evaluation of more than 1,000 patients, with no mortality and low complication rates (Dracup et al., 1994).

PA performance of cardiac catheterization has also been studied. Using a prospective database of patients undergoing cardiac catheterization, a cardiology team compared the outcomes of procedures performed by supervised PAs with those performed by supervised cardiology fellows-in-training. Outcome measures included procedural length, fluoroscopy use, volume of contrast media, and complications including myocardial infarction, stroke, arrhythmia requiring defibrillation or pacemaker placement, pulmonary edema requiring intubation, and vascular complications. Class 3 and 4 congestive heart failure was more common in patients who underwent procedures by fellows compared with those undergoing procedures by PAs. PA cases tended to be slightly faster with less fluoroscopic time. The incidence of major complications within 24 hours of the procedure was similar between the two groups (0.54% in PA cases and 0.58% in fellow cases). The authors conclude that under the supervision of experienced attending cardiologists, trained PAs can perform diagnostic cardiac catheterization, including coronary angiography, with complication rates similar to those of cardiology fellows-in-training (Krasuski et al., 2003).

Correctional Medicine

Correctional medicine is the medical management of individuals who are incarcerated. Although commonly listed as a specialty, in reality, correctional medicine is a primary care discipline that is practiced under extenuating circumstances and involves challenging behavior, ethical considerations, and certain legal constraints.

Like most large cities, each county and state has a jail or prison system—many with employment opportunities for PAs. The mission statement of correctional institutions is the same as other healthcare systems: to provide essential healthcare for inmates consistent with acceptable community standards. The Department of Justice recruits PAs to staff the federal correctional system, better known as the Federal Bureau of Prisons, either as civil service employees or public health service officers. For new and experienced PAs, opportunities abound in the Bureau of Prisons. PAs often work independently and deliver a number of primary care and specialty services, depending on the size of the institution. The great diversity of the inmates provides a challenging clinical experience, and the types of settings are unique.

Although the United States has a large incarcerated population, there are two aspects that are important to note about the types of facilities. First is the difference between a prison and a correctional facility, or jail. Prisons are usually located outside of a major city, preferably in remote regions of the state. They provide housing for inmates who have been convicted and sentenced to serve for a period of 12 months of more. Jails, on the other hand, are usually located within close proximity of city limits and tend to have access to major trauma centers and hospitals of the respective city.

With respect to the healthcare systems, inmates of jails have access to a number of healthcare services, including but not limited to normal sick calls, ongoing treatment for chronic illnesses, and limited prenatal care. In addition, because the locations of jails are close to major trauma centers and hospitals, emergency care can be attended to at any given time if such services are not immediately available within the jail facility.

Inmates of prisons are faced with a totally different set of healthcare facilities, primarily because of their remote locations and, more often than not, because of the limited number of healthcare providers assigned to the respective prison. Therefore, the prison system is where PAs are most needed and called for, simply because the available senior physicians alone cannot handle all of the health needs of the prison inmates.

Tasks and Procedures

Prisons allow PAs to follow through with their patients longitudinally while monitoring compliance. According to one estimate, PAs perform more than 80% of the tasks of the senior physician in the prison setting. The tasks and procedures performed by PAs in correctional medicine spans a number of medical specialties. These tasks may include conducting physical examinations, treating illnesses, diagnosing patients, ordering and interpreting tests results, and, sometimes, assisting in surgery. In some settings, the medical officer (doctor or PA) may be involved in stabilizing patients with psychiatric illnesses.

With a number of safeguards in place, correctional medicine PAs may hold sick call in the morning, see scheduled patients throughout the day, and perform some minor procedures. In some instances, they communicate with medical and surgical specialists and follow through with recommendations for treatment.

Professional Society

The American Correctional Health Services Association's (ACHSA's) mission is to be the voice of the correctional healthcare profession and serve as an effective forum for communication addressing current issues and needs confronting correctional healthcare. The ACHSA provides support, skill development, and education programs for healthcare personnel, organizations, and decision-makers involved in correctional healthcare, resulting in increased professionalism and a sense of community for correctional healthcare personnel and positive changes in health for detained and incarcerated individuals.

Dermatology

Dermatologists specialize in the diagnosis and treatment of diseases and tumors of the skin and its appendages. There are a variety of medical and surgical dermatological subspecialties.

Like many specialties, dermatology is faced with physician shortages, resulting in patients experiencing long waiting periods for appointments. To help alleviate this issue, PAs are increasingly being utilized in dermatology practices to increase the number of clinicians providing dermatological services. However, few data detailing the productivity and profitability of PAs in dermatology are available. Access to this information could help workforce planners and healthcare providers plan and improve patient access to dermatological care.

Of the dermatologists who responded to the American Academy of Dermatology's 2007 Practice Profile Survey, 23% reported employing a PA, a significant increase from the 15% employed in 2002 (Kimball & Resneck, 2008). Respondents seeking to hire additional dermatologists and those with surgical or cosmetically focused practices were much more likely to hire PAs or NPs. However, PAs and NPs spent the majority of their time seeing medical dermatology patients, even if the practice was surgically focused. Most dermatologists supported their PA and NP colleagues in seeing new patients and established patients experiencing new problems. This increase in utilization of PAs is likely to continue, as 36% of responding dermatologists reported that they intend to hire either PAs or NPs (Kimball & Resneck, 2008). The 2015 estimate is that at least 3.5% of all PAs work in dermatology. Females represent about 81% and 93% of all dermatology PAs work in a private office.

According to one study, the average annual revenue generated by PAs working in a dermatology practice is around $500,000, with a range of $37,000 to $1,500,000. PAs with 5 or more years of experience average $621,000 in annual revenue, whereas PAs with less than 5 years average around $375,000 annually. The median salary of a dermatology PA in 2015 was $105,000.

Tasks and Procedures

The majority of PAs in dermatology work in private dermatologists' offices and report seeing or billing for an average of 28 patients a day. PAs in dermatology assess patients' skin complaints, biopsy lesions (if necessary), and provide treatment. PAs in dermatology may medically treat common skin conditions such as acne. Some PAs with advanced skills may transpose surgical flaps, remove scars and tattoos, and assist in hair transplants (Table 6–2).

In one dermatology practice, PAs specialized in removal of suspicious moles, acne scars, port-wine stains, and other birthmarks. Lasers were used for hair removal, tattoo removal, and the treatment of hemangiomas. The procedures commonly performed by PAs in dermatology are listed in Box 6–2.

Dermatological surgeons practice skin cancer surgery (including Mohs micrographic surgery), laser surgery, cryosurgery, photodynamic therapy, and cosmetic procedures using botulinum toxin, soft tissue fillers, sclerotherapy, and liposuction. Dermatopathologists interpret tissue under the microscope (histopathology). Pediatric dermatologists specialize in the diagnosis and treatment of skin disease in children. Immunodermatologists specialize in the diagnosis and management of skin diseases driven by an altered immune system, including bullous diseases such as pemphigus. In addition, dermatologists manage wide ranges of congenital syndromes.

TABLE 6-2
Dermatology Physician Assistants, 2008

Total survey respondents	900
Age (mean years)	38
Female	703 (79%)
Solo physician practitioner	367 (41%)
Single-specialty physician group practice	372 (42%)
Multispecialty physician group practice	74 (8%)
Hospital	40 (4%)
Minor surgical procedures	94%
Years in clinical practice	8
Work in urban setting	94%
Precept PA students	34%
Work more than 32 hours per week	81%
Mean income	$104,474

Data from American Academy of Physician Assistants (AAPA). (2008). 2008 AAPA physician assistant census report. Alexandria, VA: Author.

BOX 6-2
Procedures Frequently Performed by Physician Assistants in Dermatology

- Cryotherapy of benign lesions
- Intralesional injections
- Laser surgery
- Incisional and excisional biopsies
- Wound closure of flaps and grafts
- Phototherapy
- Patch testing
- Hair transplantations
- Sclerotherapy
- Mohs' surgery
- Chemical peels

Data from Clark, A. R., Monroe, J. R., Feldman, S. R., Fleischer, A. B., Hauser, D. A., & Hinds, M. A. (2000). The emerging role of physician assistants in the delivery of dermatological healthcare. Dermatologic Clinics, 18(2), 297–302.

Professional Society

The Society of Dermatology Physician Assistants (SDPA) was founded in 1994 and is composed of members who have a medical interest in the management of dermatological conditions. The organization has over 1200 members. The *Journal of Dermatology for Physician Assistants (JDPA),* the official journal of the SDPA, premiered in 2007.

Emergency Medicine

Emergency medicine focuses on diagnosis and treatment of acute illnesses and injuries that require immediate medical attention. Emergency medicine provided within an ED must be distinguished from care provided in urgent care centers. Providers in urgent care centers offer primary care treatment to patients who desire or require immediate care, but they do not reach the acuity required for providing care in an ED.

Emergency medicine providers are tasked with seeing a large number of patients, treating their illnesses, and arranging for disposition (admitting them to a hospital or releasing them after treatment, as necessary). Emergency physicians require a broad field of knowledge and advanced procedural skills, which are commonly used in interventions such as surgical procedures, trauma resuscitation, advanced cardiac life support, and advanced airway management.

PAs have increasingly been utilized in emergency medicine as a strategy for addressing emergency physician shortages and rising costs. Most PAs in emergency medicine work as a team, although a few may be the only provider (with immediate backup by a doctor), such as in small rural hospitals. Guidelines for the scope of practice for PAs have been published; however, the role of PAs on the healthcare team can vary substantially. A common role is to treat low-acuity, or "fast-track," patients. One study suggests that in fast-track roles, PAs have greater productivity than resident physicians with similar patient satisfaction (Jeanmonod et al., 2013). However, new and innovative roles are also being developed for PAs in EDs. For example, one organization utilized a PA to perform rapid assessments, patient care procedures, patient education, and disposition planning as part of a discharge facilitator team. Others have utilized PAs in roles that assist patients transitioning between EDs and primary care or EDs and inpatient settings.

The incorporation of PAs into EDs has expanded to other countries in North America and Europe. In Canada, PAs and NPs are also employed in EDs in Ontario, New Brunswick, and Manitoba. The PAs are all formally trained and are a mix of Canadians and Americans. Outcome studies in Ontario are comparing the care PAs, NPs, and doctors provide.

Tasks and Procedures

PAs in emergency medicine tend to be highly skilled in advanced cardiac life support, advanced trauma life support, toxicology, orthopedics, trauma, pediatrics, and neurology. They may be the provider directing a code for a cardiac arrest or assisting in polytrauma stabilization.

A few studies have described the range of services PAs provide in ED settings. An analysis of the results of the National Ambulatory Hospital Medical Care Survey that began in 1992 found that PAs and NPs managed 3.5 million (4%) of the approximately 90 million nonfederal ED visits in the United States. The analysis concluded that few differences exist in the type of patient seen at PA and NP visits compared with

physician visits for gender, reason for visit, diagnosis, and prescribed medications.

In another study, Arnopolin and Smithline (2000) compared patient encounters between PAs and physicians and reached a conclusion that the distribution of diagnostic groups between PAs and physicians was similar. Some differences that emerged were the time for patients and the total charges (Table 6–3). Overall, visits were 8 minutes longer and total charges were $8 less when a PA treated a patient. Patients who had headache, otitis, respiratory infection, asthma, a gastrointestinal or genitourinary disorder, cellulitis, laceration, or a musculoskeletal disorder had a longer visit when seen by a PA. The difference in visit time ranged from 5 minutes to 32 minutes longer than a visit with a physician (Arnopoline & Smithline, 2000). Innovative programs that utilize PAs in EDs have included laceration management. In one example, the PA was on call to manage all lacerations that presented to an ED. The results indicated improved care and outcome, decreased cost, and satisfied patients.

A 10-year trend analysis of the tasks of PAs and NPs in emergency medicine found the most frequently seen diagnoses were abdominal pain, otitis media, upper respiratory infections, chest pain, and acute pharyngitis (Table 6–3). The mean number of prescriptions written by doctors, PAs, and NPs over this same period was very similar (Figure 6–5), suggesting convergence of approaches to similar patients.

In a review of 35 emergency medicine PA studies, the authors concluded the use of PAs in EDs is increasing. This expansion is due to necessity in staffing and economy of scale. Although the tasks performed seems to be expanding, this assessment identified gaps in deployment research using appropriate outcome measures in the area of clinical effectiveness of PAs (Hooker, Klocko, & Larkin, 2011).

Safety and Effectiveness

Few studies comparing the outcomes of ED care provided by PAs versus those provided by physicians have been undertaken. One prospective, nonrandomized descriptive study compared the traumatic wound infection rates in

TABLE 6-3
Most Frequently Seen Diagnoses by Type of Prescriber, 1995 to 2004

	Physician	PA	NP	*p**
Abdominal pain, unspecified	33,215,742 (3.47%)	1,552,137 (2.65%)	341,470 (1.93%)	.0001
Otitis media	31,146,225 (3.25%)	1,862,565 (3.18%)	796,764 (4.51%)	.039
Upper respiratory infection	27,731,523 (2.89%)	1,759,089 (3.00%)	589,812 (3.34%)	.594
Chest pain, unspecified	25,041,151 (2.61%)	951,978 (1.62%)	300,080 (1.70%)	.0001
Acute pharyngitis	19,970,835 (2.08%)	1,655,613 (2.82%)	589,812 (3.34%)	.0001

*p value from design-corrected Pearson chi-square.
Data from Hooker, R. S., Cipher, D. J., Cawley, J. F., Herrmann, D., & Melson, J. (2008). Emergency medicine services: Interprofessional care trends. *Journal of Interprofessional Care, 22*(2), 167–178.

FIGURE 6-5
Mean Number of Prescriptions Written by Type of Emergency Medicine Provider, 1995–2004

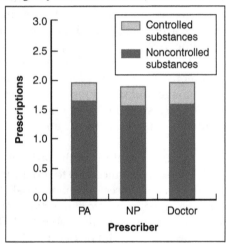

Data from Hooker, R. S., Cipher, D. J., Cawley, J. F., Herrmann, D., & Melson, J. (2008). Emergency medicine services: Interprofessional care trends. *Journal of Interprofessional Care, 22*(2), 167–178.

TABLE 6-4
Level of Training, Wound Care Practices, and Infection Rates

Emergency Department Practitioner	Wounds Per No. of Cases Sutured	Wound Infection Rate (%)
Medical student	0/60	0
All resident physicians	17/547	3.1
PAs	11/305	3.6
Attending physicians	14/251	5.6
Junior practitioners (medical students and interns)	8/262	3.1
Senior practitioners (PAs, residents, attending physicians)	34/901	3.8

Modified from Singer, A. J., Hollander, J. E., Cassara, G., Valentine, S. M., Thode, H. C., Jr., & Henry, M. C. (1995). Level of training, wound care practices, and infection rates. *American Journal of Emergency Medicine, 13*(3), 265–268.

patients based on level of training in ED practitioners. Wounds were evaluated in 1,163 patients using a wound registry and a follow-up visit or phone call. Table 6–4 demonstrates the results on wound care. The study found no significant difference in level of training and wound care rates between medical students, interns, PAs, resident physicians, and attending physicians. The authors concluded that the delegation of wound management to PAs is safe and that PAs perform similarly to physicians in the same setting.

Patient satisfaction with PAs in the ED seems to be as high as that for physicians. A 1999 study of patients who were seen in a fast-track ED were surveyed about their experience with the PA who took care of them. A total of 111 survey results were analyzed. The mean response was 93 (on a scale of 0–100). This result demonstrates a high degree of satisfaction with ED PAs. Only 12% of the patients said they would be willing to wait longer to be seen by a physician (Counselman et al., 2000).

Professional Society
Over 13% of all PAs work in emergency medicine since 2015 or about 290 PAs per emergency physicians. Fifty-eight percent are female and the median income was $115,000. The Society of Emergency Medicine Physician Assistants (SEMPA) has a membership of more

than 3,000 PAs. SEMPA works to continually support the professional, clinical, and personal development of emergency medicine PAs. It also works to educate the public about the role, importance, and value of PAs in the ED. A subset of PAs in this file are those that identify urgent care as their primary specialty; estimates from AAPA data show that they are an additional 4% of PAs in this specialty category.

Endocrinology

Endocrinology involves the study of the biosynthesis, storage, chemistry, and physiological function of hormones and the cells of the endocrine glands and tissues that secrete them. Such organs include the thyroid, parathyroid, pancreas, ovaries, testes, adrenal, pituitary, and hypothalamus. Most endocrinology work involves diabetes, thyroid disorders, or bone metabolism. However, little is known about the types and distribution of PAs in this specialized role.

Tasks and Procedures

Almost all PAs in endocrinology work with an endocrinologist. They may manage patients with thyroid disease, metabolic syndrome, vitamin deficiencies, and bone mineral metabolism or may choose to focus on patients with type 1 or type 2 diabetes mellitus. Some work specifically as diabetology PAs; although diabetes is an endocrinopathy, some diabetology PAs are part of internal medicine practices. Their role varies depending on the setting. They may be involved in monitoring severely brittle diabetics; overseeing patients with mixed endocrinopathies, such as hypothyroidism and diabetes; and managing type 2 diabetes.

Safety and Effectiveness

One study evaluated the effectiveness of PAs in endocrinology. It involved diabetes management of several hundred non–critically ill hospitalized patients. The care of diabetes patients by standard medical teams was compared with the care directed by an NP/PA endocrinology team. Despite the hospital implementing system-wide staff education and computerized insulin orders with built-in algorithms, patients cared for by the NP/PA team were nearly four times more likely to receive a *basal-bolus* regimen of insulin than patients in the standard care teams. The NP/PA patients had significantly lower glucose levels in the 24 hours before discharge. This research suggests that expertise in diabetes management can help offset hospitalizations and PAs in this role are often the ones called to manage such patients. Less than 1% of PAs work in endocrinology.

Forensic Medicine

Forensic medicine is a broad spectrum of sciences used by the judicial system to answer questions concerning a crime or a civil action. It is a multidisciplinary specialty that provides impartial scientific evidence for use in the courts of law. As a discipline, it draws principally from chemistry, biology, physics, geology, psychology, and the social sciences.

Forensic medicine is a discipline common to multiple positions, including investigator, coroner, and medical examiner:

- A medical legal *investigator* tracks the circumstances that led to a violent, unexpected, suspicious, or unattended death; the death of a child; or the death of someone in government custody. Sometimes the death could affect public health, such as with deaths caused by the bubonic plague or tuberculosis, or the victim is involved in a "medical misadventure," such as poisoning.
- A *coroner* is an appointed official responsible for investigating deaths and determining the cause of death. Depending on the jurisdiction, the coroner may determine the cause himself or herself, or act as the presiding officer of a special report conducted by other appointed experts dictated by the case.
- The term *medical examiner* is a frequently used alternative title for *coroner*; however, unlike a coroner, a medical examiner is typically a licensed pathologist. The role of a forensic medical examiner can be broad and involves solving crimes, protecting public health, exposing unsafe consumer products, and addressing questions related

to insurance claims. Other roles that come into play involve assisting clergy, funeral directors, and embassies. The examiner is called to answer who, what, when, where, and why.

That PAs would be attracted to forensic medicine is interesting because there seems to be little emphasis on forensic pathology as a potential area of practice in the current PA education curriculum. As one coroner put it, "Forensic medicine requires many of the same skills looked for in applicants to PA school. It has to be someone who is interested in medicine, someone with the ability to make decisions, someone who can communicate and is compassionate, firm, and fair. And, of course, you have to have the ability to understand scientific data" (Wright & Hirsch, 1989).

Tasks and Procedures

Forensic medicine PAs are employed as investigators in a number of jurisdictions. Examples include the medical examiner offices in Suffolk County, New York; Pueblo, Colorado; New Hampshire; Washington, DC; and New York City. For some PAs, these jobs are full time; for others, their role is part time.

Qualifications vary by state, but it is not unusual for a public coroner to be a PA, although the role of coroner is largely investigative in many jurisdictions. The coroner examines the crime scene, records what is present at the scene, and then makes determinations as to whether an autopsy, judicial hearing, or coroner's inquest is necessary. Whereas a board-certified pathologist (preferably a forensic pathologist in criminal cases) undertakes the autopsy, the medical examiner can be a PA with a good background in pathology.

Gastroenterology

Gastroenterology is the study and management of the digestive system and its disorders from the mouth to the anus. Although principally an internal medicine specialty, important advances have contributed to the enteroscopic management of esophageal, intestinal, liver, pancreatic, and biliary tree diseases (hepatology or hepatobiliary medicine). As a consequence, an overlap exists between medicine and surgery with regard to some endoscopic procedures undertaken by gastroenterologists (doctors, PAs, and NPs).

Tasks and Procedures

PAs working in gastroenterology are part of a rapidly widening internal medicine field. They may have procedure-oriented roles, such as performing endoscopies (primarily flexible sigmoidoscopies and colonoscopies) and liver biopsies. Other tasks include assessing and managing patients with celiac sprue, esophagus disease, gastric disease, biliary disease, inflammatory bowel diseases, irritable bowel syndrome, and other intestinal disorders. Additionally, hospitals with large gastroenterology centers may use PAs for performing procedures, monitoring treatment of patients with hepatitis C, and performing routine maintenance for certain diseases.

The potential for PAs to improve the delivery of care in gastroenterology is recognized, but the process of defining and evaluating PA roles within the gastroenterology team has not yet been completed. One study conducted in a single organization in Ireland stated that the role of PAs was to manage established patients with stable disease and estimated that this role could reduce the salary expenses of a clinic by 17% (Donnellan et al., 2010).

Another study that evaluated data from 9500 screening procedures concluded that, in comparison with gastroenterologists, trained PA and NP endoscopists performed screening flexible sigmoidoscopy with similar accuracy and safety but at a lower cost. The implications were that screening flexible sigmoidoscopy performed by PAs and NPs increased the availability and lowered the cost of flexible sigmoidoscopy for colorectal cancer screening.

Professional Society

Approximately 1.5% of all PAs work in gastroenterology (not including hepatology). Over 80% are female and the median salary is $95,000. Founded in 2000, the Gastroenterology Physician Assistants (GIPA) is the voice representing PAs who practice gastroenterology and hepatology. The mission of GIPA is to provide improved healthcare and access to patients with gastrointestinal and hepatobiliary disease through professional and educational support.

Geriatric Medicine and Gerontology

Geriatrics is the branch of internal medicine that focuses on health promotion and the prevention and treatment of disease and disability in later life. Gerontology is the study of the aging process and the research surrounding the delivery of services to elders.

Although only a small percentage (<0.5%) of PAs identify geriatric medicine as their primary specialty area, a significant number (1,170, or 5.6%) of all clinically active PAs report that they see patients in a nursing home or other long-term facility (American Academy of Physician Assistants, 2011). A large number of PAs report treating elderly patients, defined as those 65 years of age or older (Cherry, Woodwell, & Rechtsteiner, 2007). However, it is necessary to distinguish between those PAs who care for people older than age 65 years and those PAs who provide comprehensive geriatric care. A geriatric care model has a holistic perspective, focusing on function, cognition, and the special needs of older patients, typically 75 years of age or older.

The demographic shift toward an aging population has created a great need for PAs competent in caring for the elderly. A study that analyzed data from the 2005 National Ambulatory Medical Care Survey revealed that 32% of all patients seen by PAs for outpatient visits were age 65 or older (Cherry et al., 2007). Segal-Gideon, a PA in geriatric practice, notes that:

> Despite it being an issue that has been recognized for years, preparing a healthcare workforce for the "aging" of the population in the United States has not been well planned. The elderly represent a large group of Americans with unmet healthcare needs (Alliance for Aging Research, 2006).

Recruiting and training PAs to provide services to geriatric populations is recognized as an avenue to address the currently unmet healthcare needs of the elderly population.

PAs are well positioned to function on interdisciplinary teams because they are trained to provide care in a team model. The American Geriatric Society's position paper on geriatric rehabilitation supports an interdisciplinary approach, and specifically includes the PA as a provider along with the doctor and NP.

Caring for elders usually requires greater clinician time than that needed for other patient populations. In addition, past reimbursement constraints and low levels of reimbursement for PA services set by the Centers for Medicare and Medicaid Services (CMS) may have constrained PAs from choosing to practice geriatric medicine. However, recent gains in reimbursement and practice authority for PA services by the CMS have helped improve the climate for PA geriatric practice. Services provided by PAs are reimbursable by Medicare and Medicaid in all patient care settings, including home visits.

Tasks and Procedures

PAs working in geriatrics may team with a geriatrician or in a nursing home or other long-term care setting. PAs in nursing homes frequently care for patients with neuropsychiatric and acute diagnoses was well as long-stay status. Typically, they perform geriatric assessments and elicit significant information regarding living situations, activities of daily living, and psychosocial and other functional status information that may be helpful to rehabilitation professionals. They may provide the therapy team (which may include a physical therapist, an occupational therapist, a physiatrist, a rehabilitation nurse, and a psychologist) with an overview of the patient's chronic and acute medical problems, level of disability, level of cognitive impairment, drug history (including current therapy), and other factors that may affect formulation or progress of a rehabilitation program. Rehabilitative team members working in geriatrics may encounter a PA acting as a primary medical caregiver using (or not using) a geriatric care model; a specialty care provider working with an orthopedist, a neurologist, or a physiatrist; an administrator; a clinical researcher; or a direct member of a rehabilitation team in a multidisciplinary approach.

Providing care to geriatric patients presents many unique clinical challenges, in part because these patients require a substantial amount of coordination of care. "The healthcare of elders in the United States presents the clinician with social, medical, spiritual and political challenges that cut across the full spectrum of race, religion, and social standing" (Alliance for Aging Research, 2006, page 3). Multisystem medical problems become even more challenging in the context of ethical and social dilemmas of providing compassionate care. PAs need to know when to refer patients for physical and occupational therapy services as well as what information to provide to help therapists effectively provide rehabilitative services. Contact with families, lengthy discussions surrounding end-of-life care, and the coordination of care between many specialists is time consuming and critical in appropriate medical management of geriatric patients. Physicians commonly lack the time required to perform these vital functions. PAs could be very effective at this coordination and liaison role, especially in a solo or small group medical practice.

PAs can also perform important preventive functions in the care of geriatric patients. Most nursing homes and long-term care facilities do not have a full-time medical staff. Physicians typically visit such facilities on a weekly basis. Patients with acute problems are generally treated over the phone or sent to an ED. Having a full-time PA on staff at a nursing home or long-term care facility can translate into patients being evaluated sooner and can prevent transfer to a hospital in many cases. In fact, one study supports that employment of PAs and NPs in nursing homes is associated with a lower hospitalization rate.

Safety and Effectiveness

PAs were recognized as effective providers of quality care in geriatric care facilities as early as 1979. More than one study has demonstrated shorter hospitalization and overall lower medical costs using PAs in geriatric institutional settings. Caprio (2006) argues that only by utilizing PAs and NPs in nursing homes will the needs of this special population be met.

In a study on the impact of adding a PA to a large nursing home, the hospitalization rate was dramatically altered. A 6-year case series examined hospital events of one nursing home before and after a PA joined a 92-bed teaching hospital in central Georgia. After the PA started, the number of annual hospital admissions fell by 38%, and the total number of hospital days per 1000 patient years fell by 69%. The number of nursing home visits increased by 62% (Figure 6–6) (Ackerman & Kemle, 1998).

Global Medicine

Although global medicine is not an official specialty designation for doctors or PAs, the diverse opportunities for a PA who wants to travel abroad to work with international populations must be mentioned. More than 40 agencies recruit volunteer PA, physician, nurse, and allied health personnel to work in underdeveloped countries. Most stints range from 1 to 2 years. Usually, transportation and a small stipend are provided for the volunteer. Employers of PAs include the US government, with agencies such as the Peace Corps, US Agency for International Development, and the State Department; nongovernmental organizations (NGOs), such as Doctors Without Borders; and private corporations.

One of the easiest ways for PAs to work outside the borders of the United States is through corporations that specifically employ PAs along with other health workers. For example, Seavin is a health unit that employs over a dozen PAs in Egypt who work in remote areas to provide healthcare to American and Egyptian personnel.

Obstacles and advantages to working in global medicine are outlined in Tables 6–5 and 6–6, respectively.

Tasks and Procedures

PAs in global medicine become skilled in administering immunizations, handling refugees, dealing with sanitation, providing rural remote health and primary care, and treating diseases unique to endemic areas. Various countries have been recruiting PAs for roles in PA demonstration projects. Some of these PAs are assisting educators and healthcare analysts to implement PA programs.

FIGURE 6-6
Hospital Use Rate Before and After Introduction of a Physician Assistant in a Nursing Home

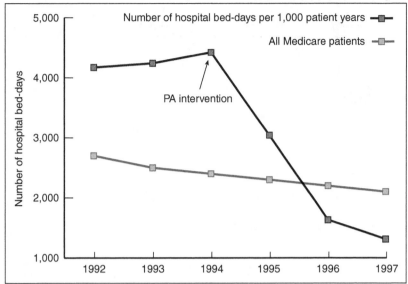

Data from Ackermann, R. J., & Kemle, K. A. (1998). The effect of a physician assistant on the hospitalization of nursing home residents. *Journal of the American Geriatrics Society, 46*(5), 610–614.

Professional Society

PAs for Global Health (PAGH) is a grassroots nonprofit organization working to meet the needs of PAs interested in working in medically underserved areas around the globe. It is the only PA organization of this type and volunteers work to support individual PAs in their efforts. PAGH is a completely volunteer-run and member funded.

Hospitalist

See Chapter 7, "Physician Assistants in Hospital Settings."

Infectious Disease, Immunology, Immunodeficiency

Infectious disease specialists address disease-causing organisms likely to be transmitted to people through the environment. Most of these specialists are trained in internal medicine and work in hospital and outpatient settings.

Tasks and Procedures

PAs who are infectious disease specialists commonly work in both inpatient and outpatient settings. Some PAs have assumed the role of the communicable disease nurse in hospital settings. Others consult with patients seeking advice regarding travel or see patients with immune deficiencies. This latter group commonly cares for patients with infectious disorders such as HIV and acquired immunodeficiency syndrome (AIDS). The way in which the tasks and procedures of these PAs become formalized into roles has not been detailed in the literature.

Safety and Effectiveness

Evidence related to the safety and effectiveness of PAs caring for patients in infectious disease specialty care is limited. A single study has compared the quality of care provided by NPs and PAs with that provided by physicians at 68 HIV care sites in 30 states. These care sites were funded by the Ryan White Comprehensive AIDS Resources Emergency (CARE) Act Title III. The authors surveyed 243 clinicians (177 physicians and 66 NPs and PAs) and reviewed medical records of 6651 persons with HIV or AIDS. Eight quality-of-care measures were assessed by medical record review. After adjustments for

TABLE 6-5
Significant Obstacles of International Physician Assistant Work

Obstacles Listed by Respondents	Percentage of Respondents
Language barriers	37.0
Substandard facilities	10.9
Lack of equipment or medicine	21.7
Competition with local doctors	2.2
Financial support	15.2
Transportation to medical facilities	2.2
Lack of knowledge of the PA profession	23.9
None	2.2
Lack of follow-up	4.4
New medicines	2.2
Governmental security	4.4
Patients' limited education in Western medicine	2.2
Lack of supervising doctors	4.4
Cost of travel	2.2
Cultural beliefs	4.4
Finding a medical team	2.2
No support from the American Academy of Physician Assistants	2.2
Lack of respect for female clinicians	2.2
Getting time off work	4.4
Time away from family	2.2

Data modified from Rogers, S. E. (2002). *Physician assistants working and volunteering abroad: A survey.* Unpublished doctoral dissertation, Arizona School of Health Sciences Physician Assistant School, Mesa, AZ.

TABLE 6-6
Significant Advantages of International Physician Assistant Work

Significant Benefits Listed by Respondents	Percentage of Respondents
Learning about another culture	37.0
Giving healthcare to those in need	37.0
Self-growth	15.2
Appreciation for the United States	4.4
New friends	10.9
Patients' eagerness for help	4.4
Travel	8.7
Challenge of clinical skills	19.6
Learning a new language	6.5
More medicine and practice options	6.5
Teamwork	2.2
Demonstrating compassion	4.4

Data modified from Rogers, S. E. (2002). *Physician assistants working and volunteering abroad: A survey.* Unpublished doctoral dissertation, Arizona School of Health Sciences Physician Assistant School, Mesa, AZ.

patient characteristics, six of the eight quality measures did not differ between NPs and PAs and infectious disease specialists or generalist HIV experts. Adjusted rates of purified protein derivative testing and Papanicolaou smears were statistically significantly higher for NPs and PAs than for infectious disease specialists and generalist HIV experts. NPs and PAs had statistically significantly higher performance scores than generalist non-HIV experts on six of the eight quality measures. For the measures examined, the quality of HIV care provided by NPs and PAs was similar to that of physician HIV experts and generally better than physician non-HIV experts. The authors concluded that NPs and PAs provide high-quality care for persons with HIV. Preconditions for this level of performance include high levels of experience, focus on a single condition, and either participation in teams or other easy access to physicians and other clinicians with HIV expertise (Wilson et al., 2005).

Maritime Physician Assistant

Maritime medicine is the care of sick and injured patients on various seafaring vessels in remote areas of the world. The scope of this field of medicine is broad and includes patients of all ages, with every conceivable form of illness or traumatic injury. The unique aspects of maritime medicine are a result of the characteristic problems encountered by those at sea, the logistical difficulties of assessing and treating patients on a vessel, and the difficulties of arranging and monitoring definitive care.

PAs serving as a ship's medical officer have two basic responsibilities: to care for passengers and to care for the crew. Anecdotal reports are that few medical problems came up that a PA was unable to handle. Overall, however, PAs who have served as medical officers on ships such as luxury ocean liners found the experience interesting despite some technical challenges (e.g., having to obtain an unusual medication that a passenger forgot).

PAs have also worked for Maritime Medical Access, an institution that provides a link to appropriate medical care for shipping vessels, aircraft, yachts, and teams in remote locations. In operation since 1989, Maritime Medical Access offers worldwide telemedicine advice in addition to clinical case management, repatriation, training, and recommendations for medical equipment and medicine chests. The institution is affiliated with The George Washington University and provides 24-hour access to teams of board-certified emergency physicians and PAs, which has enabled companies to reduce unnecessary medical expenses and the risk of liability. Such formal arrangements with an academic emergency medical center ensure current, state-of-the-art medical practices and case management for ill and injured crewmembers.

Nephrology

Nephrology is a subspecialty of internal medicine that involves the study and clinical care of kidney diseases. It is based in the inpatient hospital setting, the office setting, as well as in specialized settings such as transplant units and outpatient dialysis clinics.

Tasks and Procedures

PAs in nephrology provide a wide variety of clinical tasks, including staffing of chronic kidney disease clinics, end-stage renal disease (ESRD) dialysis management, vascular access for dialysis management, hospital rounds and reports, and transplant patient management.

Recent evidence suggests that PAs contribute significantly to education of patients with advanced chronic kidney disease. One study reported that one-third of individual classes and two-thirds of group classes are taught by PAs or NPs.

Neonatology

Neonatology is a subspecialty of pediatrics that involves the medical care of neonates, especially premature neonates and neonates who require special medical care because of conditions such as low birth weight, intrauterine growth retardation, congenital malformations, sepsis, or birth asphyxia. It is a hospital-based specialty and is usually practiced in neonatal intensive care units (NICUs). The use of PA and NP providers in the neonatal unit has been endorsed in some form since the early 1980s. In 1999, the Committee on Fetus and Newborn of the American Academy of Pediatrics published a statement on the roles of the NP and PA in the care of hospitalized children, which strongly supported their roles as members of a care team in the neonatal intensive care unit (NICU).

Tasks and Procedures

Most neonatal PAs work in large hospitals or medical centers as full-time employees, oftentimes supervised by neonatologists. They may take charge of a baby's case immediately based on the baby's birth weight or condition and hospital policies. For example, most hospitals with NICUs have a policy that says something along the lines of, "If the baby is sick enough to need intensive care or is significantly premature, it must be taken care of by the hospital neonatologist." Typically, PAs working in neonatology do not see patients in a private office outside of a hospital, although there are exceptions. The role of the neonatal PA has rapidly expanded since the early 1990s because neonatal units have grown faster than the number of pediatric staff members qualified to work on them.

Safety and Effectiveness

Evidence suggests that using neonatal PAs and NPs in the intensive care setting is an effective alternative to using pediatric residents, with no significant differences in management, outcome, or charge variables among providers. At the Bronx Municipal Hospital Center, the phasing in of PAs and neonatal NPs overlapped the phasing out of pediatric residents. A study on survival by birth weight of neonates managed by pediatric residents and those managed by neonatal PAs and NPs failed to find any difference between the providers in outcomes. Additionally, after a period of adjustment, work rounds required less time with the PA and NP staff than they did with the residents (Schulman et al., 1995).

Neurology

Neurology is a branch of medicine that deals with disorders of the nervous system. Physicians in neurology investigate, diagnose, and treat neurological disorders of the brain and peripheral nervous system. Pediatric neurologists work with children with congenital disorders, attention-deficit disorders, and convulsive disorders. The number of neurologists in the United States has not substantially increased over the past decade, but the demand for neurology services has exceed the supply. This has produced a welcoming attitude in the American Academy of Neurology for PA and NP membership and expand their role in neurology.

Tasks and Procedures

A telephone survey of 46 full-time neurology PAs working in neurology offices (mostly group practices) undertaken in 1995 found that the range of conditions seen by neurology PAs was similar to that of neurologists (Table 6–7; Box 6–3). Most PAs performed lumbar punctures (63%) and initiated multiple sclerosis therapy (50%). Other procedures that were usually reserved for neurologists were also done by PAs (Table 6–8). Half were involved in clinical research studies.

Less than 1% of all PAs in 2015 listed neurology as their specialty. Of those in neurology the median age was 38, half worked in private physician offices, 78% were female, and the median salary was $95,000.

Obstetrics and Gynecology

Obstetrics and gynecology (OB/Gyn), also called *women's health,* is the specialty that deals with health of the female reproductive system (uterus, vagina, and ovaries), with obstetrics being the surgical specialty that deals with the care of a woman and her offspring during pregnancy, childbirth, and the puerperium. Midwifery is equivalent to a nonsurgical specialty of this discipline. Most family practitioners are trained in obstetrics and gynecology.

In this specialty, PAs have practiced in teams with physicians for more than 40 years, providing a broad range of obstetric and gynecological care to women in outpatient and inpatient settings. PAs' general medical education allows them to provide the primary care services many obstetricians and gynecologists seek to offer their patients in this era of proliferating managed care. PAs in OB/Gyn tend to practice in outpatient settings. Many work in practices in which women would be likely to receive their primary medical care.

Tasks and Procedures

PAs in OB/Gyn provide care regarding routine health matters and evaluate for complaints.

TABLE 6-7
Practice Setting Characteristics of Neurology Physician Assistants, 1998

Practice Setting	Number
Group practice	26
Hospital-based practice	12
Solo practice	6
Health maintenance organization	2
TOTAL	46

Characteristics	Mean	Range	N
No. of years as a PA	13.5	1–25	46
No. of years working in neurology	7.2	1–25	46
No. of years employed in current neurology practice	5.7	2–19	46
No. of neurologists in your practice	4.2	1–20	46
If you see hospitalized patients, how many do you see in a typical week?	26	4–120	36
If you are in an outpatient practice, how many patients do you see in a typical week?	43	12–100	33
Hours employed to see patients	43.8	16–55	46
Do you see patients in nursing home?	Yes = 7	—	—
Do a you "take call?"	Yes = 17	—	—

Data from Taft, J. M., & Hooker, R. S. (1999). Physician assistants in neurology practice. Neurology, 52(7), 1513.

BOX 6-3
Conditions Managed by Neurology Physician Assistants in Order of Frequency

- Headaches (all types)
- Cerebral vascular accidents
- Parkinson's disease and other movement disorders
- Seizure disorders
- Multiple sclerosis
- Low back pain
- Peripheral neuropathies
- Chronic pain syndromes (fibromyalgia, focal myofascial pain, and others)
- Dementia, Alzheimer's disease, and others
- Head injuries

NEUROMUSCULAR DISORDERS (CONGENITAOL AND ACQUIRED)

- Neurovascular disorders
- Motor neuron disease
- Myasthenia gravis
- Muscular dystrophies
- Hereditary sensory motor neuropathy
- Radiculopathies (cervical and lumbar)
- Neck pain
- Spinal cord injuries
- Postpolio syndrome

Data from Taft, J. M., & Hooker, R. S. (1999). Physician assistants in neurology practice. *Neurology, 52*(7), 1513.

TABLE 6-8
Procedures Performed by Neurology Physician Assistants by Percentage (*N* = 46)

Procedure	Percent
Lumbar punctures	63
Initiate multiple sclerosis therapy	50
Tender point injection	14
Nerve conduction studies	14
Initiate and monitor tissue plasminogen activator	11
Nerve blocks	11
Evoked potentials	7
Quantitative sensory testing	2
Botulism injections	2
Interpret electroencephalograms	2

Data from Taft, J. M., & Hooker, R. S. (1999). Physician assistants in neurology practice. *Neurology, 52*(7), 1513.

Obstetric and gynecological care provided by PAs includes comprehensive annual reproductive organ examinations. They evaluate and manage common gynecological conditions, such as vaginal infections, sexually transmitted diseases, and menopausal issues. They also provide prenatal, intrapartum, and postpartum care. Many PAs are included on teams that evaluate and treat infertility. PAs also provide patient education and counseling on contraception, breast self-examination, lactation, and other topics.

PAs perform many obstetric and gynecological procedures, including but not limited to ultrasound, colposcopy, cryotherapy, intrauterine device insertion and removal, insemination, endometrial and vulvar biopsies, and loop excision electrocoagulation. In addition, many women's health PAs who work in ambulatory practices have hospital privileges to first assist in surgeries such as hysterectomies and cesarean deliveries.

Safety and Effectiveness
The Collaborative Practice Advisory Group of the American College of Obstetricians and Gynecologists surveyed patients to ascertain their satisfaction level with care provided in practices that used physicians and PAs, NPs, or clinical nurse specialists. The responses indicated that patients felt these team practices provided quicker appointments (80.6%), more time with their provider (82.2%), and more health information (86%). In addition, patients perceived PA and NPs as being less rushed and spending more time with them than physicians. However, they perceived physicians as providing more complete information (Hankins et al., 1996).

Goldman, Occhiuto, Peterson, Zapka, and Palmer (2004) compared complication rates after surgical abortions performed by PAs with rates after abortions performed by physicians. They conducted a 2-year prospective cohort study of women undergoing surgically induced abortion. Ninety-one percent of eligible women (1363) were enrolled. The total complication rates were 22.0 per 1000 procedures performed by PAs and 23.3 per 1,000 procedures performed by physicians ($P = 0.88$). The most common complication that occurred during PA-performed procedures was incomplete abortion; during physician-performed procedures, the most common complication was infection not requiring hospitalization. A history of pelvic inflammatory disease was associated with an increased risk of total complications. The authors concluded that surgical abortion services provided by experienced PAs were comparable in safety and efficacy to those provided by physicians.

In another study involving Planned Parenthood affiliates and Kaiser Permanente of Northern California, PAs, NPs, and CNMs were compared with physicians in a study of early aspiration abortions. Of the 11,487 aspiration abortions analyzed, 1.3% ($n = 152$) resulted in a complication: collectively 1.8% for NP-, certified nurse-midwife (CNM)-, and PA-performed aspirations and 0.9% for physician-performed aspirations. Complications were clinically equivalent between newly trained NPs, CNMs, and PAs and physicians. The findings support the adoption of policies to permit these providers to perform early aspirations to expand access to care (Weitz et al., 2013).

Professional Society

Approximately 1.0% of all PAs work in OB/Gyn. Almost all (98%) are female, almost two-thirds work in private physician offices. The median salary in 2015 was $85,000. Founded in 1991, the Association of Physician Assistants in Obstetrics and Gynecology (APAOG) is a support organization whose mission is to improve the healthcare of women. APAOG promotes physician/PA teams who provide cost-effective, quality care to female patients and promote a network of communication and education between providers dedicated to women's health.

Occupational and Environmental Medicine

Occupational and environmental medicine (also known as *occupational medicine, industrial medicine,* and *corporate medicine*) is a cross-disciplinary area concerned with the safety, health, and welfare of workers. Occupational and environmental medicine is one of the three subspecialties of

preventive medicine; the other two are general preventive medicine and aerospace medicine.

Occupational and environmental medicine included PAs as early as 1971. One early use of PAs in this field was on the Alaska Pipeline Project in the 1970s. Involvement of PAs in occupational and environmental medicine escalated in 1978 as industry responded to cost-containment pressures. Work settings initially focused on underserved areas; today, they include plant sites, private industrial medicine clinics, and corporate medical administration. In Canada, retired military PAs from the Canadian Forces work in such industrial settings as oil and gas extraction sites and refineries. Many of these industries are located in remote areas, such as Northern Alberta.

Tasks and Procedures

PAs in occupational and environmental medicine deliver physical, mental, and emotional healthcare and practice preventive medicine. Activities include occupational health and safety, stress reduction, smoking cessation, and wellness. These PAs also perform annual employee physical examinations, exercise stress testing, occupational health education, drug screening, and treatment of work-related injuries.

One administrative study compared PA and physician activities in a large industrial medicine clinic. The results revealed that PAs work more hours and thus see more patients per year than physicians do. The patients seen by each type of provider were similar in age, gender ratio, and severity of injury. Physicians saw, on average, 2.8 patients per hour; PAs saw 2.5. The average charge per patient visit and total charge for an episode of care were similar. The salary of a physician was approximately twice as much as that of a PA. The conclusion of this study was that the use of PAs in occupational and environmental medicine might represent a cost-effective advantage from an administrative standpoint (Tables 6–9 and 6–10).

An editorial identified approximately 3,000 doctors in US occupational medicine and 1,500 PAs. Because PAs are demonstrating their ability to manage relatively uncomplicated cases presenting to occupational medicine, the authors

TABLE 6-9
Comparison of Occupational and Environmental Medicine Physician Assistants and Physicians by Outcomes of Episodes of Care

	PA Average	Physician Average	Overall Average	p	SD	95% CI
Average no. of days of limited activity assigned	15.6	17.4	16.8	.015	48.2	16.1–17.5
Likely to refer a patient to an outside provider	19.7%	17.4%	18.2%	.0001		17.6–18.7
Average no. of patient visits per hour	2.5	2.9	2.8	.008	1.9	2.8–2.8
Average charge per visit	$284.77	$302.53	$296.72	NS		294.50–298.93
Average total charges for episode of care	$565.98	$608.13	$594.33	NS		583.91–604.75
Average severity score of problems treated (mild, 1; moderate, 2; severe, 3)	1.92	1.93	1.93	NS	0.33	1.93–1.94
% of male patients	74.3%	72.5%	73.1%	.007		72.5–73.2
Average age of patients	35.3	35.5	35.5	NS	11.2	35.3–35.7
Probability patients likely to keep their appointment	81%	76%	79%	.0024	1.04	78.0–80.9

CI = confidence interval; NS = not significant.
Data from Hooker, R. S. (2004). Physician assistants in occupational medicine: How do they compare to occupational physicians? *Occupational Medicine (Oxford, England), 54*(3), 153–158.

TABLE 6-10
Occupational and Environmental Medicine Provider Characteristics

	No.	Average Age	Gender	Average Salary	Average No. of Visits per Day
Physicians		50	18 males, 6 females	$143,056	
PAs		45	7 males, 5 females	$74,208	
Average	32.72				23.31

Data from Hooker, R. S. (2004). Physician assistants in occupational medicine: How do they compare to occupational physicians? *Occupational Medicine (Oxford, England), 54*(3), 153–158.

offered that opportunities are present to create new roles of doctors in overseeing PA-directed activities and to improve productivity and efficiency (Bunn et al., 2004).

Professional Society
Approximately 1.2% of all PAs worked in occupational medicine in 2015 and half are female. The average age was 38 and the median salary was $95,000. PAs can become affiliate members of the American College of Occupational and Environmental Medicine (ACOEM). The College meets twice per year and has 20 special interest sections.

Oncology

Oncology is the branch of medicine that studies cancers and seeks to understand their development, diagnosis, treatment, and prevention. Many oncologists are also hematologists. The options for oncology PAs are diverse and divided into four categories: medical (adult), pediatric, radiation, and surgical (Table 6–11). These PAs, depending on their specialization, may be employed in large centers or smaller outpatient group practices. In almost all instances, oncology PAs are part of a broad-based team that includes doctors, nurses, social workers, pharmacists, and others. Such team approaches to care result in

TABLE 6-11
Distribution of Oncology Physician Assistants at M. D. Anderson Cancer Center by Departments

	Number	Percent
Surgical oncology	9	16.7
Gastrointestinal medical oncology	8	14.8
Radiation oncology	6	11.1
Leukemia	5	9.3
Anesthesiology and pain management	3	5.6
Cardiology	3	5.6
Head and neck surgery	3	5.6
Lymphoma	3	5.6
Bone marrow transplantation	2	3.7
Melanoma medical oncology	2	3.7
Plastic surgery	2	3.7
Urology	2	3.7
Cardiovascular surgery	1	1.9
Dermatology	1	1.9
Head and neck medical oncology	1	1.9
Orthopedics	1	1.9
Genitourinary medical oncology	1	1.9
Gynecological radiation oncology	1	1.9
TOTAL	54	100.0

Ross A. C. (2008). The role of physician assistants in oncology. *ADVANCE for Physician Assistants, 12*(3), 46–49.

divisions of labor and economy of scale that provides the environment for PAs to add value in the delivery of complex care.

The Lewin Group assessed the market for chemotherapy and radiation therapy and the impact of health reform on capacity and demand. When fully implemented, an expanded insured population could increase the demand for oncologists and radiation oncologists by 500,000 visits per year, increasing the shortage to 2,393 FTEs in 2025. Unless oncologist productivity can be enhanced, the anticipated shortage will strain the ability to provide quality care (Yang et al., 2014). This shortage will likely increase the demand for PAs in oncology as well.

Safety and Effectiveness
Evidence suggests that PAs in oncology improve efficiency and quality of care. According to a survey of members of the American Society of Clinical Oncology, 54% of oncologists already work with PAs or NPs. On average, the

practice was able to handle a higher volume of weekly visits because of the collaboration with PAs and NPs. Results also indicated that productivity is highest for physicians who regularly use PAs and NPs for such advanced activities as assisting with new patient consults, ordering routine chemotherapy, and performing invasive procedures. Additionally, the practitioner survey suggested that physicians who work with PAs and NPs believe that using PAs and NPs improves efficiency and patient care as well as professional satisfaction.

Professional Society
Approximately 1% of all PAs work in oncology as of 2015. The majority, 86%, are female. The median salary was $95,000. The Association of Physician Assistants in Oncology (APAO) is a nonprofit specialty organization affiliated with the AAPA. It consists of PAs and NPs working in the field of oncology, in both clinical and research settings. Its website is http://www.apao.cc.

Ophthalmology

Ophthalmology is the branch of medicine that deals with diseases of and surgery for the visual pathways, including the eye, brain, and areas surrounding the eye, such as the lacrimal system and eyelids. Most ophthalmologists are surgeons.

Tasks and Procedures
PAs in ophthalmology tend to be office-based more than surgically based, but all such PAs work with ophthalmologists. They deal with acute injuries; diseases of the eye such as infections, uveitis, and glaucoma; débridement of foreign bodies; surgical excision of lid ptosis; and postsurgical wound dressings. They also prepare patients for surgery and care for patients postoperatively. Some states have provisions that prohibit PAs from performing duties that overlap with optometry. Less than 0.1% work in ophthalmology.

Psychiatry and Mental Health

Psychiatry is a branch of medicine that involves the treatment of mental disorders. The clinical application of psychiatry has been considered a bridge between the social world and those who are mentally ill. Because psychiatry's research and clinical applications are considered interdisciplinary, various subspecialties and theoretical approaches exist. Psychiatrists specialize in the doctor–patient relationship, using unique classification schemes, diagnostic tools, and treatments.

PAs in psychiatry expand access to mental health services. They often work in community mental health offices, psychiatric offices, corrections institutions, and in behavioral health facilities and psychiatric units of rural and public hospitals, where psychiatrists are in short supply. They also work as outpatient workers associated with psychiatric hospitals. Trained mental health PAs have demonstrated value in filling critical shortages in state hospitals and correctional institutions. Additional PA practice areas include assertive community treatment teams, psychiatric emergency departments, geriatric psychiatry, addiction medicine, and care for patients with posttraumatic stress.

Tasks and Procedures
PAs in the mental health setting are unique because they can see patients who need psychiatric or psychological services, prescribe psychotropic medication, and provide general medical services. Most mental health PAs collaborate with psychiatrists.

In private practices, PAs regularly conduct initial assessments and perform maintenance checkups for patients on psychiatric medications.

Professional Society
Only about 1% of PAs are in mental health or psychiatry. Two-thirds are female and 27% are in private offices. The median salary is $95,000. The Association of Physician Assistants in Psychiatry (APAP) is an organization committed to the advancement of PAs working in psychiatry and mental health.

Public Health and Preventive Medicine

Public health is the study and practice of addressing threats to the health of a community. This field pays special attention to the social context of health and disease and focuses on

improving health through nonmedical measures, such as immunizations and the fluoridation of drinking water. Public health PAs work in various clinic settings and in field offices for the various branches and agencies of state and federal government. For example, many PAs are employees of the US Public Health Service (USPHS).

The USPHS is organized under the US Department of Health and Human Services (DHHS). The Commissioned Corps is the only uniformed service comprised solely of commissioned officers and is currently more than 6,750 strong. The officers consist of public health professionals from every discipline within the medical arena, serving the most vulnerable and underserved populations, domestically and abroad. About 100 PAs serve the in the USPHS in diverse roles, including outbreak investigation at the Centers for Disease Control and Prevention, primary care policy analysis at the Agency for Healthcare Research and Quality, drug regulation at the Food and Drug Administration, clinical service in the Indian Health Services, and national defense in the Coast Guard.

Tasks and Procedures
Public health PAs perform a wide variety of tasks, including epidemiological research, public health promotion, and disease prevention. They work for the Indian Health Service, Bureau of Prisons, National Center for Health Statistics, National Institutes of Health, and Centers for Disease Control and Prevention.

Professional Society
US public health system PAs are eligible to join the Veterans Affairs Physician Assistant Association (VAPAA), a society for federally employed PAs. This organization advocates for federally employed PAs.

Radiology
Radiology is the medical specialty that uses imaging technologies to diagnose and, sometimes, treat diseases. Originally, radiology was the aspect of medical science dealing with the use of electromagnetic energy emitted by x-ray

machines and other such radiation devices for the purpose of obtaining visual information. Today, another aspect of radiology—interventional radiology—involves using fine catheters to reach organs for diagnosis and treatment. The addition of PAs in this specialty has shown decreases in the mean length of stay for patients undergoing various procedures and increased the capacity for interventional procedures.

Tasks and Procedures

As interventional radiologists develop busier and busier practices, they have less time to spend with individual patients. PAs represent an excellent way to improve clinical patient care. Stecker, Armenoff, and Johnson (2004) described what PAs are and how they work together with radiologists at Indiana University. The authors illustrated differences between PAs and other providers and described the duties that may be delegated to PAs in the interventional radiology setting. The authors described how PAs provided an opportunity to improve clinical patient care. The interventional radiology PAs were involved in daily morning inpatient rounds with the radiology fellows and residents rotating on the radiology service. In this capacity, they evaluated abscess, urinary, and biliary drainage catheters to ensure proper function and monitored patient progress. They also performed and monitored compliant chart documentation for all inpatients being followed by the interventional radiology service. In conjunction with the house staff, the PAs communicated with referring services as needed and helped triage queries and consultation requests during these rounds (Box 6–4). In addition, the interventional radiology PAs provided a major role in billing for inpatient evaluation and management services, a process that tended to be overlooked by the staff. The authors concluded that revenue generated by two interventional radiology PAs at this academic medical center covered the costs of their employment (Stecker et al., 2004).

Less than 1% of PAs are in radiology and two-thirds are female. The median salary is $95,000.

BOX 6-4

Procedures of Interventional Radiology Physician Assistants

- Venous access
- Temporary central venous catheters (infusion, apheresis, dialysis)
- Peripherally inserted central catheters
- Tunneled catheters (infusion, apheresis, dialysis)
- Troubleshooting of venous access devices
- Drainage catheters (biliary, urinary, abscess, and other)
- Catheter exchanges
- Troubleshooting of drainage catheters
- Resuturing of dislodged catheters

OUTPATIENT VISITS

- New patient consultations (including history and physical examination)
- Vascular malformations
- Symptomatic uterine fibroids
- Liver tumors
- Portal hypertension
- Established patient follow-up
- Wound checks (port placement, removal)
- Post-(chemo)embolization follow-up
- Post–arterial angioplasty/stent treatment
- Valuation and tracking of dialysis access performance
- Evaluation and management billing

INPATIENT CARE

- Daily patient visits
- Morning rounds
- Communication with other medical service teams
- Evaluation and management billing

Rheumatology

Rheumatology is a subspecialty of internal medicine and pediatrics involved in the diagnosis of and therapy for rheumatic diseases. Rheumatologists mainly deal with problems involving the joints and the allied conditions of connective tissue as well as pathogenesis of major rheumatological and autoimmune disorders. Better understanding of the genetic basis of rheumatological disorders makes rheumatology a specialty that is rapidly developing based on new scientific discoveries. New treatment modalities are based on scientific research on immunology, cytokines, T lymphocytes, and B lymphocytes. Future therapies may be directed more toward gene modulation. With the demand for rheumatology service increasing and the number of training programs for rheumatologists relatively flat, this specialty seems to be an unfilled niche for PAs (Deal et al., 2007).

Tasks and Procedures

Rheumatology PA tasks focus on the diagnosis and management of autoimmune and inflammatory diseases. Although the majority of these diseases are systemic, PAs in rheumatology are also skilled in medical orthopedics. They provide a broad range of services, including evaluating new patients, monitoring drug administration, performing procedures such as joint injections and muscle biopsies, and performing rounds in the hospital. Some PAs expand their functions to include pain management, sports medicine, bone metabolic disorders, and primary care.

One small study evaluated the roles of these rheumatology PAs. Women comprised 71% of both the survey participants. The mean number of years in rheumatology practice was 7.5 (range, 2–21 years). The mean number of years since graduating from a PA program was 23 (range, 2–28 years). All but three of the respondents acquired their skills through on-the-job training and continuing medical education; three were graduates of a 12-month postgraduate fellowship (Hooker & Rangan, 2008).

Questions about job and career satisfaction were the few areas that did not produce full participation. Of those who answered, the vast majority (93%) was satisfied or very satisfied with their current clinical role in rheumatology, yet only two-thirds (68%) were satisfied/very satisfied with their current career. The difference between clinical role and career satisfaction results was primarily about dissatisfaction with salary, benefits, office structure, or relationships, but not on being in rheumatology as a discipline (Hooker & Rangan, 2008). Industry sources in early 2008 said they had identified 367 rheumatology PAs and NPs; about one-third being PAs.

Professional Society

Only about 75 PAs are in rheumatology. The Society of Physician Assistants in Rheumatology was formed in 2003 and represents PAs who provide rheumatology services.

Urology

Urology is the branch of medicine that focuses on the urinary tracts of males and females and on the reproductive system of males. Urologists diagnose, treat, and manage patients with urological disorders. The organs covered by urology include the kidneys, ureters, urinary bladder, urethra, and the male reproductive organs (testes, epididymis, vas deferens, seminal vesicles, prostate, and penis).

One of the first descriptions of an American PA was of a technician who functioned as a PA in a urology practice (Crile, 1987). Later, a role for the PA in urology was developed at a time when a number of emerging technologies were requiring a special person trained to manage the tools and instruments of this specialty. In 1970, a program in Cincinnati, Ohio, trained PAs in urology to administer intravenous pyelograms, obtain detailed voided specimens, assist in methods to snare renal stones, perform cystoscopies, and analyze renal calculi. Although the opportunities for PAs to continue in this vein are plenty, a new role of the outpatient urology PA (an office-based PA who does not participate in surgery) has emerged.

Tasks and Procedures

PAs who work in urology tend to be more office-based than surgical. They often provide initial consultations, perform cystoscopies, evaluate and perform biopsies on the prostate, and manage impotent patients. An expanded role for PAs in this field is in sexology.

Urology PAs tend to work in an office with one urologist or a group of urologists but sometimes extend into the surgical suite to perform lithotripsy procedures and assist in other roles. Women are increasingly becoming employed in this traditionally male-dominated field, which has increased the availability and choice of providers for patients.

FURTHER RESEARCH ON PHYSICIAN ASSISTANT SPECIALIZATION

The literature about the deployment of PAs in specialties outside of family medicine is mixed; in some areas, it is developing, whereas in other areas, almost nothing is known. Gradually, orthopedic and rheumatology PA roles are being revealed, whereas almost nothing is known about urology PAs. A review of this literature reveals large areas missing and large questions unanswered. The following is a brief list of areas in need of research attention:

- **Role delineation in team-based care:** How are PA roles defined on healthcare teams in each specialty? How much do those roles vary, and what are factors that predict those roles?
- **Safety and effectiveness:** What are the safest and most effective roles for PAs in each specialty?
- **Economics:** What is the overlap among the doctor, PA, and NP in each specialty role? Is the outcome a substitution or a complementary effect?
- **Breadth of knowledge:** How does a specialty PA obtain his or her knowledge set once in practice? Does the acquisition of knowledge have different trajectories depending on age, gender, and experience?
- **Career selection:** Do PAs in some specialty area have different expectations and aspirations than those in other specialties?
- **Procedures:** What are the procedures that a PA in anesthesia (or any other specialty) needs to know to be considered competent?
- **Ratios:** What are the ratios of PAs and NPs to doctors in various specialties? What contributes to these differences?
- **Retention:** What are the factors that contribute to retention or attrition of PAs in orthopedics (or any other specialty)?

- **Education:** How do PAs in a specialty come to that specialty, and how are they trained to carry out their roles? Do they build on some fundamental set of skills, or do they have a formal indoctrination?

SUMMARY

One of the major rationales for the development of the PA profession was to augment the supply of medically trained providers in those specialties in greatest need of assistance. The diversity of employment settings for PAs is an indication of the maturity of the profession. Although the primary care role of the PA is the root of the profession and remains the basis of PA education, the profession has become much more specialized since the mid-1990s, primarily as a result of economic pressures. These areas of specialization are where the jobs are and where the role of the PA may be more enhanced. Specialty PAs are widely dispersed throughout the spectrum of medical disciplines and have become well integrated. Specialty practice areas expected to remain strong for PAs in nonprimary care roles include emergency medicine, cardiovascular surgery, orthopedic surgery, dermatology, and a large number of internal medicine subspecialties. Many PAs enjoy membership status in physician specialty societies or in professional specialty societies of their own making. Specialization will remain an important component of the PA program and, with the exception of surgery, no one specialty is likely to dominate.

References

The following citations are key to supporting this chapter's content. You can find a complete list of citations for all chapters at www.fadavis.com/davisplus, keyword *Hooker*.

Albert, N. M., Fonarow, G. C., Yancy, C. W., Curtis, A. B., Stough, W. G., Gheorghiade, M., et al. (2010). Outpatient cardiology practices with advanced practice nurses and physician assistants provide similar delivery of recommended therapies (findings from IMPROVE HF). *American Journal of Cardiology, 105*(12), 1773–1779.

Alliance for Aging Research. (2006). *Ageism: How healthcare fails the elderly.* Washington, DC: Author.

Arnopolin, S. L., & Smithline, H. A. (2000). Patient care by physician assistants and by physicians in an emergency department. *Journal of the American Academy of Physician Assistants, 13*(12), 39–40, 49–50, 53–54, 81.

Bunn, W. B., III, Holloway, A. M., & Johnson, C. E. (2004). Occupational medicine: The use of physician assistants and the changing role of the occupational and environmental medicine provider. *Occupational Medicine, 54,* 3145–3146.

Caprio, T. V. (2006). Physician practice in the nursing home: Collaboration with nurse practitioners and physician assistants. *Annals of Long Term Care, 14*(3), 17–24.

Cherry, D. K., Woodwell, D. A., & Rechtsteiner, E. A. (2007). National Ambulatory Medical Care Survey (NHAMCS): 2005 summary. *Advance Data from Vital and Health Statistics, 387.* Hyattsville, MD: Centers for Disease Control and Prevention, National Center for Health Statistics.

Counselman, F. L., Graffeo, C. A., & Hill, J. T. (2000). Patient satisfaction with physician assistants (PAs) in an ED fast track. *American Journal of Emergency Medicine, 18*(6), 661–665.

Crile, G., Jr. (1987). Cleveland Clinic: The supporting cast 1920–1940. *Cleveland Clinic Journal of Medicine, 54*(4), 344–347.

Deal C. L., Hooker R. S., Harrington T., Birnbaum N., Hogan P., Bouchery E., Klein-Gitelman M., & Barr W. (2007). The United States rheumatology workforce: supply and demand, 2005-2025. *Arthritis Rheumatism, 56*(3): 722-729.

DeMots, H., Coombs, B., Murphy, E., & Palac, R. (1987). Coronary arteriography performed by a physician assistant. *American Journal of Cardiology, 60*(10), 784–787.

Donnellan, F., Harewood, G. C., Cagney, D., Basri, F., Patchett, S. E., & Murray, F. E. (2010). Economic impact of prescreening on gastroenterology outpatient clinic practice. *Journal of Clinical Gastroenterology, 44*(4), e76–e79.

Dracup, K., DeBusk, R. F., De Mots, H., Gaile, E. H., Sr., Norton, J. B., Jr., & Rudy, E. B. (1994). Task force 3: Partnerships in delivery of cardiovascular care. *Journal of the American College of Cardiology, 24*(2), 296–304.

Estes, E. H. (1993). Training doctors for the future: Lessons from 25 years of physician assistant education." In D. K. Clawson & M. Osterweis (Eds.), *The roles of physician assistants and nurse practitioners in primary care.* Washington, DC: Association of Academic Health Centers.

Goldman, M. B., Occhiuto, J. S., Peterson, L. E., Zapka, J. G., & Palmer, R. H. (2004). Physician assistants as providers of surgically induced abortion services. *American Journal of Public Health, 94*(8), 1352–1357

Hankins, G. D., Shaw, S. B., Cruess, D. F., Lawrence, H. C., III, & Harris, C. D. (1996). Patient satisfaction with collaborative practice. *Obstetrics and Gynecology, 88*(6), 1011–1015.

Hooker, R. S. (2004). Physician assistants in occupational medicine: How do they compare to occupational physicians? *Occupational Medicine (Oxford, England), 54*(3), 153–158.

Hooker, R. S., Klocko, D. J., & Larkin, G. L. (2011). Physician assistants in emergency medicine: The impact of their role. *Academic Emergency Medicine, 18*(1), 72–77.

Hooker, R. S., & Rangan, B. V. (2008). Role delineation of rheumatology physician assistants. *Journal of Clinical Rheumatology, 14*(4), 202–205.

Jalperneanmonod, R., DelCollo, J., Jeanmonod, D., Dombchewsky, O., & Reiter, M. (2013). Comparison of resident and mid-level provider productivity and patient satisfaction in an emergency department fast track. *Emergency Medicine Journal, 30*(1), e12.

Kimball, A. B., & Resneck, J. S., Jr. (2008). The US dermatology workforce: A specialty remains in shortage. *Journal of the American Academy of Dermatology, 59*(5), 741–745.

Krasuski, R. A., Wang, A., Ross, C., Bolles, J. F., Moloney, E. L., Kelly, L. P., et al. (2003). Trained and supervised physician assistants can safely perform diagnostic cardiac catheterization with coronary angiography. *Catheterization and Cardiovascular Interventions, 59*(2), 157–160.

National Commission on Certification of Physician Assistants, Inc. (2016, June). 2015 Statistical Profile of Certified Physician Assistants by Specialty: An Annual Report of the National Commission on Certification of Physician Assistants. Retrieved from http://www.nccpa.net/research

Sadler, A. M., Jr., Sadler, B. L., & Bliss, A. A. (1972). *The physician's assistant: Today and tomorrow.* New Haven, CT: Yale University Press.

Schulman, M., Lucchese, K. R., & Sullivan, A. C. (1995). Transition from housestaff to nonphysicians as neonatal intensive care providers: Cost, impact on revenue, and quality of care. *American Journal of Perinatology, 12*(6), 442–446.

Sigurdson, L. (2007). Meeting challenges in the delivery of surgical care. Clinical & Investigative Medicine, 30(Suppl. 4), S35–S36.

Stecker, M. S., Armenoff, D., & Johnson, M. S. (2004). Physician assistants in interventional radiology practice. *Journal of Vascular and Interventional Radiology, 15*(3), 221–227.

Weitz, T. A., Taylor, D., Desai, S., Upadhyay, U. D., Waldman, J., Battistelli, M. F., & Drey, E. A. (2013). Safety of aspiration abortion performed by nurse practitioners, certified nurse midwives, and physician assistants under a California legal waiver. *American Journal of Public Health, 103*(3), 454–461.

Wilson, I. B., Landon, B. E., Hirschhorn, L. R., McInnes, K., Ding, L., Marsden, P. V., et al. (2005). Quality of HIV care provided by nurse practitioners, physician assistants, and physicians. *Annals of Internal Medicine, 143*(10), 729–736.

Wright, W. K., & Hirsch, C. S. (1987). The physician assistant as forensic investigator. *Journal of Forensic Science, 32*(4), 1059–1061.

Yang, W., Williams, J. H., Hogan, P. F., Bruinooge, S. S., Rodriguez, G. I., Kosty, M. P., et al. (2014). Projected supply of and demand for oncologists and radiation oncologists through 2025: An aging, better-insured population will result in shortage. *Journal of Oncology Practice, 10*(1), 39–45.

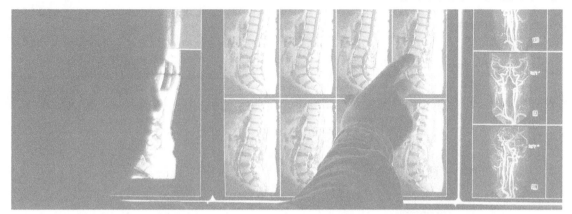

CHAPTER 7

PHYSICIAN ASSISTANTS IN HOSPITAL SETTINGS

CHRISTINE M. EVERETT ■ JAMES F. CAWLEY ■ RODERICK S. HOOKER

"How many desolate creatures on the earth have learnt the simple dues of fellowship and social comfort, in a hospital?"
— *Elizabeth Barrett Browning, English poet, political thinker, and feminist (1806–1861)*

When the role of the physician assistant (PA) emerged in the United States, characterized by its clinical flexibility, it was in many respects a natural fit for hospital practice. Since the start of the new millennium, a variety of social and economic forces—such as a decreasing number of residents, an increasing number of hospital beds, and hospitalists—have raised the demand for PAs in hospital settings. The intent is to increase the supply of hospitalists and other providers at the same time maintaining quality of care for patients. A variety of approaches to integrating PAs into hospital services have emerged, and their value in hospital settings continues to increase.

Dispersed widely, PAs work in major teaching hospitals, medium-size hospitals, small community and rural hospitals, and other types of inpatient care institutions. As of 2015, at least one-third of American PAs had a connection with a hospital in some capacity.

Because the American and Canadian medical nomenclature may differ from the terminology used in other countries, a brief taxonomy is offered in Box 7–1.

THE IMPORTANCE OF HOSPITALS IN HEALTHCARE SYSTEMS

In his masterful history of the US hospital system, *The Care of Strangers: The Rise of America's Hospital System*, Charles Rosenberg (1987) argues that it is not possible to understand medicine and the medical care system without a full appreciation of the role played by hospitals. Hospitals are a major workplace for many healthcare professionals, including PAs.

At the start of the new millennium, there were a little more than 6,000 hospitals in the United States; by 2014, the number of registered hospitals had decreased to 5,723 (American Hospital Association, 2014). The major explanation for this decrease is economy of scale; small hospitals have not survived, as newer, modern, and bigger tertiary medical centers thrived due to marketing, economy of scale, and other pressures. Hospitals also needed reengineering for

Because some confusion arises when using terms for hospitals and their employees, following is a brief set of definitions and terms used for hospitals in North America.

Attending doctors: The journeyman doctors employed by a hospital to have ultimate responsibility for patients. They are the senior doctors in charge of the residents and are involved with their education. Generally, they countersign the notes of trainees.

Chief resident: A member of the medical staff who is employed, usually for 1 year, to oversee residents. This person is not a trainee and may take a fellowship after serving in the position as chief resident.

Hospitalist: An attending physician who devotes at least three-quarters of his or her time overseeing acutely ill, hospitalized patients.

House staff/house officers: Doctors in postgraduate training. The term is held over from when resident house staff was given room and board to live in a hospital for their internship and additional training.

Internship: The first year of postgraduate training. A residency may follow the internship year or include the internship year as the first year of residency. At one time, only graduates of medical school did an internship before starting a general medical practice.

Medical students and PA students: Students who are assigned to a team of doctors. The team may be composed of an attending doctor, a senior resident, an intern, and a student.

Medical staff: Physicians and other clinicians who are granted privileges to admit patients to a hospital and perform a range of defined duties and responsibilities in patient care, such as surgery and obstetrics.

Residency: A stage of postgraduate medical training certification in a primary care or referral specialty. In the United States and Canada, a resident physician has received a medical degree (MD, MBBS, MBChB, or DO) and mainly cares for hospitalized or clinic patients, mostly with direct supervision from senior physicians.

efficiency and safety. Despite the shrinking number of hospitals, the number of beds has increased significantly. In 2014, US hospitals had 920,829 hospital beds that were associated with 36,156,245 admissions (American Hospital Association, 2014). Each bed represents a patient who requires a physician, a nurse, and a large cadre of other healthcare professionals to oversee the benefit of the patient and to have some responsibility for the outcomes of care. As in many other places in the world, the demand for physician services in US hospitals has exceeded

the supply. This predicament has opened the door for PAs in ways unexpected.

The financial impact of hospitals on the US healthcare system is significant. In 2014, the United States spent more than $800 billion on hospital admissions—more than 30% of its annual healthcare expenditures (Figure 7–1).

FACTORS THAT AFFECT HOSPITAL SERVICES

Given the United States' investment in hospital care and the impact it has on the lives of patients, the cost and quality of care delivered in hospitals has become a major focus of policy makers. As a result, hospitals have considered and implemented alternative organizational approaches, such as new staffing arrangements, in response to a variety of competitive, economic, and social pressures. Some of the key forces driving these actions and the effects of these actions on PAs are discussed next.

Supply of Physicians

The supply of physicians fluctuates over time and is a function of medical school enrollment, immigration, emigration, and retirement patterns. The number of US medical (allopathic and osteopathic) graduates in 2015 approached 25,000, with most entering into graduate medical education (residency). Taking into account entrants and attrition, as of 2015, there were approximately 850,000 MD/DOs (approximately 710,000 were clinically active), 100,000 PAs, and 125,000 nurse practitioners (NPs) considered clinically active. Given the 2015 numbers, the Association of American Medical Colleges estimates a shortage of more than 90,000 physicians in all specialties by 2020. Although that specific number is debated, most believe that the United States is likely to experience shortages in some places, and such shortages are likely in other countries as well.

Another key factor that has had a big effect on the supply of physicians in hospitals is resident work-hour restrictions. Although residents are still trainees, they contribute significantly to the clinical care provided in US hospitals. Effective 2004, the Accreditation Commission on

FIGURE 7-1
Distribution of Medical Expenditures in the United States

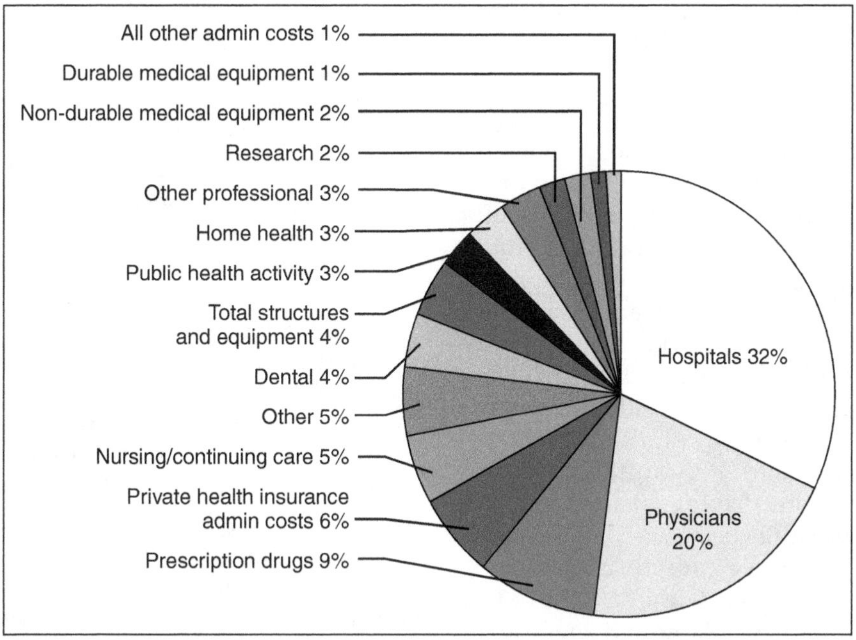

All other admin costs 1%
Durable medical equipment 1%
Non-durable medical equipment 2%
Research 2%
Other professional 3%
Home health 3%
Public health activity 3%
Total structures and equipment 4%
Dental 4%
Other 5%
Nursing/continuing care 5%
Private health insurance admin costs 6%
Prescription drugs 9%
Hospitals 32%
Physicians 20%

Data from Centers for Medicare and Medicaid Services. (2014). National Health Expenditure Data. Retrieved January 13, 2016, from https://www.cms.gov/Research-Statistics-Data-and-Systems/ Statistics-Trends-and Reports/NationalHealthExpendData/index.html?redirect=/NationalHealth ExpendData/

Graduate Medical Education imposed a limitation on the number of hours resident physicians could work. This restriction was placed in an effort to increase patient safety by decreasing the number of errors caused by residents' lack of sleep. The result was that, although the supply of physicians remained constant, the clinical work that each resident physician could complete was significantly reduced. As a result, more clinicians were needed to cover the same amount of clinical work.

Efficiency

The drive for increased efficiency in the delivery of hospital services is long-standing and the result of a variety of influences. In the recent past, two factors significantly influenced the drive for efficiency: specialization (or the partition of care to highly skilled experts) and managed care. Each sector has improved the delivery of care by organizing services for maximum effect with minimum resource use. For example, specialized care for conditions as acute myocardial events provide a greater survival rate as the result of cardiologists and intensivists being involved. Traumatologists can reduce the mortality rate of casualties through the use of broad resources concentrated under one roof.

In addition, the efficient use of assets has improved with the development of health maintenance organizations. Previously, primary care providers were responsible for providing outpatient services as well as inpatient care for their hospitalized patients. However, decreasing hospitalization rates made staying current on inpatient care challenging. Annual productivity was affected by the need for a single provider to be in two locations, often miles apart. Managed care, a common payment model in the 1980s and 1990s, placed a high premium on efficient care delivery. Having a provider occupy an ambulatory care setting 5-6 days a week meant that a hospitalist could be assigned to care for patients all in one hospital. One hospitalist could manage a larger number of inpatients, and a family physician could see a larger number of outpatients annually by remaining in his or her office.

Quality of Care

The impact of the quality of hospital care on patients and society is large. Quality in this regard is based on outcomes, costs, benefits, and patient perceptions of their encounters. Meeting the needs of a patient and improving the outcomes of an acute event means rehabilitating the patient quickly but also effectively in an effort to reduce hospitalization readmission, or rehospitalization (defined as a hospital admission within 30 days after an original admission). Per capitated hospitalization rates are driving quality and efficiency in ways unexpected.

One area of grave concern is medical errors. Errors in hospital care affect nearly 1 out of every 10 patients. Although these errors range in severity, the Institute of Medicine (IOM) estimates that between 44,000 and 98,000 Americans die each year as a result of hospital-related medical errors—more than the number who die of motor vehicle accidents, breast cancer, and acquired immunodeficiency syndrome. Of the nearly 1 million Medicare beneficiaries discharged from hospitals in October 2008, about one in seven experienced an adverse event that met at least one criteria during their hospital stays (13.5%). This rate projects to an estimated 134,000 Medicare beneficiaries experiencing at least one adverse event in a hospital during a 1-month study period (US Department of Health and Human Services, 2010).

However, these numbers have improved in recent years. A 2013 study by the Agency for Healthcare Research and Quality (AHRQ, 2015) identified a 9% decline in the rate of hospital-acquired conditions (HACs) from 2012 to 2013, and a 17% decline, from 145 to 121 HACs per 1000 discharges, from 2010 to 2013. Hospital patients experienced a cumulative total of 1.3 million fewer HACs over the 3 years (2011, 2012, 2013) relative to the number of HACs that would have occurred if rates had remained steady at the 2010 level. The AHRQ

estimates that approximately 50,000 fewer patients died in the hospital as a result of this reduction in HACs, and approximately $12 billion in healthcare costs were saved from 2010 to 2013.

Rehospitalizations account for much of societal costs of poor quality hospital care. Almost 20% of Medicare beneficiaries who are discharged from a hospital are rehospitalized within 30 days; these unplanned rehospitalizations result in $17.4 billion in additional costs per year to Medicare. For conditions with both large numbers of stays and high readmission rates, Medicare and especially Medicaid patients are more likely to be readmitted than privately insured or uninsured patients. For example, heart failure readmission rates are 30.1% for Medicaid, 25.0% for Medicare, 19.5% for privately insured, and 17.1% for uninsured patients.

Value is defined as the quality of care received for a given amount of money spent. A growing body of evidence supports the conclusion that spending more money does not necessarily result in the delivery of higher quality care. To encourage the delivery of high-quality care at a reasonable cost, the Affordable Care Act initiated a number of payment reforms, referred to as "pay for performance." An example of one payment reform that has particularly affected hospitals is the rule related to costly, excess readmissions. In 2012, the Centers for Medicare and Medicaid Services (CMS) reduced Medicare payments to hospitals with excess readmissions; in addition, the reimbursement for readmission is less than that for the initial episode of care. At some point, the evaluation of this rule will determine whether such policies are successful in improving the quality of care delivered.

HOSPITAL INNOVATIONS

Hospitals have responded to the changing economic and social forces that shape their services for a number of reasons and in a variety of ways. The most compelling reason is quality. The reputation of a hospital hangs on quality of services in terms of outcomes and perception of quality of care. The other reason is cost. In terms of strategy, two of the more innovative and influential approaches hospitals have taken to address these issues are discussed here.

Hospitalists

Hospitalists are physicians, PAs, and NPs who specialize in the practice of hospital medicine. Just as primary care physicians are responsible for managing the outpatient care of patients, hospitalists are specialists in inpatient medicine who are responsible for managing the care of hospitalized patients. Although physicians with this expertise have existed since the creation of hospitals, the formal recognition of this specialty did not occur until 1996. Since then, the use of hospital-employed providers has grown substantially and the percentage of physicians in general internal medicine who are identified as hospitalists has steadily increased. Similarly, the number of patients who receive care from hospitalists also increased. Evidence suggests that these providers have contributed to reductions in the length of hospital stays, with associated cost reductions and equivalent or better quality of care.

Accountable Care Organizations

Although policy changes aimed at specific problems such as rehospitalization are helpful, the IOM posits that value-based care will not be achievable unless the US healthcare system is restructured (IOM, 2001). The contention is that the system is overly fragmented, with uncoordinated care delivered in a range of inpatient and outpatient settings. The IOM argues that this lack of coordination largely explains the costly, low-quality care delivered in the United States.

The Affordable Care Act established multiple programs to improve the structure of the US healthcare system to reduce fragmentation and improve coordination. The initiative that is most relevant to hospitals is the Accountable Care Organization (ACO). An ACO is an integrated group of healthcare providers, which may include a hospital, that assume responsibility for all aspects of care for a defined population of patients. Examples of defined populations might be the members of an insurance group in a region of the country, the population served by a

Veteran's Affairs medical center, or some other group of people who are tied in a particular way to a provider system.

Assuming responsibility for a patient population involves two aspects:

1. Meeting quality of care reporting requirements and standards
2. Reducing costs

Of the ACOs that participated in the CMS ACO program, 46% include hospitals. The Medicare Shared Savings Program is a voluntary CMS program designed to incentivize care redesign in a way that results in high-quality, efficient healthcare. If a participating ACO meets quality standards and demonstrates cost reductions, they "share in the savings" by receiving a portion of the savings in payment. As of 2014, most of the hospitals associated with ACOs were large, nonprofit teaching hospitals located in the Northeastern and Midwestern United States.

HOSPITAL-BASED PHYSICIAN ASSISTANTS

The previously discussed economic and social forces, and their resulting innovations, have created a promising environment for PA hospital employment. The number of PAs in inpatient settings continues to increase. At the same time, the proportion of PAs in critical care units remains steady and the proportion of PAs working in hospital operating rooms is decreasing (Table 7–1). Moreover, as of 2014, approximately 48% of all PAs first time certified by the National Commission on the Certification of Physician Assistants (NCCPA) reported that they worked primarily in a hospital (NCCPA, 2015).

Physician Assistants as Substitutes for Residents

The use of PAs has been particularly widespread in hospitals to fill positions once filled by residents. Taking surgery as an example, some residency programs lost accreditation because they lacked sufficient cases to provide adequate clinical experience. Thus, PAs have

TABLE 7-1
Trends in Physician Assistants Working in Hospital Settings, 2003 to 2013

	Percentage (and Number) of all American Academy of Physician Assistants Survey Respondents*				
	2003 (N = 18,155)	*2005* (N = 19,951)	*2006* (N = 21,023)	*2008* (N = 25,174)	*2013* (N = 15,798)
All hospital work settings	17.9%	18.1%	18.6%	19.0%	18.2%
Intensive care/critical care unit	1.5% (280)	2% (403)	2.1% (446)	2.3% (590)	2.3% (326)
Inpatient unit	7.4% (1,335)	9.3% (1,848)	9.8% (2,059)	10.3% (2,595)	10.6% (1,674)
Operating room	9% (1,629)	6.8% (1,350)	6.7% (1,408)	6.4% (1,608)	6.0% (872)

*Respondents working in hospital outpatient units and emergency departments were not included.
Data from American Academy of Physician Assistants Census Reports, 2003–2013.

been employed to provide essential preoperative and postoperative care, thereby freeing residents to obtain the required operative case experience necessary to meet residency requirements. Increasingly in modern medicine, PAs are assuming considerable clinical responsibility for providing preoperative and postoperative care, obtaining histories, conducting physical examinations, and performing invasive as well as noninvasive clinical procedures. One early example of an institution adopting widespread employment of PAs as house staff was Butterworth Hospital in Grand Rapids, Michigan, where PAs served in cardiothoracic surgery, neurosurgery, urology, orthopedics, and numerous other medical and surgical specialties. Large PA house staffs, with numbers of PAs anywhere from 100 to 250, are now seen in major academic teaching institutions, such as the Johns Hopkins Hospital, the Cleveland Clinic, the University of Iowa Hospitals and Clinics, Yale–New Haven Hospital, Brigham and Women's Hospital, Grady Memorial, Duke University Hospital, Wake Forest University/Baptist Hospital, M.D. Anderson Hospital, and numerous other major centers.

To analyze the effects of replacing medical residents with PA hospitalists in a community hospital, Dhuper and Choksi (2009) compared prospective data for 2 years of PA service with 2 years of retrospective data from the medical residents' model. For PAs versus medical residents models, all-cause and case mix index-adjusted mortality was 107/5,508 (1.94%) and 0.019 versus 156/5,458 (2.85%)

and 0.029, respectively. The adverse event cases were nine versus five, and the readmission rate within 30 days was 64 versus 69. Patient satisfaction was 95% versus 96%. Quality of care provided by the PA model was equivalent. All-cause and case mix index-adjusted mortality was significantly lower during the PA–hospitalists period. Although the application of these findings to other institutions requires further study, the authors found no intrinsic barriers that would impede implementation elsewhere.

An earlier study addressed the clinical potentials for several types of PAs and NPs to fulfill resident roles (Table 7–2). Although the estimates of PA-specific capacities for resident substitution are not precise, these data offer insight by comparing the proportion of levels of PA capabilities to assume physician resident inpatient clinical duties in teaching hospitals. The exercise was useful in addressing workforce issues related to PA roles in the downsizing of graduate medical education programs.

Perceived Barriers to Integration of PAs into Hospitals

Clinical, financial, and practical criticisms have been raised about using PAs in place of residents. Although PAs may work well as substitutes for first- and second-year residents, some suggest they may require additional training to assume responsibility for more complex cases that call for more advanced medical decision-making or greater technical skill. However, one

TABLE 7-2
Personnel Who Could Perform Physician Resident Activities: Two Staffing Scenarios, by Percent Time

	Traditional Model		PA/NP Model	
	N	%	N	%
Physician only	6,248	46.7	2,693	20.0
None (education activities)	2,778	20.7	2,778	20.8
None (personal time)	1,800	13.3	1,800	13.4
Nurse	588	4.5	449	3.4
Laboratory technician	160	1.2	160	1.2
Unskilled personnel	822	6.1	822	6.1
PA/NP	988	7.4	4,681	35.0
TOTAL	13,384	100.0	13,383	100.0

Modified from Knickman, J. R., Lipkin, M., Jr., Finkler, S. A., Thompson, W. G., & Kiel, J. (1992). The potential for using non-physicians to compensate for the reduced availability of residents. *Academic Medicine, 67*(7), 429–438.

study found that PAs and NPs were filling positions that had once been filled by both junior *and* senior residents (Table 7–3).

On the other hand, certain leaders in medical education have made the point that the complexity of modern medicine may require PAs to possess advanced educational training and skills that most don't necessarily possess. To make up for this perceived deficit, a few hospital-based postgraduate residency programs have developed opportunities for graduate PAs to obtain additional formal training in inpatient medical and surgical disciplines.

Two other barriers to using more PAs arise from time to time. One is the view that PAs are more expensive to hire than residents and work fewer hours. According to the Bureau of Labor Statistics, the 2015 median annual wage (hourly wage x 2080 hours) for PAs was $98,180 compared with an average stipend of about $55,029 for second- and third-year residents. However, after a decade of resident reform in the United States, residents and PAs now work similar hours per week and stipends for PAs in postgraduate residency programs are roughly similar to those of physician residents.

TABLE 7-3
Distribution of Departments Where Physician Assistants Are Performing Some Tasks Previously Performed by Resident Physicians

Specialty	Physician Assistant Only		Nurse Practitioner Only		Both		Total	
	N	%	N	%	N	%	N	%
General surgery	20	17.2	0	0.0	9	14.5	29	11.4
Surgical specialties	36	31.0	14	19.2	9	14.5	59	23.1
Internal medicine	16	13.8	11	14.3	11	17.7	38	14.9
Pediatrics	1	0.9	13	16.9	4	6.5	18	7.1
Other primary care	5	4.3	8	10.4	7	11.3	20	7.8
Emergency	14	12.1	2	2.6	3	4.8	19	7.5
Neonatal	0	0.0	15	19.5	2	3.2	17	6.7
Other specialty	14	12.1	6	7.8	5	8.1	25	9.8
Unspecified	10	8.6	8	10.4	12	19.4	30	11.8
TOTAL	116	100	77	100	62	100	255	100

Data from Riportella-Muller, R., Libby, D., & Kindig, D. (1995). The substitution of physician assistants and nurse practitioners for physician residents in teaching hospitals. *Health Affairs, 14*(2), 181–191.

Another argument against using PAs is reimbursement. One of the chief financial issues when trading resident services for PA services in the United States is remuneration. Physicians in training, or residents, bring graduate medical education (GME) payments (through Medicare) to the institution. Conversely, hospitals do not always receive an explicit payment for the services of a PA, depending on their process for billing insurers. Medicare pays practices and services employing PAs for hospital-delivered services under Medicare Part B when such services would be covered if furnished by a physician, including assistant-at-surgery services, inpatient hospital care, and assisting-at procedures. Specifically, for all billable service in a hospital, Medicare covers PAs at 85% of the physician fee schedule for any service that would have been covered if a physician performed it.

Benefits of Hospital-Based Physician Assistants

Counterarguments to these perceived barriers are offered by hospital employers of PAs. These counterarguments center on satisfaction, economics, resident education, and quality of care.

Satisfaction with PA Services

Satisfaction of PA services has to do with many components; role satisfaction from the provider or employer standpoint is foremost. A growing body of literature documents that teaching hospitals have favorable experiences using PAs in a growing variety of inpatient units and specialties. In fact, under certain circumstances, PAs may be preferable to residents.

The perceptions of faculty, other hospital staff, and patients are also important. Some research suggests that faculty and hospital staff would rather work with PAs due to their lower turnover rates, greater familiarity with departmental procedures, and more clinical experience than first- and second-year residents. One study of nurses' attitudes toward PAs found that nurses who have experience working with PAs or have an understanding of the role of the PA in the healthcare system have more positive attitudes toward them than nurses without such knowledge or experience (Figure 7–2). Other

FIGURE 7-2
Physician Assistants at the Johns Hopkins Hospital

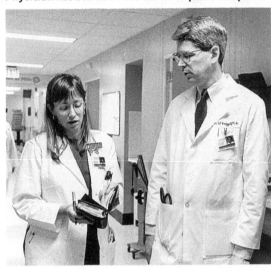

Courtesy of American Academy of Physician Assistants.

research finds that nurses report that having one person who is visible long-term is better than having a new resident every month or two.

Economics of PA Service for Resident Services

The main economics argument is that PAs employed by hospitals may be more economical than salary figures suggest because they may be more efficient than residents, use fewer resources than residents, and require less faculty supervision. In the long run, cost-effectiveness to the institution may be increased when the PA house officer, as a permanent employee, does not need to be retrained each year (or every few months), is knowledgeable about the system, and operates at a higher level of visibility with the staff. An annual transition to new staff and scheduling, which is required for resident arrangements, is costly in administration and supervision.

Some argue that the services residents provide are an economic benefit. However, economists generally regard the services of a resident as "neutral" or "negative" because the educational commitment to train and pay a resident is expensive with efficiency less than that of a permanent staff house officer. On the other hand, some hospitals pay salaries to PA house officers that are greater than those of physician residents. This trade-off is made with the expectation that greater continuity and coordination of care will contribute to better outcomes, shorter lengths of stay, and savings.

An example of the benefits of the PA-as-house-staff trade-off is found in one randomized trial comparing two inpatient-staffing models. The study was undertaken to compare the clinical and financial outcomes for general medicine inpatients assigned to resident (teaching) or staff (nonteaching) services. The staff service used a PA and four physicians. When the unit was fully staffed and operational, patients admitted to the staff service had a 1.7-day lower average length of stay than patients admitted to the resident service, lower average total charges, and significantly lower laboratory and pharmacy charges. No differences emerged in mortality rates or readmission rates. Although the personnel costs were higher on the staff service, the staffing arrangement

was financially viable because of the more efficient pattern of care. Shorter length of stay translated into cost savings and increased revenue that offset the higher salary costs (Simmer, Nerenz, Rutt, Newcomb, & Benfer, 1991).

In a similar but retrospective study, van Rhee and colleagues (2002) compared the use of resources and length of stay between patients cared for by PAs and residents. This study drew its sample from patients admitted to the internal medicine service attended by physicians who rotated between PA and resident services over 1.5 years. A mixed-model analysis was used for each of the five diagnosis-related groups (DRGs) to test for significant differences in resources used and length of stay (Table 7–4). The results of this study revealed no significant differences in usage of resources except for those used in the care of patients with pneumonia, which were

TABLE 7-4
Outcomes of Patients Managed by Physician Assistants and Medical Residents

Diagnosis-Related Group	Variable	PA Service Mean (SD)	Resident Service Mean (SD)
CVA/stroke	Total RVUs	695.41 (389.53)	803.63 (475.42)
	RAD RVUs	192.37 (207.24)	241.63 (281.18)
	LAB RVUs	149.13 (83.39)	182.30 (96.67)*
	LOS	5.93 (2.15)	5.75 (2.68)
Pneumonia	Total RVUs	480.41 (331.89)	626.31 (378.73)†
	RAD RVUs	79.69 (71.81)	98.35 (82.29)
	LAB RVUs	208.77 (102.83)	271.01 (145.73)†
	LOS	5.80 (2.68)	6.16 (2.21)
AMI, discharged alive	Total RVUs	785.46 (300.96)	789.95 (279.05)
	RAD RVUs	33.28 (21.46)	30.68 (31.97)
	LAB RVUs	188.17 (83.31)	200.55 (94.43)
	LOS	5.05 (1.76)	4.97 (1.42)
Congestive heart failure	Total RVUs	454.67 (260.75)	501.53 (245.50)
	RAD RVUs	67.69 (75.71)	62.81 (52.25)
	LAB RVUs	200.43 (87.95)	236.97 (111.87)†
	LOS	5.12 (2.42)	5.44 (2.41)
GI hemorrhage	Total RVUs	506.86 (310.50)	491.45 (244.58)
	RAD RVUs	48.31 (100.42)	53.02 (77.16)
	LAB RVUs	246.71 (146.00)	240.94 (101.31)
	LOS	3.96 (2.00)	3.84 (1.77)

*$P < 0.05$
†$P < 0.01$

AMI = acute myocardial infarction; CVA = cerebrovascular accident; GI = gastrointestinal; LAB = laboratory; LOS = length of stay; RAD = radiology; RVU = relative value unit; SD = standard deviation.

Data from Van Rhee, J., Ritchie, J., & Eward, A. M. (2002). Resource use by physician assistant services versus teaching services. *JAAPA: Official Journal of the American Academy of Physician Assistants, 15*(1), 33–38, 42 passim.

significantly lower in the PA group than in the resident group. No significant differences in the length of stay were found.

With multiple changes occurring in the staffing and cost arrangements of hospitals in the 21st century, hospitals (at least teaching hospitals) might want to consider incorporating PAs to serve as adjuncts to staff services and teaching services. By doing so, they can promote team management of patients and provide a level of skill residents might not have obtained.

Resident Education

PAs can also be employed to enrich the educational experiences of residents. For example, in some cases, residents are spending time performing tasks and procedures that can safely and effectively be done by PAs, such as inserting catheters and drawing blood. Because these tasks lose their pedagogical value after a certain number of repetitions, delegating them to PAs can free residents to focus on more complex cases. In fact, incorporating PAs allows in-house coverage of patients, preserves the educational integrity of physician residency programs, allows time for residents' conferences and clinics, and prepares junior doctors for practice on multidisciplinary teams.

Quality of Care

Research on the use of PAs on inpatient staffs also centers on quality of care. While helping to meet service needs brought about by the limitation of resident working hours, PAs must maintain the standards of hospital care. PAs are not only capable of fulfilling a substantial portion of the clinical duties required on inpatient services; they also provide patient care continuity.

Models for PA Integration

At least three models exist for integration of PAs into hospital settings:

1. **Fully integrated model**—In the fully integrated model, PAs and physicians and/or residents sharing responsibilities for the same group of patients.
2. **Separate-but-equal model**—In this model, PAs have one wing or ward of patients that they care for with minimal supervision and residents have another wing or ward in which care is more closely supervised by attending physicians.
3. **Partially integrated model**—The partially integrated model has PAs working some set hours during the week and residents taking over other hours.

One example of PA integration into a community hospital setting is presented in Box 7–2.

Expanding and contracting work demand creates job inequality. Physicians with limited exposure to PAs and their capabilities may view PAs as their assistants and relegate tasks that do not fully utilize PAs' skills. Thus, the fully integrated model is subject to whim and misuse or underuse of skills. At the other end of the labor spectrum is the separate-but-equal PA and resident model. With this model, services are often duplicated and separate policies and skills apply to different types of providers. The partially integrated model has residents and PAs "cross-cover" for each other when needed and stratifies junior and senior resident services. Over time, the residents and the PAs come to see the advantages of each other's roles and seek the availability of each other's services when the hospital census is high. The main difference in roles is that the resident's role is to learn and move on; the PA's is a career role.

One major teaching institution in the northeastern United States also incorporates three grades of PAs into its model of PA integration. These grades are based not on the PAs' clinical experience but on the nonclinical responsibilities they take on in addition to their work with patients. Some work on continuing education programs, whereas others work on hospital-wide PA grand rounds. One PA works in the organizational area of patient satisfaction and has been doing quality improvement projects related to satisfaction with the PA program. Another PA conducts chart reviews and looks at readmission rates, and one PA works as a liaison between the hospital and the group, working on qualifications and credentialing issues.

Rural Hospitals

The employment of PAs and NPs by rural hospitals is rising. In 1991, approximately 10% of nonmetropolitan hospitals employed

BOX 7-2
A Community Hospital Model of Physician Assistant Utilization

Northwest Hospital Center (NWHC) is a 240-bed, nonteaching community hospital located in the Baltimore, Maryland metropolitan area. The hospital is part of the LifeBridge Health System, which also contains a large tertiary academic medical center, Sinai Hospital of Baltimore. NWHC serves a suburban and urban patient-base and treats primarily adult patients. The institution is one of the more successful hospitals in Maryland from both a financial and growth perspective.

The hospital opened in the late 1960s and employed its first PA in 1974 to serve as an assistant in the operating room. NWHC also served as one of the first preceptor sites for the then newly formed Essex Community College PA program (now the Towson/CCBC PA Program). Over the next several years, additional PAs were employed to provide operating room assistance, admission support, and coverage of the acute care floors in performing minor procedures such as inserting nasogastric tubes and catheters. The impetus to provide these services was in part due to the growth of the facility but also occurred at the request of the attending medical staff, who expected services at par with facilities having resident staff.

In 1984, changes in Medicare policy prohibited hospitals from including physician charges in their rates, and the clearer distinction of Part A and Part B billing caused many facilities to rethink the roles of their house staff. NWHC, which in addition to PAs had a number of house doctors, recognized that they would not be able to recoup those expenditures through the new physician charge system. The decision was made to decrease the component of physician staff serving in this role and to expand PA coverage around-the-clock, giving PAs more responsibilities for assisting with patient management. Initial skepticism that PAs could replace physicians faded as communication improved and customer service satisfaction rose, due in large part to the PA staff.

Throughout the 1990s, PAs at NWHC continued to gain experience and respect from many skeptical physicians. During this time, under new leadership, PAs at NWHC were cross-trained in the medical and surgical disciplines. Capitalizing on this PA plasticity model provided management efficiency by requiring flexibility of the PA staff. Shifting staff to the areas of greatest need without being restricted by specific discipline boundaries is considered a highly principled management tool. As a consequence, management, under a PA manager, developed into a department of PAs (as opposed to having PAs in departments). As additional staff members were hired, the PA division's responsibilities grew to include employee health and occupational health services.

Another period of growth followed the federal Balanced Budget Act in 1997, which allowed for reimbursement of PA services. NWHC significantly increased its operating room PA staff, at the same time recovering the majority of expenses through "first-assisting" fees. As the PA program at NWHC grew, the attending surgical staff endorsed this improved service by redirecting their patients to NWHC. The reason most often cited was the reliability of and satisfaction with the surgical service.

At the turn of this century, NWHC employed a prominent healthcare consulting firm to perform a rigorous internal analysis of its staffing and expenses. As a result of this analysis, and after extensive review and piloting of programs, the PA department was one of the few areas that increased staff. By assigning a PA directly to each patient zone (20 beds), NWHC demonstrated improved efficiency with a reduction of length of stay by nearly one-third.

In 1999, a hospitalist program was inaugurated at NWHC. PAs were quickly incorporated into teams with doctors. The service integrated the hospitalist physicians with PAs to afford greater efficiency of both components. After a decade of experience, the hospitalist/PA service alone accounts for the management of 75% to 80% of all hospital admissions.

In summary, NWHC is a metropolitan hospital with a sizeable PA staff. It has grown from having four PAs in the 1970s to having 40 full-time equivalent PA staff. The constant pulse-taking of its operation, using 360-degree analysis techniques, allowed the assessment of the facility's services and quality. The high results from patients, staff, management, and employees endorse this staffing strategy. The hospitalist team consistently outperforms other services in terms of quality, Hospital Consumer Assessment of Healthcare Providers and Systems, and other performance metrics. The PA relationship with nursing and other professional staff remains "outstanding." PA employment retention is high and job satisfaction is equally high. Finally, the trust of the attending physicians and administration suggests the strategy of utilizing a flexible and talented team of doctors, nurses, and PAs has spelled financial and management success at NWHC.

Source: R. Rohrs, PA-C, Senior Fellow in Hospital Medicine, Director of LifeBridge Medicine, Northwest Hospital; personal communication; January 2016.

a full-time PA and almost 9% employed an NP. In 2014, approximately 37% of PAs said they had a relationship with a hospital, either as an employee or with privileges (NCCPA, 2015). This rise in employment may be because of the need to improve or maintain access to healthcare services and the inability to recruit or retain primary care physicians. (For more information, see Chapter 8, "Physician Assistants in Rural Health.")

PAs and NPs are considered cost-effective or more economical medical staff for rural areas and are used by rural hospitals to enhance their delivery of outpatient services. In addition, the employment of PAs and NPs in rural areas is a requirement of the federal rural health clinic program. One study on rural hospital PA employment described and compared 407 sites spread over eight states (Minnesota, North Dakota, South Dakota, Iowa, Montana, Idaho, Oregon, and Washington). The results showed that rural hospitals are important employers of PAs and NPs and that these settings have a greater demand for than supply of these providers as well as physicians (Table 7–5).

Another role PAs are playing is in staffing critical access hospitals (CAHs), which are hospitals certified to receive cost-based reimbursement from Medicare. This reimbursement value added is intended to improve their financial performance and reduce hospital closures. Each hospital is responsible for reviewing its own situation to determine whether CAH status would be advantageous. CAHs are certified under a different set of Medicare conditions of participation that are more flexible than the acute care hospital conditions of participation. As of 2014, the United States had 1,326 CAHs, many with PAs and NPs on their medical staff.

COSTS AND FINANCING ISSUES

It is no coincidence that the period of rapid growth of hospital employment of PAs, beginning in the early 1980s, closely parallels the time when hospitals were coming under increasing pressure to contain costs. Even before the introduction of DRGs in 1982, many hospitals were faced with the problems of inadequate staffing, rising costs of physician and nursing staffing, and loss of physician residency training programs. For many hospital administrators, the use of PAs in a restructured staffing pattern was an attractive solution to these problems.

TABLE 7-5
Characteristics of Rural Hospitals That Use Physician Assistants and Nurse Practitioners

Hospital and Community Characteristics	Physician Assistants*		Nurse Practitioners*	
	Use (N = 5,216)	Do Not Use (N = 5,191)	Use (N = 5,125)	Do Not Use (N = 5,282)
Hospital beds	49 (45)	42 (34)	60[†] (53)	39 (31)
Full-time hospital employees	122[‡] (150)	96 (102)	164[†] (177)	86 (94)
Physicians on active staff	20 (32)	15 (22)	30[†] (39)	12 (19)
No. of specialty types on active staff	4 (4)	4 (4)	6[†] (5)	3 (3)
Primary care physicians on active staff[§]	9 (11)	8 (8)	12[†] (13)	7 (7)
Hospital admissions	1,509[‡] (1,962)	1,183 (1,334)	2,101[‡] (2,362)	1,026 (1,170)
Outpatient visits (emergency and other)	22,621 (25,033)	18,544 (21,566)	31,283[†] (31,655)	16,020 (16,910)
Surgical procedures (inpatient and outpatient)	1,138 (1,739)	867 (1,232)	1,654[†] (2,079)	725 (1,092)
Percent of revenue from Medicare	54% (14.5)	54% (13.4)	51%[‡] (13.9)	55% (13.8)
Owns or manages a rural health clinic	35%[†]	16%	30%	24%
Education site for PA/NP/CNM/CRNAs	28%	14%	22%	21%
Currently recruiting for a physician	66%	68%	74%	64%
Population of the hospital's service area (38,914)	26,731 (33,571)	23,558 (44,993)	35,559[†] (31,056)	20,690
Road miles to a city of 50,000 population	92 (60)	92 (65)	95 (60)	90 (63)

*Mean values with standard deviations in parentheses.
[†]$P < .001$ (compared with hospitals that do not use the practitioner).
[‡]$P < .05$ (compared with hospitals that do not use the practitioner).
[§]*Primary care* is defined as general practice, family practice, internal medicine, and pediatrics.
Modified from Krein, S. L. (1997). The employment and use of nurse practitioners and physician assistants by rural hospitals. *Journal of Rural Health, 13*(1), 45–58.

Billing in Hospital Settings

Medicare Part A (also known as *hospital insurance*) covers inpatient hospitalization, nursing facility care, home healthcare, and hospice care (such as facility fees and supply costs). Part B (supplemental medical insurance) covers professional services provided by physicians, PAs, and certain other authorized practitioners in an office, clinic, hospital (including emergency department), and nursing facility. In the past, Medicare gave hospitals two options for covering services by hospital-employed PAs. Services provided by PAs could be billed under Medicare Part B as a professional service, or a PA's salary could be included in the hospital's cost reports and covered under Medicare Part A. Because of Medicare's shift to prospective payments, the option of including a PA's salary in the hospital's cost reports is no longer an appropriate method of coverage. Still, it appears some Medicare carriers are not aware of this policy change and continue to allow Part A coverage.

Rules for Evaluation and Management Services

Traditionally, Medicare rules for hospital (inpatient, outpatient, or ED) billing required that the practitioner who provided the majority of professional service to a patient be the one to bill for the service. That is, if a PA did the majority of the work for a patient, the service should be billed under the PA's personal identification number (PIN) and reimbursement would be at 85% of the fee schedule. Some believed mistakenly that the physician could bill the service at 100% if the physician was on-site, cosigned the patient's chart, and/or provided some minor service to the patient.

From September 2001 through September 2002, Medicare suggested that a concept known as "split billing" be used to separately bill for evaluation and management (E/M) services provided by PAs and physicians when both provided care to the same patient on the same day in the hospital setting. However, after being made aware of the administrative and billing difficulties this concept would cause for both practitioners and Medicare carriers, the split billing concept was rescinded.

New rules championed by the American Academy of Physician Assistants (AAPA) and enacted by the CMS give PAs and their physicians increased latitude in hospital billing for E/M services. These new rules allow PAs and physicians who work for the same employer or entity to "share visits" made to patients with the combined work of both billed under the physician at 100% of the fee schedule. That is, if the physician provides any face-to-face portion of the E/M encounter, even if the PA provides the majority of the service for a patient, the entire service may be billed under the physician. This new rule does not extend to procedures performed in hospital settings. In those cases, the practitioner who does the majority of the procedure is the person under whom the procedure should be billed.

For reimbursement of a PA's E/M services, the following guidelines must be in place:

- The PA and the physician must work for the same entity (e.g., same group practice, same hospital, or PA employment by a solo physician).
- The regulation applies to E/M services but not to procedures or consultations.
- The PA and the physician must see the patient on the same calendar day.
- The physician must provide at least some face-to-face part of the E/M visit. Simply reviewing or signing the patient's chart is not sufficient. (If the physician does not provide some face-to-face portion of the E/M encounter, then the service is appropriately billed at the full fee schedule amount under the PA's PIN with reimbursement paid at the 85% rate.)

PHYSICIAN ASSISTANTS IN SURGICAL SPECIALTIES

The inclusion of PAs in surgical practices occurred early in the professions' development and continues to increase. With cost-containment, unfilled surgical residency positions, advancements in surgical techniques, shortage of surgeons, resident work hour restrictions and the acceptance of PAs, the field of surgery for PAs continues to grow.

In surgery, there are three distinct aspects

- Preoperative or postoperative outpatient care
- The operating room
- The hospital care that occurs immediately before and after a surgical procedure

As a result, some surgical PAs are inpatient providers who do not provide care in outpatient clinics. Others provide medical management before as well as after surgical procedures. Still others predominantly function in the surgical theater. However, many have roles that may include inpatient, outpatient, in-theater, and discharge management.

Cardiovascular and Thoracic Surgery

Cardiovascular surgery and thoracic surgery are separate surgical specialties but are frequently grouped together as cardiothoracic surgery (primarily in the United States). *Cardiovascular surgery* generally refers to surgery of the heart and great vessels, and *thoracic surgery* generally refers to surgery of parts of the chest other than the heart.

Tasks and Procedures

PAs in cardiovascular and thoracic surgery commonly fill the role of first assistant in surgery, provide preoperative and postoperative care in the hospital, and see patients in the medical office. Tasks frequently include performing a pulmonary and circulatory examination, explaining the surgical procedure to the patient and family members, and answering questions. PAs may insert and remove vascular lines and monitoring devices, such as central artery catheters and PIC lines; insert and remove wound drains; and regulate the metabolic needs of the patient. Procedures include heart or lung transplantation, liver transplantation, cardiac vessel bypass grafts, and heart valve replacement. Technical skills involve placing and monitoring intra-aortic balloon pumps, right and left ventricular assist devices, cardiopulmonary support systems, and extracorporeal membrane oxygenators. In many cases with these procedures, PAs may be the

ones to open and close the chest and assist the surgeon with a second set of hands.

Postoperatively, cardiothoracic PAs manage patient care in intensive care units (ICUs) and hospital wards and watch for early postsurgical complications. Providing optimal patient care includes managing the patient's surgical condition as well as other disease processes the patient may have, such as hypertension and diabetes. Other roles include overseeing cardiac rehabilitation, teaching about diet, and discharging patients. PA involvement with patients continues in the form of answering telephone calls regarding their concerns after returning home and seeing them in the office for postoperative visits.

Safety and Effectiveness

Only a few studies have examined the safety of cardiothoracic PAs. In one 3-year retrospective examination of 1,226 central venous cannulations in 732 patients undertaken by PAs in a vascular surgery section of Geisinger Medical Center, seven patients experienced a pneumothorax as a complication. Six of the seven procedures were performed by different PAs. Although statistics were not included for physicians, the less than 1% incident of pneumothorax for this procedure is considered low compared with the 4% overall major complication rate of surgical house officers, anesthesiologists, and other house officers (Marsters, 2000).

Another study evaluated the effectiveness of a physician assistant home care (PAHC) program. The intention of the intervention was to decrease hospital readmission rates for patients who underwent cardiac surgery by incorporating house calls provided by PAs. Home interventions included adjustment of medications, ordering of imaging studies, and administration of direct wound care. The overall readmission rate for the control group was 16% and 12% for the PAHC group, a 25% reduction in the rate of readmissions. The rate of infection-related readmissions was reduced by almost half (Nabagiez, Shariff, Molloy, Demissie, & McGinn, 2016).

Professional Society

The Association of Physician Assistants in Cardiovascular Surgery (APACVS) includes PAs who participate in the surgical treatment of cardiovascular disease that encompasses three specialty areas: general thoracic surgery, surgery for congenital heart disease, and surgery for acquired heart disease. The APACVS began as an educational organization and represents the professional interests of the CVPA. Its primary objectives are to promote the clinical and academic excellence of its members and enhance the quality of medical care to their patients. Today, the APACVS is the educational, scientific, and political subspecialty organization representative of surgical PAs practicing in the field of cardiovascular and thoracic surgery. The APACVS is recognized and endorsed by the Society of Thoracic Surgeons and the American Association for Thoracic Surgeons.

General Surgery

General surgery focuses on surgical treatment of abdominal organs such as the intestines (including esophagus, stomach, colon, liver, gallbladder, and bile ducts), the thyroid gland (depending on the availability of head and neck surgery specialists), hernias, and, sometimes, the breast.

PAs have significantly reduced the workload of general surgeons in training (residents) during the period the 80-hour workweek was initiated in the United States. Their positive influence on graduate surgical education programs involves decreasing surgery resident work hours and improving resident work outlook.

Tasks and Procedures

PAs in general surgery often serve as first assistants. They may create the surgical opening, close a patient's wound, and follow the patient into the surgical ICU or recovery area, where they may write the orders for a patient's immediate care and accompany the doctor on rounds. Postoperatively, PAs may dictate the operative report, apply and remove monitoring devices, and regulate the pharmaceutical management of the patient. Additional procedures and tasks may include placing and removing temporary pacemakers; applying and removing casts, sutures, and skin clips; and relieving the surgeon of many routine matters. Some

serve as permanently employed staff working closely with the chief resident in surgery to maintain continuity of care for patients as residents rotate through the service.

Professional Society

The American Association of Surgical Physician Assistants (AASPA) was established in 1972. It maintains an active relationship with the AAPA as well as with the American College of Surgeons (ACS).

Neurosurgery

Neurosurgery is the surgical discipline focused on treating the central and peripheral nervous system as well as spinal column diseases amenable to mechanical intervention.

Tasks and Procedures

PAs in neurosurgery function in all areas of surgical practice, from closing deep and superficial wounds and assisting with all neurosurgical procedures, including craniotomies, spinal procedures, fine instrumentation of nerves, and microscopic procedures. Other procedures commonly include brain or peripheral nerve surgery, spinal cord surgery, and routine neurological procedures. Neurosurgical PAs sometimes perform minor procedures, such as carpal tunnel releases, on their own.

Neurosurgical PAs perform appropriate laboratory and diagnostic studies, such as lumbar punctures, ventriculostomies, and myelograms, and may place tong traction or halo fixation devices on the cranium.

Office duties for neurosurgical PAs include seeing patients and completing a thorough history and physical examination that is oriented for neurosurgical conditions. They present patients to the attending neurosurgeons, help formulate a treatment plan, order appropriate radiographic studies, and perform office procedures such as local nerve blocks. Other tasks include evaluating postoperative patients, handling routine follow-up visits, and being available to see those patients who require same-day office visits. Neurosurgical PAs also evaluate, screen, and counsel patients on health maintenance.

Orthopedic Surgery

Orthopedic surgery is concerned with acute, chronic, traumatic, and overuse injuries and other disorders of the musculoskeletal system. Orthopedic surgeons manage most musculoskeletal ailments, including trauma, congenital deformities, and the effects of arthritis. The discipline uses surgical and nonsurgical interventions.

There is some confusion about PAs who work in orthopedic settings and technicians who call themselves orthopedic PAs (OPAs). Formally trained and NCCPA-certified PAs who work in an orthopedic setting differ from another group of technicians trained to assist orthopedic surgeons. Both groups have *orthopedic* in the title, and each may refer to themselves as *OPAs*. However, the educational qualifications of the two groups—OPAs and PAs—differ substantially. Consequently, Medicare does not pay for services provided by OPAs.

OPAs have been in the United States since at least 1954 in some capacity, whether assisting with cast application or holding a retractor, and many developed expertise while in the military. It is unclear when the first formal orthopedic technical program started; however, the American Medical Association (AMA) House of Delegates first adopted minimum educational standards for OPA education in 1969 upon a recommendation from the American Academy of Orthopedic Surgeons (AAOS). The orthopedic assistant programs were confined to training technical orthopedic tasks without the substantial background in the basic medical sciences that the primary care PA programs stressed.

Tasks and Procedures

The range of tasks and procedures performed by PAs in orthopedics is, in contrast, much broader than that of OPAs (Table 7–6). PAs in orthopedic practice perform history taking and physical examinations and prescribe medications. In addition, most interpret x-rays, apply casts, suture wounds, assist in surgery, and reduce simple long-bone fractures. Out of 10,000 orthopedic PAs only 50 or so are postgraduate-trained (Chalupa & Hooker, 2016).

Larson (2011) found that orthopedics is the third most common specialty practiced by

TABLE 7-6

Tasks Performed by Physician Assistants in Orthopedic Surgery

Task	Percent
History taking	99.0
Physical examination	99.0
Interpretation of x-ray studies	94.2
Cast application	94.5
Wound suturing	93.8
Assistance in surgery	92.9
Joint aspiration/injection	80.8
Brace application	76.0
K-wire removal	73.4
Wound incision and drainage	67.5
Fracture reduction	57.1
Dislocation reduction	54.5
Hardware removal	50.3
Compartment pressure measurements	31.2
Administer regional anesthesia	22.1
Tendon repair	22.1
Percutaneous pinning of fractures	21.4

Data from Broughton, B. (1996). A delineative study of physician assistants in orthopaedic surgery: Tasks, professional relationships, and satisfaction [PhD dissertation]. Columbia Pacific University, California.

PAs. From a representative sample between 2005 and 2007, a majority completed a 4- to 8-week rotation in orthopedic surgery during PA school, but most did not complete any advanced postgraduate orthopedic training. Orthopedic group practices were the most commonly reported employer type. Respondents performed an average of 59 outpatient visits per week and 16 inpatient visits per week. More than 87% participated in surgery on a regular basis, most often working as first assistants. Many orthopedic generalists and specialists performed a broad range of clinical activities, including ones suggestive of general, rather than close and direct, physician supervision, such as closing surgical incisions independently and taking first call.

PAs in orthopedic surgery (as distinguished from orthopedic technicians who refer to themselves as PAs but are not NCCPA certified) provide a host of roles that closely juxtapose the orthopedic surgeon. They provide preadmission physical examinations; write admitting orders, first assist in surgery, and conduct fracture clinics. A comprehensive listing of tasks commonly performed by PAs in orthopedic surgery is in Table 7–7.

In hospital settings, some PAs work in surgery as the first assistant in joint reconstruction. They may write preoperative and postoperative orders and may close deep and superficial wounds when assisting with surgical procedures (including joint reconstructions, joint prostheses, spinal procedures and instrumentations, and microscopic procedures). PAs in orthopedic surgery conduct hospital rounds of all patients, including those on ICUs, on a daily basis. Tasks include writing orders and progress notes; performing all admission history and physicals; and ordering appropriate laboratory and radiographic tests, such as MRIs, myelograms, and CT scans as needed or indicated. PAs also perform appropriate laboratory and diagnostic studies, such as joint aspirations and injections and placement of traction devices. They evaluate and clarify clinical conditions, formulate and implement treatment and therapeutic plans for hospitalized patients, write discharge planning, and dictate discharge summaries.

Some PAs are primarily employed in outpatient settings, evaluating acute bone and joint injuries, stabilizing bone fractures, removing hardware and sutures, and placing patients in rehabilitation programs (inpatient or outpatient). Other PAs in orthopedics move between the two settings (surgical and outpatient) as the surgeon or surgical group may need them.

Professional Society

Physician Assistants in Orthopaedic Surgery (PAOS) is an organization created by and for PAs who are NCCPA-certified and are licensed to work in orthopedics. This official specialty organization of the AAPA has an official liaison with the AAOS.

Otorhinolaryngology (Head and Neck Surgery)

Otorhinolaryngology is the specialty responsible for the diagnosis and treatment of ear, nose, throat, and head and neck disorders. The full name of the specialty is *otolaryngology-head and neck surgery*. Practitioners are called *otolaryngologists-head and neck surgeons*, or sometimes *otorhinolaryngologists*. A commonly used term for this specialty, although somewhat out of favor, is *ENT* (ear, nose, and throat).

Evidence suggests that otolaryngology is a specialty with limited, although growing, PA involvement. According to AAPA census data,

TABLE 7-7
Orthopedic Physician Assistants Select Roles and Activities, n (%)*

	2009	2010	2011	2012	2013	2014	2015
Cast/splint application	94 (37)	119 (41)	337 (50)	428 (49)	471 (44)	477 (43)	520 (44)
Assistance with surgery	197 (78)	243 (83)	572 (85)	719 (82)	923 (86)	961 (86)	1011 (85)
Administration of digital blocks	49 (19)	55 (19)	158 (24)	171 (20)	203 (19)	203 (18)	231 (20)
Administration of regional blocks	14 (6)	17 (6)	50 (7)	37 (4)	52 (5)	53 (5)	67 (6)
Closed fracture reduction	42 (17)	66 (22)	151 (23)	191 (22)	214 (20)	253 (23)	284 (24)
Measurement of compartment pressure	6 (2)	16 (3)	18 (3)	20 (2)	22 (2)	23 (2)	26 (2)
Tendon repair	15 (6)	16 (6)	63 (9)	84 (10)	106 (10)	99 (9)	107 (9)
Percutaneous pinning of fractures autonomously	6 (2)	5 (2)	18 (3)	23 (3)	23 (2)	28 (3)	24 (2)
Traction pin insertion autonomously	5 (2)	8 (3)	14 (2)	31 (4)	33 (3)	33 (3)	23 (2)
Phone calls	150 (61)	178 (63)	399 (60)	506 (58)	654 (59)	590 (57)	641 (54)
Supervising physician does not see any of the PA's patients unless asked	93 (38)	116 (41)	283 (42)	400 (46)	525 (48)	564 (49)	671 (61)

* Multiple responses were allowed, so results do not total 100%.
Data from Chalupa, R., & Hooker, R. S. (2016). Physician assistants in orthopedic surgery: Education, role, distribution, compensation. *Journal of the American Academy of Physician Assistants, 29*(3), in press.

only 52 (0.5%) PAs were employed in this specialty in 1996. By 2001, the number had risen to 104 (0.6%); in 2015 it was 859 (1.0%). This steady increase over several years suggests that PAs are fulfilling an important role within the specialty.

A study of PA involvement in outpatient otolaryngology practice suggests that PAs are involved in approximately 5% of outpatient visits and more commonly provide care for established patients, rather than perform visits for new patients.

Tasks and Procedures

Office procedures may include cleaning ear canals and mastoid cavities, performing electrocautery for the control of epistaxis, inserting nasal packing, and providing immediate postoperative care of patients in the inpatient and outpatient setting. They may also perform rhinopharyngolaryngoscopy, videostroboscopy, and vocal/voice recordings.

Professional Society

The Society of Physician Assistants in Otorhinolaryngology-Health and Neck Surgery (SPAO-HNS) was founded during the American Academy of Otorhinolaryngology-Head and Neck Surgery's annual meeting in 1991. The society was developed to enhance the professional growth development of PAs who work in the field of ear, nose, and throat diseases and now serves as an opportunity to meet and interact with PAs who share a common interest and to obtain continuing medical education specific to their field.

Plastic and Reconstructive Surgery

Plastic surgery is a specialty that uses a number of surgical and nonsurgical techniques to change the appearance and restore the function of a person's body. Procedures involve cosmetic enhancements (also referred to as *cosmetic surgery*), functionally reconstructive operations, or both.

Plastic surgeons employ PAs in a variety of ways. In fact, reconstructive microsurgery has relied on trained PAs in this area to reduce operating time in the United States since the 1970s. Sigurdson (2007) had used PAs extensively and theorizes that the introduction of a reconstruction surgical PA in a Canadian practice could improve productivity by 37%.

Tasks and Procedures

PAs in plastic and reconstructive surgery work in a variety of settings and with a variety of medical issues that encompass cosmetic surgery, burn management, and reconstruction of congenital and trauma-related injuries. Because many plastic surgeons practice in office-based operating rooms and "surgicenters," PAs must be able to first assist on all cases, provide suture skills equal to that of the surgeon, and be knowledgeable in anatomy and the latest surgical techniques. Perioperatively, PAs in plastic and reconstructive surgery perform physical examinations and discharge planning, oversee rehabilitation, communicate with various members of the surgical team, and are knowledgeable about surgical supplies and prostheses. In clinic settings, PAs may see postoperative patients. They may order routine laboratory tests, dictate discharge summaries, monitor patients, and change dressings.

Trauma Surgery

Trauma personnel concentrate their practice on the care of injured and critically ill patients. In the United States, trauma surgeons generally work in large urban hospitals specifically designated as trauma centers by the ACS (Oswanski, Sharma, & Shekhar, 2004).

Tasks and Procedures

Perioperatively, PAs in trauma surgery perform physical examinations and discharge planning, oversee rehabilitation, communicate with various members of the surgical team, and are knowledgeable about surgical supplies and prostheses.

Because trauma surgery PAs interface with emergency departments, they must be able to quickly assess a patient's needs in the absence of a surgeon. For example, a PA may be the first member of the trauma team to evaluate an injured victim and institute immediate therapy. Trauma PAs may also assist in the operating room and with postoperative management, following the patient through the critical care portion of recovery. They often attend to patients closely on the hospital surgical ward. In most trauma centers, patient follow-up occurs in the trauma surgery clinic, where PAs may provide continuity of care not usually possible with surgical residents. Trauma surgery PAs may also make rounds with the attending surgeon and report on pertinent issues regarding patient care. Other responsibilities include dealing with patient calls after hospital discharge and answering general follow-up questions. These responsibilities may include triaging patients to the ED or trauma clinic.

Safety and Effectiveness

Several studies have evaluated quality of care when PAs were included on trauma surgery teams. The Oswanski et al study (2004) was undertaken to assess the quality of patient care during transition from a resident-assisted to a PA-assisted trauma program (without residents). Focused analysis showed 100% participation of PAs during the trauma alert compared with 51% by residents. Additional analysis indicated that mortality and transfer time were similar between resident and PA teams, but length of stay (LOS) significantly decreased by 1 day. The authors stated that trauma programs benefit from collaboration of residents and PAs inpatient care (Oswanski et al., 2004).

Another study evaluated the impact of introducing PA and NPs to trauma teams on resource utilization at a level I trauma center. Mean daily admissions increased after introduction of PA and NPs. Reductions in hospital and ICU length of stay and incidence of complications were also observed. The authors concluded that PA and NPs offer a clinically effective and resource-efficient alternative to residents on a trauma service (Gillard et al., 2011).

The use of PAs was also examined in a large trauma center in Flint, Michigan. Over the 3 years spanning 1994 through 1996, the use of a team of trauma surgeons and PAs was introduced in an effort to off-load some of the surgeon's workload. During this period of PA use,

the injury severity scores increased 19%, transfer time to the operating room decreased 43%, transfer time to the ICU decreased 51%, and transfer time to the floor decreased 20%. The length of stay for admissions decreased 13%, and the length of stay for neurotrauma ICU patients decreased 33%. Some of the procedures performed by PAs included chest tube insertion, admit and discharge summaries, central venous and pulmonary artery catheter placements, and subclavian catheterizations. The authors concluded the decreased length of stay in critical care units and in the hospital as a whole resulted in significant savings by the employment of these two trauma PAs (Miller, 1998).

Reviewing medical records and trauma registry data for a level I trauma center, another study evaluated the safety and effectiveness of PAs performing procedures commonly used on trauma teams. They monitored placement of intracranial pressure (ICP) monitors by neurosurgeons (105), PAs (97), and general surgery residents (13) and remained in place a mean of 4 days. No major complications attributable to ICP monitor placement occurred. However, 19 minor complications (malfunction, dislodgment) were noted. Of the ICP placements that resulted in minor complications, 11 monitors were placed by neurosurgeons (10%), 7 placed by PAs (7%), and 1 placed by a resident (8%). The authors concluded that ICP monitor placement by PAs is safe and may aid neurosurgeons in providing prompt monitoring of patients with head injuries (Kaups, Parks, & Morris, 1998). A similar study focused on complications concluded that ICP monitors could be safely inserted by PA/NPs.

Professional Society

The AASPA includes trauma surgery PAs. It advances information about the needs of membership by marketing the profession, offering quality cost-effective hands-on continuing medical education, assisting with professional issues, and providing a forum for networking and the exchange of ideas. In addition to serving surgical PA professionals, AASPA represents PA students—both students and PA residents—in a wide variety of academic settings.

PHYSICIAN ASSISTANTS IN HOSPITAL-BASED MEDICAL SPECIALTIES

Inpatient PAs are on staff in many medical and surgical specialties and subspecialties (e.g., cardiology, pulmonary medicine, gastroenterology, nephrology, rheumatology, infectious disease, and oncology), in addition to pediatrics, internal medicine, and geriatrics. This section focuses on PAs who work in specialties that provide the majority of their care in inpatient settings, namely neonatal intensive care PAs, acute and critical care PAs, and hospitalists. A discussion of the work of PAs in the remaining principal medical specialties appears in Chapter 6, "Physician Assistant Specialization: Nonprimary Care."

PAs who have the principal role of hospital-based employment (including intensivists and critical care specialists) are a growing presence in American medicine and elsewhere. Their professional focus is the general medical (and surgical) care of hospitalized patients. Their roles are constantly evolving, largely because of house officer shortages and growing demand for highly efficient team-based care. These unique roles include activities of patient care, teaching, research, and management. Many of the activities of patient care can cross over from the outpatient setting to the inpatient setting, and PAs in these positions sometimes follow their patients through the medical care process. The roles of these specialty PAs are also delineated in Chapter 6.

Neonatal Intensive Care

PAs and NPs are increasingly being recruited to fill roles traditionally performed by neonatal residents and fellows. The work required to care for babies who need intensive medical attention requires skill and is labor intensive, yet studies have shown that such care can be safely transferred to PAs and NPs. For example, downsizing of a pediatric residency program prompted a phased-in replacement of house staff in a 26-bed neonatal intensive care unit (NICU) in the Albert Einstein College of Medicine–Montefiore Medical Center in Bronx, New York. Subsidized education for neonatal NPs, recruitment of PAs, and leadership took place over 18 months, at which time all house staff functions were assumed by PAs or NPs. The cost to establish the program at the Albert Einstein College of Medicine–Montefiore Medical Center was evaluated under New York's prospective reimbursement system. Ongoing costs of the program were estimated at $1.2 million per year (including salaries, off-hours medical backup, recruitment, administrative overhead, and loss of indirect and direct medical education reimbursement, partially offset by recaptured house staff salaries and ancillary expense reductions). At a glance, PAs and NPs may appear more expensive in comparison with house staff when only salary is taken into consideration. The study showed, however, that revenue was minimally affected. The upside is PAs and NPs are present when there is turnover of new physicians in postgraduate training.

Safety and Effectiveness

Safety and effectiveness are key components of quality measures. Several studies have evaluated the effectiveness of PAs in NICUs and demonstrated that access to care was maintained. In one study, quality of care was assessed during the last 6 months of house staff being in service and during the first 6 months of full PA and NP staffing; the results revealed similar rates of survival of low-birth-weight neonates and an improvement in documentation and compliance with immunization and blood-use guidelines during the PA and NP period. The authors concluded that, in the context of work hour reform (resident duty hour restrictions per week), the employment of PAs are an answer to staffing problems (Schulman, Lucchese, & Sullivan, 1995).

Another study was undertaken to compare patient care delivery by neonatal PAs and NPs with that of pediatric residents in the intensive care unit (ICU) setting. Charts for 244 consecutive admissions to an NICU in Jacksonville, Florida, were reviewed. Patients were cared for by one of two teams: one staffed by residents and the other staffed by neonatal PAs and NPs. The two teams cared for patients with similar patient background characteristics and diagnostic variables. The researchers assessed performance of the two teams by comparing patient management, outcome, and charges. Management variables included data on length of critical care and hospital stay, ventilator and oxygen use, total parenteral nutrition use, number of transfusions, and the performance of various procedures. Outcome variables included the incidence of air leaks, bronchopulmonary dysplasia, intraventricular hemorrhage, patent ductus arteriosus, necrotizing enterocolitis, retinopathy of prematurity, and infant death. Charge variables included hospital and physician charges. The results demonstrated no significant differences in management, outcome, or charge variables between patients cared for by the two teams. This study underscores other observations that neonatal PAs and NPs are effective alternatives to residents for patient care in NICUs (Carzoli et al., 1994).

Intensive/Acute Care and Critical Care

ICUs have grown steadily in the United States since their inception in the 1950s; in more recent years, their use has begun to outpace other sectors of medicine. From 1985 to 2000, the number of US hospitals decreased by 9% and the number of hospital beds decreased by 26%; yet from 1985 to 2005, the number of ICU beds increased by 32.5%. However, the increase in acute care services has not been associated with an increase in critical care physicians or intensivists. Quite the opposite is occurring. Many ICUs are short staffed, and it appears that this problem will continue to worsen; it is estimated that the intensivist workforce will have a shortfall equivalent to 22% of demand by 2020 and 35% by 2030 (Halpern et al., 2013).

A number of factors have exacerbated the declining interest of acute care medicine as a residency option. The most prevalent and related factors are staffing and workload. Aspects of intensivist workload include the number of hours worked per day, the details of nighttime and weekend coverage, the number of days worked per week and month, the number of patients cared for at a time, and the intensity of intellectual and physical effort while providing care. The concern is an increase in "workload" will lead to job burnout.

Tasks and Procedures

The tasks and procedures performed by PAs who work in intensive/acute care commonly include performing patient care management; rounding; obtaining histories and performing physical examinations; diagnosing and treating illnesses; ordering and interpreting tests; initiating orders, commonly under protocols; prescribing and performing diagnostic, pharmacological, and therapeutic interventions consistent with their education and with practice and state regulations; assessing and implementing nutrition; and performing procedures (as credentialed and privileged). Examples of procedures performed by acute care PAs include arterial line insertion, suturing, and chest tube insertion. They also assist in the operating room.

PAs who work in intensive/acute care also collaborate and consult with the interdisciplinary team, including the patient and family. They educate and promote communication among staff, patients, and families to help optimize patient care. Intensivists PAs also coordinate discharge planning, including transfer and referral consultations and patient and family education regarding the anticipated plan of care.

Some hospitals have created unique roles for PAs, such as lead positions on the rapid response team (RRT). One study assessed the effectiveness of implementing such a role. It evaluated the rates of in-hospital cardiac arrests, unplanned ICU admissions, and hospital mortality. The cardiac arrest rate, hospital mortality, and ICU admissions all decreased after implementation (Figure 7–3). Other key roles include monitoring and reinforcing practice guidelines for patients undergoing intensive care unit procedures, such as central line insertion procedures, infection prevention measures, and stress ulcer prophylaxis, and leading quality assurance initiatives, such as the ventilator-associated pneumonia bundle, sepsis bundle, and rapid response team. Research-related tasks include data collection, subject enrollment, and research study management.

Safety and Effectiveness

Research on the role and impact of PAs in the care of acute and critically ill patients has focused mostly on how PAs manage patient care.

FIGURE 7-3
Cardiac Arrests per 1,000 Discharges Versus Rapid Response Team Calls (May 2004–October 2005)

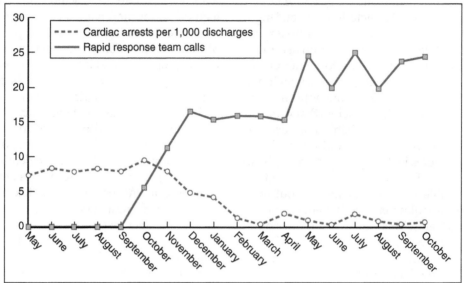

Data from Dacey, M., Mirza, E., Wilcox, V., Doherty, M., Mello, J., & Boyer, A., et al. (2007). The effect of a rapid response team on major clinical outcome measures in a community hospital. Critical Care Medicine, 35(9), 2076–2082.

Fewer studies have focused on comparing PA care with physician care, although one study that evaluated the association between PA/NP staffing and in-hospital mortality for ICU patients at 29 ICUs in 22 US hospitals found that patients in ICUs with PAs/NPs were less sick but had no differences in in-hospital mortality after accounting for patient acuity (Costa et al., 2014). Further research that examines the impact of different models of care, including multidisciplinary and outcomes management models, and explores the impact of PAs in the ICU setting on patient outcomes, including financial aspects of care, is needed. In addition, information on successful multidisciplinary models of care is needed to promote optimal use of these providers in acute and critical care settings.

Hospitalists

Hospital medicine represents a growing opportunity for PAs. The term *hospitalist* was coined by Wachter and Goldman in 1996, reflecting a major shift in hospital-based medicine with the introduction, or more precisely, the rise of this new discipline. A hospitalist is concerned with the medical care of hospitalized patients rather than with specialty care organized around a particular organ system (for example, gastroenterology), a disease (diabetes), or a patient's age (geriatrics). Some anecdotal reports identify PAs as part of many hospitalist teams, whereas others speculate a hospitalist track for physicians tends to attract recent medical graduates looking to bridge time until they find fellowships. In some cases, the turnover of these transient physician hospitalists has been significant. In an effort to stabilize this attrition, the PA-hospitalist has evolved and become the primary staff member for continuity in care.

Tasks and Procedures
Hospitalists manage patients throughout the continuum of hospital care, often seeing patients in the ED, admitting them to inpatient wards, following them as necessary into the critical care unit, and organizing postacute care. Physicians who are hospitalists are typically board certified in internal medicine, family medicine, or pulmonology. The activities of

a hospitalist may include patient care, teaching, research, and leadership related to hospital care.

Safety and Effectiveness

Two studies have been compared the safety and effectiveness of hospitalist-PA teams to hospitalist-resident teams. Both studies were single-institution studies. One study evaluated length of stay (LOS), charges, readmissions, and inpatient mortality (Singh et al., 2011). The other evaluated LOS, cost, inpatient mortality, ICU transfers, readmissions, and patient satisfaction (Roy et al., 2008). The results of this research indicate that mortality, readmission rates, costs, ICU transfers, and patient satisfaction were similar or better when care was delivered by PA teams than when care was delivered by resident teams. However, the results for LOS differed between studies. One study showed equivalent LOS between the two groups, and one showed slightly longer LOS for the PA team.

FURTHER RESEARCH ON HOSPITAL-BASED PHYSICIAN ASSISTANTS

The literature about PAs in hospitals is limited and, for the most part, outdated. A review of this literature reveals important but unanswered questions. In this section, select research questions that might contribute to the successful deployment of PAs in hospital-based operations are offered.

- **Case reports:** What are the role and responsibilities of a hospitalist PA? Case reports can show what a hospital-based PA does and what a typical day is like. Each defined role in a hospital needs a case report.
- **Task delineation:** What are the procedures that hospital-based PAs need to know to be considered competent? Task delineation studies are needed approximately every 5 years to identify the skill sets and activities required of PAs, particularly those serving in critical care medicine and hospitalist services. These studies need to be undertaken for PAs in urban and rural settings, in large and

small hospitals, and the results need to be compared.

- **Team roles:** What roles do PAs perform in different hospital-based specialties? What are the overlaps in hospitalist care by doctors, PAs, and NPs in the same setting?
- **Economics:** Does the use of PAs on a hospitalist team produce a missing synergy where two doctors are working in parallel as hospitalists? Does the addition of a PA to a team indicate substitution or a complementary effect?
- **Breadth of knowledge:** How does a PA in an ICU obtain his or her knowledge set once in practice? Does the acquisition of knowledge have different trajectories depending on age, gender, and experience?
- **Career selection:** How do PAs in NICUs come to their jobs? Do they take hospital-based care as a choice or a trade-off? How long do they remain in this career setting?
- **Procedures:** What is the range of procedures that a typical PA in a hospital setting needs to know and perform adequately?
- **Ratios:** What are the ratios of PAs and NPs to doctors in various types of hospitals? What contributes to these differences? Are the differences due to shifting policy regarding residents and fellows? Are there management advantages to using one practitioner over the other?
- **Retention:** What are the factors that contribute to retention or attrition of PAs in neonatal intensive care, orthopedic surgery, interventional radiology, or any other hospital-based specialty?
- **Education:** How do PAs in hospital-based specialties come to that specialty? How are they trained to carry out their role? Do they build on a fundamental set of skills or do they have a formal indoctrination?

SUMMARY

Expansion of the roles of PAs into the hospital setting has been the most significant recent trend in healthcare's use of these professionals. As two forces converge—a US hospital bed capacity of one million and an inadequate medical force necessary to meet the bed expectation—hospitals turn to PAs and NPs. The intent is to increase the supply of hospitalists and other providers while maintaining quality of care for patients. Initially intended to be primary care providers, PAs moved into the institutional setting with ease and in large numbers to assume roles as medical and surgical inpatient house staff and as assistants to specialists and subspecialists. This trend is a manifestation of the even larger trend of PA specialization.

The use of PAs in hospitals emerged from changing social and economic forces. Some of these forces were changing house staff policies of a workweek, frequent turnover, salary, and the available supply of PAs. Employing PAs has permitted hospitals to cost-effectively maintain the required level of patient care, has allowed residency programs to balance the number of specialty-trained physicians, and has thereby contributed to a more balanced supply of specialists in overcrowded fields. PAs in hospitals maintain or improve the existing level of quality and access to medical care, are cost-effective in the delivery of inpatient services, display extensive clinical versatility among the various medical disciplines, and enrich the quality of residency education for physicians in training.

Federal legislation amending the Medicare program has clarified and established policies so that employing hospitals are now reimbursed for services provided by PAs. The significance of these actions is the recognition by major third-party payers of the value of PAs in rendering quality clinical services in various settings. Such measures solidify the role of the PA as an important member of the healthcare team.

All of the aforementioned factors mean that health workforce experts no longer overlook PAs and that their demand in a broad variety of inpatient settings is likely to continue. Employment trends indicate a strong demand for PAs among hospitals and that there are not enough PAs to fill available positions. Much of this trend is the result of new technology, the limitation on resident work hours, and the appreciation of PA clinical adaptability and flexibility. There is every reason to believe that PAs will continue to function successfully in the hospital setting.

References

The following citations are key to supporting this chapter's content. You can find a complete list of citations for all chapters at www.fadavis.com/davisplus, keyword *Hooker*.

Agency for Healthcare Research and Quality (AHRQ). (2015). *2013 Annual hospital-acquired condition rate and estimates of cost savings and deaths averted from 2010 to 2013* (AHRQ Publication No. 16-0006-EF). Rockville, MD: AHRQ. Retrieved from: http://www.ahrq.gov/professionals/quality-patient-safety/pfp/index.html

American Hospital Association. (2014). *Fast facts on US hospitals*. Retrieved from http://www.aha.org/research/rc/stat-studies/101207fastfacts.pdf

Association of American Medical Colleges. (2012). Estimating the number and characteristics of hospitalist physicians in the United States and their possible workforce implications. *AAMC Analysis in Brief, 12*(3). Retrieved from https://www.aamc.org/download/300620/data/aibvol12_no3-hospitalist.pdf

Carzoli, R. P., Martinez-Cruz, M., Cuevas, L. L., Murphy, S., & Chiu, T. (1994). Comparison of neonatal nurse practitioners, physician assistants, and residents in the neonatal intensive care unit. *Archives of Pediatrics & Adolescent Medicine, 148*(12), 1271–1276.

Chalupa R., & Hooker R. S. (2016). Physician assistants in orthopaedic surgery: education, role, distribution, compensation. *Journal of the American Academy of Physician Assistants, 29*(5), 1–7

Costa, D. K., Wallace, D. J., Barnato, A. E., & Kahn, J. M. (2014). Nurse practitioner/physician assistant staffing and critical care mortality. *Chest, 146*, 1566–1573.

Dhuper, S., & Choksi, S. (2009). Replacing an academic internal medicine residency program with a physician assistant–hospitalist model: A comparative analysis study. *American Journal of Medical Quality, 24*(2), 132–139.

Gillard, J. N., Szoke, A., Hoff, W. S., Wainwright, G. A., Stehly, C. D., & Toedter, L. J. (2011). Utilization of PAs and NPs at a level I trauma center: Effects on outcomes. *Journal of the American Academy of Physician Assistants, 24*(7), 34–43.

Halpern, N. A., Pastores, S. M., Oropello, J. M., & Kvetan, V. (2013). Critical care medicine in the United States: Addressing the intensivist shortage and image of the specialty. *Critical Care Medicine, 41*(12), 2754–2761.

Institute of Medicine (IOM). (2001). *Crossing the quality chasm: A new health system for the 21st century.* Washington, DC: IOM.

Kaups, K. L., Parks, S. N., & Morris, C. L. (1998). Intracranial pressure monitor placement by midlevel practitioners. *Journal of Trauma, 45*(5), 884–886.

Kohn, L., Corrigan, J., & Donaldson, M. (Eds.). (2000). *To err is human: Building a safer health system.* Washington, DC: National Academies Press.

Larson, E. H., Coerver, D. A., Wick, K. H., & Ballweg, R. A. (2011). Physician assistants in orthopedic practice: A national study. *Journal of Allied Health, 40*(4), 174–180.

Marsters, C. E. (2000). Pneumothorax as a complication of central venous cannulation performed by physician assistants. *Surgical Physician Assistant, 6*(3), 18–24.

Miller, W., Riehl, E., Napier, M., Barber, K., & Dabideen, H. (1998). Use of physician assistants as surgery/trauma house staff at an American College of Surgeons–verified level II trauma center. *Journal of Trauma, 44*(2), 372–376.

Nabagiez, J. P., Shariff, M. A., Molloy, W. J., Demissie, S., & McGinn, J. T. (2016). Cost analysis of physician assistant home visit program to reduce readmissions after cardiac surgery. *The Annals of Thoracic Surgery, 102*(3), 696–702.

National Commission on the Certification of Physician Assistants (NCCPA). (2015). *2014 Statistical profile of recently certified physician assistants: An annual report of the National Commission on the Certification of Physician Assistants.* Retrieved from http://www.nccpa.net/uploads/docs/recentlycertifiedreport2014.pdf

Oswanski, M. F., Sharma, O. P., & Shekhar, S. R. (2004). Comparative review of use of physician assistants in a level I trauma center. *American Surgeon, 70*(3), 272–279.

Rosenberg, C. E. (1987). *The care of strangers: The rise of America's hospital system.* New York: Basic Books.

Roy, C. L., Liang, C. L., Lund, M., Boyd, C., Katz, J. T., McKean, S., & Schnipper, J. L. (2008). Implementation of a physician assistant/hospitalist service in an academic medical center: impact on efficiency and patient outcomes. *Journal of Hospital Medicine, 3*(5), 361–368.

Schulman, M., Lucchese, K., & Sullivan, A. (1995). Transition from housestaff to nonphysicians as neonatal intensive care providers: Cost, impact on revenue, and quality of care. *American Journal of Perinatology, 12*(6), 442–446.

Simmer, T., Nerenz, D., Rutt, W., Newcomb, C., & Benfer, D. (1991). A randomized, controlled trial of an attending staff service in general internal medicine. *Medical Care, 29*(7), JS31–JS40.

Singh, S., Fletcher, K. E., Schapira, M. M., Conti, M., Tarima, S., Biblo, L. A., & Whittle, J. (2011). A comparison of outcomes of general medical inpatient care provided by a hospitalist-physician assistant model vs a traditional resident-based model. *Journal of Hospital Medicine, 6*(3), 122–130.

US Department of Health and Human Services, Office of the Inspector General. (2010). *Adverse events in hospitals: National incidence among Medicare beneficiaries* (OEI-06-09-00090). Retrieved from https://oig.hhs.gov/oei/reports/oei-06-09-00090.pdf

CHAPTER **8**

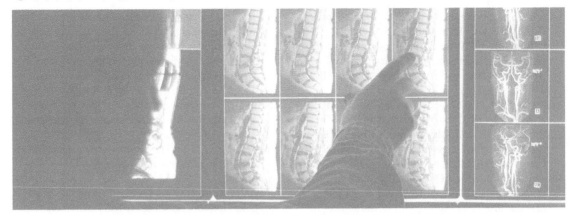

PHYSICIAN ASSISTANTS IN RURAL HEALTH

RODERICK S. HOOKER ■ CHRISTINE M. EVERETT ■ JAMES F. CAWLEY

"The public health infrastructure in rural America is not well understood but is potentially the most fragile aspect of the rural healthcare continuum."
— *Thomas C. Ricketts, 1999*

Physician assistants (PAs) play a key role in increasing access to care in rural areas, especially in North America. They are proportionally more likely to provide family medicine in rural locations than are doctors, and they do so with lower labor costs. In many of the nonmetropolitan facilities where they work, PAs provide a wide range of services for patients ranging in age from newborns to the elderly and they treat a diversity of illnesses and emergencies. Their adaptability to their surroundings and ability to fit in has endeared them to many communities in US and Canada. This adaptability will be more visible as their presence expands globally. In some instances, PAs have come from rural areas and have returned home to practice. This trend is apparent in western and southwestern communities as well as in Alaska. The federal government has used various policies to promote the employment of PAs, such as requiring rural health clinics to employ at least one PA,

nurse practitioner (NP), or nurse-midwife and offering loan repayment programs for bonded rural service. These policies have had mixed successes.

PROBLEMS ASSOCIATED WITH RURAL HEALTH

Most industrialized nations face the issue of having insufficient numbers of healthcare providers who are willing to work and live in rural areas. According to the Health Resources and Services Administration (HRSA), as of 2011, approximately 16% of North Americans live in rural areas, but less than 10% of doctors practice there. North America is hardly unique; other countries suffer similar if not worse statistics. Still, no two countries define "rural health" quite the same way. For some countries, it is a definition of geographic location or population density. For example, Australia uses the term *remote* to define a uniquely isolated community, whereas the United States uses the term *frontier counties* to designate very rural areas, such as in the far west and most of the boroughs of Alaska. Most demographers define "rural" as sparsely clustered communities that are not metropolitan. Often, the term needs to be parsed to enable publicly funded programs to assist rural populations.

For the purposes of this chapter, *rural* is defined according to the HRSA division of the US Department of Health and Human Services as encompassing "all population, housing, and territory not included within an urban area. Whatever is not urban is considered rural." Other terms sometimes used include *nonmetropolitan*, *nonurban*, and *micropolitan* (although *suburban* and *semirural* may also be included).

Access to healthcare in rural areas depends on a sufficient supply and distribution of healthcare providers. The methods employed to attempt to attain this supply and distribution also vary by country. Certain countries, including the United States, Australia, Canada, and South Africa, have been singled out as making a concerted effort toward developing PAs to manage healthcare needs in these areas (Table 8–1). Other countries, such as those in eastern Europe, sub-Saharan Africa, and Asia, have adopted policies that require doctors to serve some period of time working in rural and underserved regions or have introduced some other form of policy to help address the shortage of doctors.

Despite the efforts on four continents to meet the needs of citizens, the rural people of the world are wanting. The issues for rural healthcare delivery are fairly universal:

- Delivery of needed health resources is underserviced due to a maldistribution of resources, infrastructure, economics, and labor.
- The needed population for economic viability of a doctor or clinic is often too small.
- Specialty services tend to be scarce and people who require specialty care face economical and geographical barriers.

To understand the healthcare needs of people living in rural populations as well as the role that PAs can play in these populations, one must consider explicitly the impact of competitive forces and public policy developments on rural healthcare systems along with the patients and communities they serve.

RURAL HEALTHCARE IN THE UNITED STATES

Overview

The devolution of responsibility for healthcare, income security, employment and training programs, and social services from the US federal government to the states has been gradual but has left general and rural areas within states and provinces struggling for infrastructure to meet adequate care. Rural communities are experiencing changes caused by many of the same forces that are affecting urban areas. However, because of the structure of the healthcare system, the characteristics of the population, and other realities of rural life that differ in significant ways from those of the urban experience, the market and policy effects

TABLE 8-1
Population Statistics—Doctors and Physician Assistants (PAs), 2013

Country	Population	No. of PAs	No. of Doctors	Doctor/Population Ratio	Percent Rural* Population
Australia	23,092,132	2	47,875	3.9/1,000	7
Canada	35,141,542	270	66,583	2.1/1,000	20
The Netherlands	16,793,200	275	50,854	3.2/1,000	34
Scotland	5,062,011	12	12,738	2.5/1,000	20
South Africa	52,981,991	60	30,740	0.8/1,000	43
United Kingdom	63,181,775	226	133,641	2.8/1,000	11
United States	316,291,000	85,000	650,000	2.4/1,000	20

*Rural is defined by each country.

of these forces in rural areas can be quite different from the effects in urban areas.

The absence of a provider, whether it be a health facility or a health professional's practice, is potentially greater in rural areas. Because alternative sources of care within reasonable proximity in the community are scarce, each provider plays a critical part in maintaining access to healthcare in the community. For this reason, in most rural communities, all providers should be considered part of the healthcare safety net—if not directly through the care they provide to vulnerable populations, then indirectly through their contribution to the stability of the community's healthcare infrastructure. Moreover, the healthcare infrastructure in a rural community is likely to be a mainstay of the community's economy. In addition to the constantly evolving healthcare marketplace, factors that influence the structure and strength of the rural healthcare safety net include demography, geography, and policies at the federal, state, and local levels. The safety net in rural areas generally includes almost all local providers. Therefore, maintaining the safety net in rural communities strengthens the entire healthcare infrastructure.

In the United States, doctors, PAs, nurse practitioners (NPs), certified nurse-midwives (CNMs), dentists, and a host of other healthcare professionals play key roles in delivering care to rural populations. However, the ability of rural communities to maintain healthcare services for their residents in the changing healthcare environment is a challenge. Although maintaining physician supply and distribution have historically been the focus of this problem, in the late 1980s, attention began shifting to relying on PAs and NPs as additional providers for bolstering primary healthcare when it became apparent that many of them were successfully filling these rural provider roles.

Family/general physicians are the principal healthcare providers in rural America, as well as in rural areas of such countries as Australia, Canada, Africa, parts of Europe, Asia and Central/South America. Family medicine is the only medical specialty in which the ratio of physicians to population is greater in rural areas than in urban areas (Table 8–2). In addition, in the United States, more PAs practice family medicine than any other medical specialty; however, the percentages are falling. The medical specialties of primary care make up the majority of PA practice in general and in rural areas in particular. Approximately one-third of PAs report they practice in communities with populations of 50,000 or less and a smaller percentage report practicing in rural areas with less than 20,000 people (American Academy of Physician Assistants [AAPA], 2013). Family medicine is the predominant specialty of PA practice in rural areas.

On the state level, researchers in Texas, North Carolina, Washington State, California, Utah, and others have found that, compared with doctors, PAs are in higher levels of visibility in small communities. Jones (2008) analyzed

TABLE 8-2
Distribution of Urban and Rural Visits by Specialty of US Doctors, 1996 to 1997

	Percent of Visits All Patients			
	Family Practice	*General Practice*	*Internal Medicine*	*Pediatrics*
Urban	34.2	8.9	29.9	27.0
Rural	60.3	9.3	22.1	8.3
	Patients Ages 14 Years and Younger			
Urban	16.0	5.0	2.0	77.0
Rural	53.0	4.0	2.0	41.0

Data from Probst, J. C., Moore, C. G., Baxley, E. G., & Lammie, J. J. (2002). Rural–urban differences in visits to primary care physicians. *Family Medicine, 34*(8), 609–615.

the 254 counties of Texas by population, persons per square mile, and specialty for clinically active doctors and PAs. A total of 60 counties (24%) were populated with six or fewer people per square mile—thus meeting the federal guideline of "frontier" county. In the 60 frontier counties of Texas, there were 32 PAs and 75 primary care physicians, or 1 PA per 2.3 physicians. Fourteen of the 32 PAs (44%) were female. Seventeen Texas counties (exceeding the land mass of Connecticut, Vermont, and Rhode Island) had no licensed physician.

The distribution of PAs in other states also appears to be related to population density (Figure 8–1). Several studies have demonstrated that the smaller the community, the more likely it is to have practicing PAs and NPs.

Reasons Rural Healthcare Is Unique

Many factors associated with rural areas affect the health of rural citizens (Table 8–3). For example, lack of access to providers is a common healthcare obstacle in rural areas. Rural residents commonly have transportation difficulties with reaching healthcare providers, sometimes traveling great distances to reach a care provider or hospital.

Economic and social factors also create a unique milieu that influences healthcare in rural areas. For example:

■ Rural residents tend to be poorer. On average, the per capita income is $7,417 lower than in urban areas, and rural Americans are more likely to live below the poverty level. The disparity in incomes is even

FIGURE 8-1
Distribution of PAs in Rural US Locations (per 100,000 population)

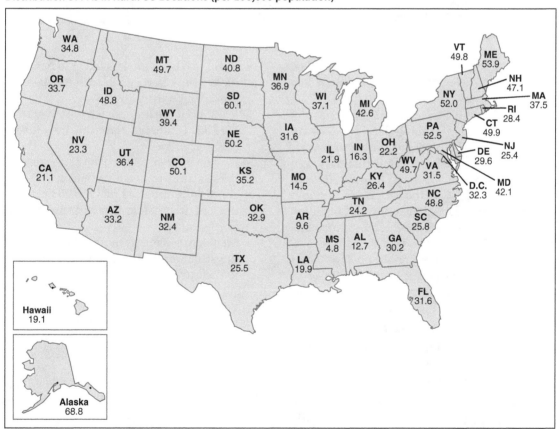

Data from *Hooker, R. S., & Muchow, A. N. (2014). Census of physician assistants: 2013.* Journal of the American Academy of Physician Assistants, 27(7), 34–40.

TABLE 8-3
A National Rural Health Snapshot, 2005

Characteristic	Rural	Urban
Percentage of US population	25%	75%
Percentage of US physicians	10%	90%
No. of specialists per 100,000 population	40.1	134.1
Population aged 65 and older	18%	15%
Population below the poverty level	14%	11%
Average per capita income	$19,000	$26,000
Population who are non-Hispanic whites	83%	69%
Adults who describe health status as fair/poor	28%	21%
Adolescents (ages 12–17) who smoke	19%	11%
Male death rate per 100,000 (ages 1–24)	80	60
Female death rate per 100,000 (ages 1–24)	40	30
Population covered by private insurance	64%	69%
Population who are Medicare beneficiaries	23%	20%
Medicare beneficiaries without drug coverage	45%	31%
Medicare spent per capita compared with US average	85%	106%
Medicare hospital payment-to-cost ratio	90%	100%
Percentage of poor covered by Medicaid	45%	49%

Statistics used with permission from the Rural Wisconsin Health Cooperative, *Eye on Health,* from an article titled "Rural Health Can Lead the Way" by former NRHA President, Tim Size; Executive Director of the Rural Wisconsin Health Cooperative.

greater for minorities living in rural areas. Nearly 24% of rural children live in poverty.

- People who live in rural America rely more heavily on the federal food stamp program. The National Rural Health Association's analysis found that although 22% of Americans lived in rural areas in 2013, a full 31% of the nation's food stamp beneficiaries lived there. In all, 4.6 million rural residents received food stamp benefits in 2013.
- The health professional shortage areas (HPSAs) in rural and frontier areas of all states and US territories number 2,157, compared with 910 in urban areas.

Certain healthcare-related factors also make rural healthcare unique. These factors range from issues of access and availability to issues of payment and coverage. For example:

- Only about 10% of physicians practice in rural America despite the fact that nearly one-sixth of the population lives in these areas.

- Rural residents are less likely to have employer-provided healthcare coverage and prescription drug coverage.
- Rural poor are less likely to be covered by Medicaid benefits than are their urban counterparts.
- Anywhere from 57% to 90% of first responders in rural areas are volunteers.
- Dentists number 60 per 100,000 populations in urban areas versus 40 per 100,000 in rural areas.
- Medicare payments to rural hospitals and physicians are dramatically less than those to their urban counterparts for equivalent services. This statistic correlates closely with the fact that more than 470 rural hospitals have closed since 1990.
- Mental health services are lacking in 20% of nonmetropolitan counties versus only 5% of metropolitan counties. In 1999, 87% of the 1669 mental health professional shortage areas in the United States were in nonmetropolitan counties and home to more than 30 million people (Gamm et al., 2003).

Research has also shown that certain healthcare issues tend to be more prevalent in rural areas. For example:

■ Cerebrovascular disease is 1.45 higher in rural areas than it is in urban areas.

■ Hypertension is higher in rural areas than it is in urban areas (128.8 per 1,000 individuals in rural areas versus 101.3 per 1,000 individuals in urban areas).

■ The suicide rate among certain populations in rural areas is significantly higher than that in urban areas. In particular, adult men and all children under the age 18 are at higher risk for suicide than their urban cohorts.

■ The suicide rate among rural women is approaching that of men.

■ Medicare patients with acute myocardial infarction (AMI) who are treated in rural hospitals are less likely to receive recommended treatments than are those treated in urban hospitals. They also have significantly higher adjusted 30-day post-AMI death rates from all causes.

■ Although only one-third of all motor vehicle accidents occur in rural areas, two-thirds of the deaths attributed to these accidents occur on rural roads.

■ Death and serious injury accidents account for 60% of total rural accidents versus only 48% of urban accidents. One reason for this increased rate of morbidity and mortality is that, in rural areas, prolonged delays can occur between a crash, the call for emergency medical services (EMS), and the arrival of an EMS provider. Many of these delays are related to increased travel distances in rural areas and personnel distribution across the response area. National average response times from motor vehicle accident to EMS arrival in rural areas was 18 minutes, which is 8 minutes greater than in urban areas (Gamm et al., 2003).

■ Rural residents are nearly twice as likely to die of unintentional injuries other than motor vehicle accidents than are urban residents.

■ Rural residents have a significantly higher risk of death by gunshot than do urban residents.

■ Abuse of alcohol and tobacco is a significant problem among rural youth. The rate of driving under the influence arrests is significantly greater in nonurban counties; 40% of rural 12th graders reported using alcohol while driving compared with 25% of their urban counterparts. Rural eighth graders are twice as likely to smoke cigarettes (26.1% vs. 12.7% in large metropolitan areas; Gamm et al., 2003).

Improving Rural Healthcare Access

Primary care and rural health were the two driving reasons for the original development of the PA concept. Early on, the central government thought PAs could be a vital part of the healthcare infrastructure that supports ambulatory and institutional care in rural areas. In 1977, the US Congress enacted the Rural Health Clinics Act (Public Law [PL] 95-210) to encourage the use of PAs, NPs, and CNMs in rural areas. This decision was based on a growing realization that many small communities could no longer support a sufficient number of physicians. PL 95-210 facilitated this goal by entitling various healthcare providers to receive reimbursement from Medicare and Medicaid on a cost basis. This policy continues into the 21st century with various modifications that enable rural health clinics (RHCs) to remain in operation as characteristics of staffing and populations change.

RURAL HEALTH PHYSICIAN ASSISTANTS

Characteristics

A rural health PA is one who identifies his or her location of employment, either by a policy definition or the characteristics of his or her employer (designation, geographic location, etc.), as "rural." PAs who work in rural health do not necessarily need to live in rural locations. In its annual census, the AAPA (2013) identifies PAs by population density and notes that between 9% and 10% of PAs practice in rural areas (census <20,000), depending on specialty (Table 8–4).

In Pennsylvania, the state with the largest rural population, a survey revealed significant differences in socioeconomic, demographic, and practice profile parameters between rural and urban providers. For example, providers in rural areas are more likely than their urban counterparts to practice in a primary care setting, they see more patients per week, and they are the principal provider of care for a higher percentage of their patients. Moreover, a rural PA is more likely than an urban PA to practice in an underserved area—at least in Pennsylvania (Table 8–5). For rural and urban PAs who practice primary care, significant differences were noted in their willingness to practice in a rural underserved area compared with PAs who do not practice in primary care.

Little is known about the propensity of PAs to care for underserved populations, but research evidences this trend. One study compared the numbers of primary care clinicians in two states that have significant rural populations and a long history of using PAs and NPs in rural areas (California and Washington). This study found that PAs ranked first or second in each state in the proportion of their members practicing in rural areas and HPSAs. In California, the number of PAs who were working with

TABLE 8-4
Distribution of US Physician Assistants in Rural Primary Care, 2013

	Family Medicine	General Internal Medicine	Pediatrics	Obstetrics and Gynecology (Women's Health)
Number who responded to survey	5,572	1,497	516	485
Percent of all PAs	23.8	6.4	2.2	2.1
Mean age	42	42	40	39
Percent female	62	67	76	96
Percent Rural Distribution of Primary Care Physician Assistants				
Nonmetropolitan population 20,000–1 million	10.4	9.0	8.6	7.2
Nonmetropolitan population 2,500–20,000	14.5	6.4	7.8	3.8
Nonmetropolitan population <2,500	5.2	1.4	0.4	0.2

Data reprinted with permission from American Academy of Physician Assistants (AAPA). (2013). *2012 AAPA Physician Assistant Census Report.* Alexandria, VA: Author.

TABLE 8-5
Characteristics of Rural and Urban Physician Assistant Respondents

Characteristic	Urban (N = 491)	Rural (N = 190)	Test of Differences Between Samples	Statistical Significance (P)
Age	39.40 (7.87)*	39.29 (8.14)*	$F = 0.030$	.863
Gender			Chi-square = 10.603	
Male	37.6 (183)[†]	51.3 (97)[†]		.001
Female	62.4 (304)	48.7 (92)		
Race			Chi-square = 6.395	
White	92.1 (452)[†]	97.4 (185)[†]		.011
Nonwhite	7.9 (39)	2.6 (5)		
Income	$53,545 ($17,188)*	$49,534 ($12,255)*	$F = 8.215$	.004

*Mean (SD).
[†]Percentage (number).
Data from Martin, K. E. (2000). A rural-urban comparison of patterns of physician assistant practice. *Journal of the Academy of Physician Assistants, 13*(7), 49–72.

vulnerable populations was also greater than those of other clinicians (Table 8–6).

In a study of Texas community health centers, the researchers probed as to why medical providers and support staff chose to work with the medically indigent and economically disadvantaged. They concluded that the level of care they were able to provide and the gratitude of patients seemed to make a difference. Overall PAs like their role, their coworkers, enjoy the collegiality of each other, are recognized for their skills and tasks that contribute to positive health outcomes for patients, and are trusted by clinical staff and patients (Henry & Hooker, 2014).

Clinical Activities

The scarcity of doctors in rural environments has increased the role of PAs. The literature on rural PAs holds that they provide cost-efficient and supplemental medical services to underserved rural populations and that these services are valued. Rural PAs also appear to possess a larger scope of practice than do urban PAs. This broad range of skills and procedures may be necessary to match the extensive healthcare needs of underserved rural populations. It appears that PAs are well adapted to rural health. Important issues regarding the recruitment and retention of PAs to rural populations also emerged. In the end, the progressive improvement in enabling legislation contributes to the utilization of PAs in America.

What PAs do and how often they provide care has been based more on assumption and less on documentation. However, some literature suggests that PAs are adept at procedures. A survey of Iowa family practice PAs identified the clinical activities, skills, and procedures of these practitioners and compared them with those of family practice physicians in the same state. The undertaking was an effort to understand the skill set a PA would require when entering rural healthcare. Iowa PAs reported a wide range of activities, including providing patient education, prescribing and dispensing medication, interpreting radiographs, and evaluating and referring patients (Table 8–7). The study documented that PAs possess a wide

TABLE 8-6
Percentage of Clinicians Practicing in Underserved Areas, by Type of Underserved Area

	Rural Area	Vulnerable Population Area	Primary Care Health Professional Shortage Area
CALIFORNIA	**13.0**	**39.0**	**28.0**
Family physician	13.2	30.5	24.2
General pediatrician	6.2	31.0	18.6
General internists	5.9	31.5	17.9
Obstetricians/gynecologists	6.3	28.3	16.9
Nurse practitioner	15.0	34.4	26.3
Physician assistants	21.7	47.7	35.2
Certified midwives	15.5	41.1	35.3
WASHINGTON	**24.0**	**40.0**	**38.6**
Family physician	23.6	45.6	43.5
General pediatrician	14.3	43.5	32.8
General internists	13.8	54.5	28.4
Obstetricians/gynecologists	13.7	52.9	31.6
Nurse practitioner	19.7	51.8	37.3
Physician assistants	27.8	50.3	42.1

Data from Grumbach, K., Hart, L. G., Mertz, E., Coffman, J, Palazzo, L. (2003). Who is caring for the underserved? A comparison of primary care physicians and nonphysician clinicians in California and Washington. *Annals of Family Medicine, 1*(2), 97–104.

TABLE 8-7
Activities Performed by Iowa Family Practice Physician Assistants by Frequency (N = 55)

Clinical Skill	Mean*	(SD)	Clinical Skill	Mean*	(SD)
Patient education	3.95	(0.30)	Neonatal checks	1.19	(1.02)
Dispense medication	3.44	(1.23)	Primary treatment of psychiatric illness (e.g., bipolar disorder, schizophrenia)	1.16	(1.10)
Make patient referrals directly to specialists	3.39	(0.68)			
X-ray film interpretation	3.19	(1.18)	Nasal packing for epistaxis	1.13	(0.71)
Electrotherapy or cryotherapy of the skin	2.92	(0.81)	Incise and drain external hemorrhoid	1.07	(0.77)
Counseling for contraception	2.91	(0.83)	Provide care to patients in a home setting (house calls)	1.00	(1.03)
Manage depression by drug therapy	2.82	(0.88)			
Counseling for smoking cessation	2.80	(0.88)	Perform audiometry	0.87	(1.18)
Repair and close laceration	2.75	(0.83)	Low-risk prenatal care	0.85	(1.15)
Counseling for stress management	2.61	(0.76)	Bladder catheterization	0.79	(0.57)
Electrocardiographic interpretation	2.60	(0.87)	Administer pulmonary function test	0.78	(1.15)
Manage depression by counseling	2.53	(1.03)	Joint injection	0.68	(0.83)
Removal of small skin lesions	2.43	(0.82)	Perform cardiopulmonary resuscitation	0.65	(0.62)
Psychological counseling	2.42	(1.13)	Perform advanced cardiac life support	0.65	(0.73)
Fluorescein eye examination or foreign body removal from eye	2.36	(0.65)	Bartholin cyst drainage	0.64	(0.52)
			Reduce fractures and dislocations	0.64	(0.73)
Perform vision screening	2.33	(1.39)	Diaphragm fitting	0.57	(0.64)
Use a microscope	2.15	(1.60)	Arthrocentesis	0.55	(0.72)
Incision and drainage of abscess	2.09	(0.66)	Perform advanced trauma life support	0.55	(0.69)
Counseling for alcohol abuse	1.93	(0.80)	Nasogastric tube placement	0.33	(0.58)
Provide care to patients in nursing homes	1.85	(1.47)	Endotracheal intubation	0.32	(0.51)
			Arterial blood gas draw	0.31	(0.63)
Evaluate wet mounts or potassium hydroxide stains	1.84	(1.50)	Use a slitlamp	0.30	(0.64)
			Perform breast mass aspiration	0.28	(0.49)
Involved in personal management activities	1.81	(1.49)	Norplant insertion/removal	0.25	(0.43)
			Perform Gram stain	0.11	(0.37)
Splinting and casting	1.78	(0.88)	Central venous line placement	0.06	(0.23)
Skin biopsy	1.73	(0.99)	Chest tube placement	0.04	(0.19)
Removal of ingrown toenail	1.71	(0.99)	Paracentesis or thoracentesis	0.04	(0.19)
Counseling for human immunodeficiency virus testing	1.63	(0.94)	Lumbar puncture	0.02	(0.14)
			Suprapubic tap on infants	0.02	(0.14)
Perform urinalysis	1.56	(1.74)	Colposcopy	0.00	(0.00)
Regional block with local anesthesia	1.49	(1.20)	Flexible sigmoidoscopy	0.00	(0.00)
Counseling for drug abuse	1.46	(0.88)	Obstetric ultrasonography	0.00	(0.00)
Venipuncture	1.25	(1.24)			

*Mean frequency of reported activity on a relative scale of 0 to 4. *Never* = 0; *a few times a year* = 1; *at least once a month* = 2; *at least once a week* = 3; *daily* = 4.

Data from Dehn, R., & Hooker, R. S. (1999). Procedures performed by Iowa family practice physician assistants. *Journal of the American Academy of Physician Assistants, 12*(4), 63–77.

range of skills and procedures and seem to use them frequently. One of the other findings of this study was that rural PAs regard themselves as generalists and place a fair amount of pride in their ability to be so versatile.

One survey of PAs practicing in rural Iowa found that the most commonly performed skill was dispensing medications (Figure 8–2). This trend was due to the lack of readily available pharmacy services in the small rural

FIGURE 8-2
Most Commonly Performed Skills in Communities of Less Than 10,000 (*N* = 94)

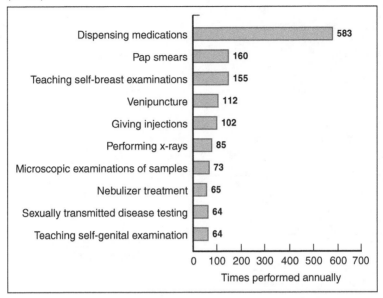

Data from *Asprey, D. (2006). Clinical skills utilized by physician assistants in rural primary care settings.* Journal of Physician Assistant Education, 17(2), 45–47.

communities in which the clinics were located. Other commonly identified skills included obtaining pap smears, teaching breast self-examinations, performing venipuncture, and providing injections. These findings suggest that PAs practicing in rural settings are responsible for providing a wide array of clinical services, including those that in many larger settings may be performed by other clinical personnel. In addition, the study determined that the rural practicing PAs considered cardiopulmonary resuscitation, suturing, and field-block anesthesia as the most important skills for their practices (Table 8–8).

Settings

Rural Health Clinics

The term *rural health clinic* refers to any outpatient medical center located in a nonmetropolitan area. As of 2015, the number of RHCs was approximately 4,084, with most located in HPSAs, medically underserved areas (MUAs), or governor-designated shortage areas (Figure 8–3). Federally certified "independent" RHCs are

TABLE 8-8
Skills Assigned Greatest Importance, Communities of <10,000 population (*N* = 94)

Rank	Skill	Average Level of Importance*
1	Cardiopulmonary resuscitation	4.9
2	Suturing	4.8
3	Field block anesthesia	4.7
3	Pap. smear	4.7
3	Sexually transmitted disease testing	4.7
3	Self-breast examination	4.7
7	Splinting of digits or extremities	4.6
7	Casting	4.6
9	Four items tied for ninth: cardioversion, intubation, incision and drainage of abscesses, microscopic wet smears	4.5

*Scale utilized is 1 = *low*, 5 = *high*.
Data from Asprey, D.P. (2006). Clinical skills utilized by physician assistants in rural primary care settings. Journal of Physician Assistant Education, 17(2), 45–47.

FIGURE 8-3
Map of Rural Health Clinics

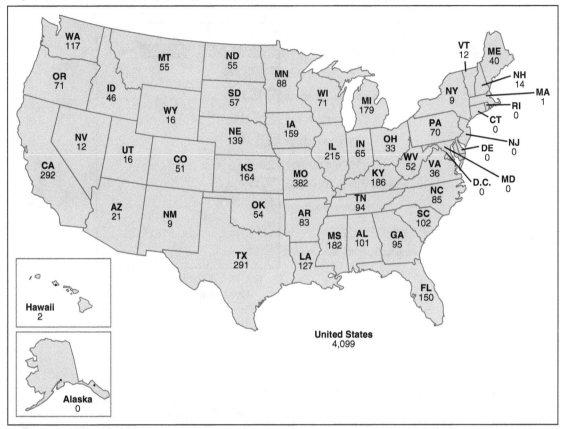

Data from *Centers for Medicare and Medicaid Services. (2013). CASPER Report 0006D Name and Address Listing for Rural Health Clinic Based on Current Survey. Retrieved from http://www.cms.gov/MLNProducts/downloads/rhclistbyprovidername.pdf*

reimbursed on a cost basis for their Medicare and Medicaid patients and are designed by the government to provide care that would not otherwise be available through enterprise or the marketplace.

Since the early 1980s, RHCs have made up one of the largest outpatient primary care programs for rural underserved communities and one of the fastest growing Medicare programs. By law, RHCs must be staffed by PAs, NPs, or CNMs at least half of the time they are open. Physician-owned facilities make up almost one-half of RHCs; hospitals and public and private companies own the rest (Figure 8–4 and Figure 8–5).

FIGURE 8-4
Distribution of Rural Health Clinic Ownership

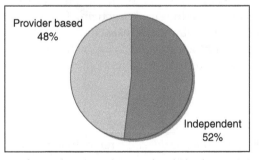

Data from *Gale, J. A., & Coburn A. F. (2003). The characteristics and roles of rural health clinics in the United States: A Chartbook. Portland, ME: University of Southern Maine, Edmund S. Muskie School of Public Service.*

FIGURE 8-5
US Rural Health Clinic Ownership

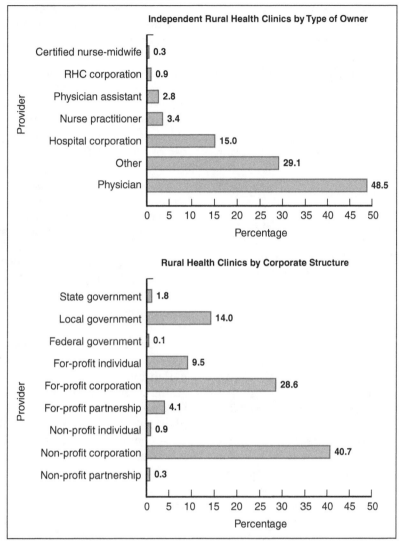

Data from *Gale, J. A., & Coburn A. F. (2003)*. The characteristics and roles of rural health clinics in the United States: A Chartbook. *Portland, ME: University of Southern Maine, Edmund S. Muskie School of Public Service.*

Although RHCs are required to employ a PA, an NP, or a CNM, they may receive a waiver of this requirement for up to 1 year. Approximately one-fifth of clinics have operated without a PA, an NP, or a CNM for some period, and many clinics have had problems retaining these practitioners. However, at the same time, more than one-third of RHCs reported they had problems retaining health-care professionals in general.

Rural Hospitals

Different markets and organizational factors tend to influence the employment of PAs and NPs by rural hospitals. A study involving an an eight-state region in the northwestern United States (Minnesota, North Dakota, South Dakota, Iowa, Montana, Idaho, Oregon, and Washington) revealed a greater demand for PAs and NPs in rural hospitals than in urban ones (Krein, 1997). Moreover, several differences exist in the characteristics of the hospitals that employ these clincians. Rural hospitals use PAs and NPs to enhance the delivery of outpatient services, and a major factor related to their employment is the RHC program. In the aggregate, rural hospitals seem to employ PAs and NPs for similar reasons:

- To extend care, assist physicians, or increase access to primary care
- Because physicians are unavailable or too difficult to recruit
- Because PA and NPs are considered cost-effective or more economical for rural areas
- For Rural Health Clinic certification

PAs and NPs appear to play a crucial role in this development and influence of provider-based RHC. The key variables that influence the establishment of rural hospitals are the measures of competitive pressures (e.g., hospital market share), physician resources, NP or PA practice regulations, hospital performance pressures (e.g., operating margin), innovativeness, and institutional pressure (i.e., the cumulative force of RHC adoption). The adoption of provider-based RHCs by rural hospitals appears to be motivated less as an adaptive response to observable economic or internal organizational signals than as a reaction to bandwagon pressures.

Another conclusion of Krein's research (1997) was that rural hospitals with limited resources tend to have an inadequate ability to fully evaluate strategic activities for remaining viable. One strategy for remaining viable is the employment of PAs and NPs, which serves as a cost-effective strategy for a hospital referral base. Additionally, because PAs and NPs are more flexible than doctors, they are easier to employ in outlying rural clinics. Although the author concluded that such activity could have a harmful effect on some providers and some rural residents, evidence of harm has not been

demonstrated in the decades since the study was conducted.

In a national study of all patient visits from 2001 to 2010 using the National Hospital Ambulatory Medical Care Survey (NHAMCS), all visits to hospital-based clinics were examined. Ten years of survey results were analyzed to estimate the total share of visits by provider type and to identify differences in patient characteristics evaluated by each primary care provider. A trend analysis identified that the use of PA and NPs almost doubled, reflecting growth of the professions and their utilization. In the aggregate, NPs (8.9%) and PAs (5.4%) attended 14% of 777 million weighted visits that were examined, with NPs and PAs managing 36% of visits in nonmetropolitan areas. Over the latter 5 years, NPs and PAs were the provider of record for one-fifth of visits involving at least one major chronic condition. For all three providers, the most common chronic disease visits were diabetes and hypertension. There were few significant differences in patient characteristics. NPs were more represented in pediatrics, women's health, and geriatric encounters than were PAs. When examining nonmetropolitan visits, hypertension was the most frequent of all diagnoses seen by physicians (3.4%) and PAs (5.4%) and the third most common diagnosis for NP visits (3.9%). PAs were proportionally more represented than NPs in nonmetropolitan clinics (Table 8–9). The authors concluded that the proportional distribution of primary care chronic disease visits is similar for PAs, NPs, and physicians. But PAs and NPs are providing a significantly larger proportion of care for patients in nonmetropolitan areas, and this is a trend that is increasing (Table 8–10).

ISSUES FOR PHYSICIAN ASSISTANTS WHO WORK IN RURAL AREAS

Retention

The issue of retaining PAs who work in rural areas is a complicated one. In one study, a team of workforce specialists and medical anthropologists visited several towns to interview the residents of the town as well as the

TABLE 8-9
Characteristics of Outpatient Department Visits, Percent Share of Visits by Provider Type, 2001 to 2010

	Physician	Physician Assistant	Nurse Practitioner	Total
CENSUS GEOGRAPHIC REGION				
Northeast	87.8	3.7	8.5	20,000,000
Midwest	85.2	5.9	8.9	24,000,000
South	83.7	5.2	11.2	24,000,000
West	86.2	7.8	6.0	10,000,000
METROPOLITAN AREA STATUS				
MSA	89.8	2.9	7.3	60,000,000
Non-MSA	64.4	17.3	18.4	13,000,000
Total	85.4	5.4	9.2	73,000,000
TYPE OF CLINIC				
General Medicine	81.9	7.7	10.4	48,000,000
Surgery	95.4	2.5	2.0	10,000,000
Pediatric	92.8	1.0	6.2	9,800,000
Obstetrics & Gynecology	82.0	1.8	16.3	6,500,000
Substance Abuse	93.5	0.3	6.2	150,000
Other	90.3	1.9	7.8	4,600,000
Total (Percentages)	85.5	5.4	9.1	100.0
Total (Visits)	62,000,000	3,900,000	6,700,000	79,000,000

Data from Hooker, R. S., Benitez, J. A., Coplan, B. H., & Dehn, R. W. (2013). Ambulatory and chronic disease care by physician assistants and nurse practitioners. *Journal of Ambulatory Care Management, 36*(4), 293–301.

TABLE 8-10
Number of Hospital Outpatient Department Visits and Percentage of Visits by Provider Type, 2001 to 2010

Data from the National Hospital Ambulatory Medical Care Survey							
Year	Physician		PA		NP/CNM		Total
	Estimated Visits	Percent Share of Visits	Estimated Visits	Percent Share of Visits	Estimated Visits	Percent Share of	Estimated Visits Visits
2001	5,800,000	87	340,000	5	510,000	8	6,700,000
2010	7,200,000	84	460,000	5	910,000	11	8,500,000
Total	68,000,000	86	4,200,000	5	7,200,000	9	79,000,000

Approximately 79 million weighted visits. Nurse practitioners (NP)/certified nurse-midwives (CNMs) and physicians assistants (PAs) 11.4 million: 24% increase in physician visits, 35% increase in PA visits, 78% increase in NP visits.
From Hooker, R. S., Benitez, J. A., Coplan, B. H., & Dehn, R. W. (2013). Ambulatory and chronic disease care by physician assistants and nurse practitioners. *Journal of Ambulatory Care Management, 36*(4), 293–301.

town PA (Box 8–1 and Figure 8–6). The results were surprising; only one of the eight PAs was raised in a small town—the rest grew up in urban areas. Those with families were there primarily for the amenities of a small town and, as one PA said, "so my child could ride his bike down the main street, and if [he was] hurt, someone would take care of him." All but one PA lived in the town where they worked (the eighth lived in a nearby town that had a high school for his children). Most of the PAs were involved with civic activity (for example, members of the Lions Club. PTA, etc.), and all socialized with the residents

BOX 8-1
Criteria for Retention of Rural Physician Assistants Study

- The PA had to be working autonomously in a rural health clinic with no more than 8 hours per week with the supervising doctor.
- The PA had to be employed as the sole primary care practitioner in the community.
- The PA had to have worked in the community for more than 24 months before being interviewed.
- The town (or census tract) was smaller than 5,000 persons and in Texas.
- Town residents had no other primary care options within a 40-km radius.
- The PA and the town leaders were willing to be interviewed.

Data from Henry, L. R., & Hooker, R. S. (2007). Retention of physician assistants in rural health clinics. *Journal of Rural Health, 23*(3), 207–214.

of the town by eating at the local diner or attending activities together. Most of the towns were quite remote (Table 8–11), and the commuting distance to a larger town was far; none were close to a major highway. Seven of the eight PAs were not bound by a contract or other links to the town and were free to move away if they wanted. Two of the PAs were

female, and all eight were married (Henry & Hooker, 2008).

Most of the PAs in this rural study were employees of a hospital system some distance away. Almost all were dissatisfied with the hospital as owner of the clinic, primarily due to inefficiencies, bureaucracies, or reimbursement errors that consumed unnecessary administrative time. Yet all of the PAs were satisfied with their careers and their relationships with their towns. They liked their clinic staff and had a good relationship with their supervising doctor. This group of rural PAs maintained contact with the supervising doctor primarily via phone, but some cited that they also used beepers or e-mail. Texas State Board of Medical Examiners policy requires the supervising doctor to work in the same clinic with the PA at least 8 hours every 2 weeks. Both the supervising physician and the PA adhered this to policy requirement and commented positively about seeing each other on a periodic basis for professional reasons. None were planning to leave their clinic or role.

The retention of PAs in some rural practices is high. In one survey, PAs listed all of the places where they had practiced since completing their PA training, making it possible to

FIGURE 8-6
Age and Years in Rural Health Location of Texas Physician Assistants

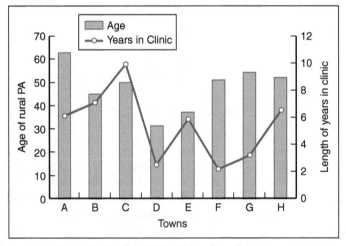

Data from *Henry, L. R., & Hooker, R. S. (2007). Retention of physician assistants in rural health clinics.* Journal of Rural Health, 23*(3), 207–214.*

TABLE 8-11
Characteristics of Rural Towns Served by Physician Assistants

	Town A	Town B	Town C	Town D	Town E	Town F	Town G	Town H
Population	637	2,235	241	2,589	844	2,424	800	740
RUCA code*	5	5	10.5	10.5	5	10	10.6	10
Distance from nearest town (miles)	30	25	60	32	25	30	80	25
Median age	40.4	39.3	46.1	37.8	38	38.7	43	42.7
Median household income	$28,333	$42,098	$28,281	$41,686	$20,278	$24,712	$23,594	$27,778

*Rural-Urban Commuting Area (RUCA, Version 2.0) codes. RUCA codes range from 1 to 10.6, with 1 being the most urban and 10.6 being the most rural. A RUCA code of 5 means that the census tract is strongly tied to a large town, with primary flow 30% or more to a large town. A RUCA code of 10 means that the town is considered an isolated small rural census tract, with less than 5% primary flow to a larger town. A RUCA code of 10.6 is slightly more rural than a code of 10.
Data from Henry, L. R., & Hooker, R. S. (2007). Retention of physician assistants in rural health clinics. *Journal of Rural Health, 23*(3), 207–214.

classify the career histories of PAs as "all rural," "all urban," "urban to rural," or "rural to urban." The study examined the retention of PAs in rural practice at several levels: in the first practice, in rural practice overall, and by predominantly rural states. PAs who started their careers in rural locations were more likely to leave their positions during the first 4 years of practice than were urban PAs, and female rural PAs were slightly more likely to leave than were their male counterparts. Those starting in rural practice had high attrition, and 41% left for urban areas; however, a significant proportion of PAs who started in urban practice settings left for rural settings (10%). Because the proportion of urban PAs is so much larger than that of rural PAs, this movement kept the total proportion of PAs in rural practice at a steady 20%. Although 21% of the earliest graduates of PA training programs have had exclusively rural careers, only 9% of PAs with 4 to 7 years of experience have worked exclusively in rural settings (Figure 8–7). At the state level, generalist PAs were significantly more likely to leave states with practice environments unfavorable to PA practice in terms of prescriptive authority, reimbursement, and insurance. Major perceived barriers to rural recruitment include low salaries, cultural isolation, poor-quality schools, limited desirable housing, and lack of spousal job opportunities. The conclusion is that some locations face substantial challenges in recruitment of clinical staff. The largest numbers of unfilled positions were for family physicians at a time of declining interest in family medicine among graduating medical students.

Community Acceptance

The issue of how PAs are perceived by rural America has also been of interest to sociologists. Before the new century, the issue of community acceptance sometimes surfaced. Interviews with townsfolk about the town PA revealed that only two-thirds had used the clinic. The main reason cited for not using the PA or the clinic was that they had a relationship with a doctor in some other town. Almost all said they would like to have a doctor instead of a PA but that a PA was better than no medical care provider. For some parents, the presence of a health clinic, regardless of the type of provider, was the reason they stayed in the town. If the clinic were not available, some parents of young children said they would move closer to an urban area.

Baldwin and colleagues (1998) also explored community acceptance of PAs and NPs in rural, MUAs. Community acceptance in the context of this study implied not only satisfaction with the care received but also willingness of the community to support an NP or a PA practice through its infrastructure and encourage members to initially seek and continue to receive care from an NP or a PA. Five focus groups were conducted in each of five rural, medically underserved communities. The two

FIGURE 8-7
Current Practice Location and Specialty by Total Experience

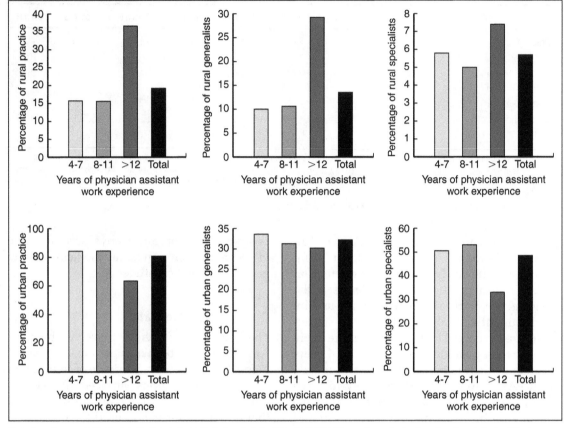

Data from *Larson, E. H., Hart, L. G., Goodwin, M. K., Geller, J., & Andrilla, C. (1999). Dimensions of retention: A national study of the locational histories of physician assistants.* Journal of Rural Health, 15(4), 391–402.

most pervasive findings were the lack of previous exposure to NPs and PAs and the general belief that PA and NPs would be accepted in these communities if certain conditions could be met. The theme of conditional acceptance included personal and system factors. Personal factors included friendliness, competence, willingness to enter into the life of the community, and the ability to keep information confidential. System factors considered critical for acceptance included service type, integration with the existing healthcare system, cost, geographic proximity, and availability.

Another study used survey data from 285 small rural hospitals and case studies of 36 of these hospitals were analyzed to answer questions about the extent to which PAs and NPs provide primary care in small, rural hospitals; the benefits that they might bring to the hospitals; and the reactions of the public to such providers. The Healthcare Financing Administration in 1993 and 1994 collected the data as part of an evaluation of the hospitals. Most of the hospitals used the following: 70% NPs, 30% PAs, and 20% both. Although some patients had negative reactions to the use of PAs and NPs, most accepted them. The hospitals benefitted in the form of reduced recruitment costs, increased revenues, and increased service offerings. The authors concluded that PA and NP practitioners are beneficial to rural hospitals and that communities should develop and implement mechanisms to encourage their acceptance (Bergeron, Neuman, & Kinsey, 1999).

Physician Acceptance

Focusing on a different perspective, Isberner and colleagues (2003) surveyed rural Illinois physicians to identify incentives and constraints that influence their receptivity to utilization of PAs. Receptive physicians reported six incentives related to appointments, workload, productivity, education/counseling, complex cases, and patient satisfaction. Unreceptive physicians identified four constraints related to perceived patient opposition, malpractice risk, overstepping authority, and continuity of care. Receptive physicians also identified perceived patient opposition as a constraint.

Reimbursement

Another important issue for rural PAs is a favorable reimbursement policy. Because state-to-state variability in compensation and Medicaid reimbursement laws affects PA deployment, increased efforts should be directed toward tailoring state policies to adequately compensate PAs. Reimbursement is also considered a critical indicator of output and is commonly used as a benchmark for productivity. Evidence based on productivity measures, salaries, and costs of medical education indicates that PAs and NPs are cost-effective employees of rural clinics.

Productivity in Rural Areas

An important issue in health workforce analysis is how to count the contribution of each provider and each provider type to patient care. Simple head counts of providers are unlikely to produce realistic estimates of the actual supply of healthcare available to a population. Differences in training, location, specialty, inpatient care activities, experience, scope of practice, and full-time versus part-time status create large differences in the number of visits that a given clinician is likely to perform during a week. If, for example, an average family physician provides 105 ambulatory patient visits each week, a general pediatrician 95, and a general internist about 65, then there is some idea of productivity by specialty. If estimates of available care include PAs and NPs, then basing estimates of available care on head counts becomes yet more

doubtful because so little is known about the productivity of PAs and NPs and their total contribution to care.

Larson and colleagues (2003) wanted to understand the contribution to generalist care made by PAs and NPs in underserved rural areas. Their study addressed the following questions:

- What is the total contribution to generalist care made by PA and NPs?
- What is the role of PAs or NPs in providing generalist care in rural HPSAs?
- What proportion of total generalist care is provided by women doctors, PAs, and NPs?

They found that women make up an increasing part of the physician and PA workforce. In fact, female PAs and NPs make up a larger share of the care provided to women than do female doctors. Combined, female PAs and NPs represented 51% of full-time equivalents provided by women.

Healthcare of Migrant Workers

The healthcare of migrant workers, and all that it entails, is another issue for PAs who practice in rural areas due to the higher population of this group in these areas. The health status of migrant farm workers is below that of the average American, and financial, cultural, and social barriers limit the availability of and accessibility to healthcare for this population. Given these facts, Henning et al. (2008) assessed the capacity of healthcare providers in selected counties in east Tennessee to provide primary care to this population. The study also examined the attitudes of providers toward migrant workers. The first half of the survey assessed the providers' opinion in three areas: awareness of migrants' health needs, options for delivering care, and desirability of migrants as patients. The second part requested information regarding the type of provider (physician or NP/PA); type of agency (private or community/public health); type of practice (primary care, obstetrics/gynecology, or pediatrics); number of encounters with migrants; and provider's ability to speak Spanish. The respondents were also given a list of primary care services and asked to identify those they provided directly, formally referred, or did not provide.

The results revealed that both groups of providers were not very knowledgeable about migrants' health needs, but providers expressed a willingness to learn more about these health needs and to support local initiatives toward the amelioration of migrants' conditions. Also, providers were in favor of extending Medicaid to migrants and accepting referrals or contractual agreements to provide the care. Physicians generally were less inclined to approve of the federal government's subsidization of this care than were PAs and NPs. Although both provider groups would treat migrants as any other patients regardless of legal status, the PAs and NPs were more willing to accommodate their schedules to fit the schedules of migrants. The majority of providers were found to deliver basic healthcare services, although deficiencies were noted in some health education areas, dental health, and issues related to pesticide exposure. The researchers concluded there was a need for major improvements in establishing linkages and cooperative agreements at the interagency level and between agencies and institutions of higher learning in meeting the health needs of migrants (Henning et al., 2008).

INNOVATIONS IN RURAL HEALTH EMPLOYMENT IN THE UNITED STATES

The deployment of PAs to US areas of medical need is primarily attributed to policies initiated by the federal government. Meeting the needs of rural populations has roots in 200 years of priorities—going back to the development of the agrarian society in the United States. At the beginning of the 20th century, 70% of the American population resided in agricultural regions and lived outside of urban centers. As of the 21st century, only 3% of Americans farm or grow items for consumption (yet this population produces almost all of the food for the rest of the country). Approximately 16% of Americans are considered rural (by HRSA definitions). The US Congress and state legislatures have created policies to address the disparities of rural

people, and those policies have direct effect on PAs. In addition, state legislation and policy enactments have also had an effect on the employment of PAs in rural areas; however, these initiatives vary widely by state.

National Health Service Corps

To combat the shortage of physicians, PAs, NPs, and other healthcare workers in rural areas, the US government created a national policy of promoting healthcare provider relocation to rural and underserved areas through the National Health Service Corps (NHSC). This federal program, which is administered by the HRSA Bureau of Primary Healthcare, implemented various strategies to place healthcare professionals in more than 500 areas (neighborhoods to rural areas) that are suffering from critical shortages of primary healthcare providers. Strategies include service commitments to a designated HPSA through loan repayment and scholarships.

Although the NHSC program has been successful in the deployment of providers to rural and medically underserved areas, the experience has not always been ideal. NHSC scholarship recipients have identified various underlying problems with the system that lead to poor PA provider retention:

1. Too few potential placement sites are made available from the outset.
2. NHSC placement deadlines do not allow enough time for making the best possible placement.
3. Many community health centers are not highly supportive of or invested in the program.
4. NHSC efforts to support the development of local medical providers from within underserved regions are inadequate.
5. NHSC officers working with nonphysician providers do not demonstrate a high degree of commitment to achieving an optimal provider-site match.

Changes in the NHSC program based on these five problems might help to improve the retention of health professionals in this important.

Rural Health Clinics Act

The Rural Health Clinics Act (PL 95-210) in 1977 was an attempt to provide for the development of federally subsidized RHCs and to staff them appropriately. One proviso provides for the reimbursement of services to Medicare patients by PAs and NPs who practice in communities that are rural or underserved. A modification to the Rural Health Clinics Act in 1997 and the creation of the National Association of Rural Health Clinics (NARHC) allowed the number of RHCs to grow from 600 in 1990 to more than 3,950 in 2012.

The Centers for Medicare and Medicaid Services (CMS) issued a rule relating to RHCs in 2003 that has had a significant impact on PAs and NPs. Much of this rule was adopted in response to statutory requirements signed into law in 1997 (under the Balanced Budget Act of 1997). Various components of the rule stipulate:

- All RHCs must be located in "currently" designated shortage areas.
- RHCs that can no longer meet the location requirements must apply for an exception to this requirement to continue to participate in the RHC program.
- There are limits for waivers of nonphysician provider staffing.

The rule also:

- Codifies the definition of a "bed" for purposes of the RHC cap exception for hospitals with fewer than 50 beds
- Codifies the RHC payment limits previously extended to most provider-based RHCs
- Codifies PA/NP/CNM staffing requirement at 50% of the time the clinic is open to see patients
- Restricts PA/NP/CNM staffing waiver requests to already certified RHCs
- Mandates the establishment of a quality assessment performance improvement initiative by RHCs.

The impact of these policies continues to be felt because of the requirement for RHCs to employ a PA, an NP, or a CNM. More importantly, these policies emphasize that PAs and NPs are valued in these settings.

State Legislation and Policy Enactments

Legislation on the state level has also been instrumental in expanding PA development and deployment into rural areas. This legislation involves three important components: supportive legislation, prescribing, and reimbursement. Expanding the authority of PAs to work with fewer restrictions than before allows for PA development in medically underserved areas.

Rarely does legislation precede experimentation in health professions. However, one of the earliest legislative measures in favor of PAs was enacted in Alaska in 1971; this preceded the introduction of PAs into Alaska in 1972. In 1973, the Trans-Alaska Pipeline System began and PAs were actively recruited to serve in the aid stations along the route (Marzucco et al., 2013).

Various strategies of state governments have resulted in proven policy initiatives for PA placement in rural areas. One strategy used in a number of states, such as Washington, California, Iowa, and New Mexico, is to underwrite public-funded PA programs that emphasize rural health. With this approach, state funds are used to subsidize the education of PAs in the hope that such students would practice in rural communities within the state upon graduation. Some states, such as Pennsylvania and Utah, have developed comprehensive health workforce plans that include PAs and other nonphysician providers as part of the strategy to improve service delivery and efficiency.

Economic Incentives

An economic incentive is another strategy used to entice PAs and other medical care professionals to rural and underserved healthcare locations. These programs include scholarships, the education loan repayment programs, and the Junior Commissioned Officer Student Extern Program (JRCOSTEP).

In exchange for qualifying service, usually in health personnel shortage areas or state-designated areas of unmet healthcare need, participants may receive funds to repay qualifying graduate-level, federal loan debt. The maximum of any state or federal loan repayment is $100,000. The loan has some obligations. Once the first payment from this program is received and processed, the participant is obligated to satisfy the minimum practice requirement or pay a penalty equal to 150% of the program benefit received. For PAs and NPs, the annual payments equal 25% of the total qualifying loan principal for a minimum service obligation of 3 years and maximum program participation of 4 years; 2 years of employment are required to avoid penalties. Students may apply for the program during the last year leading to the professional degree.

Certain states have also created a number of initiatives to encourage relocation to and retention in rural practices. These initiatives come in the form of loan repayment similar to the federal government system, tax incentives (usually in the form of deductions), mortgage assistance in the form of low-cost loans subsidized by the state, and cash incentives.

National Association of Rural Health Clinics

The NARHC is the only national organization dedicated exclusively to improving the delivery of quality, cost-effective healthcare in rural underserved areas through the RHC program. NARHC works with Congress, federal agencies, and rural health allies to promote, expand, and protect the RHC program. Through the association, NARHC members become actively engaged in the legislative and regulatory process.

Area Health Education Centers

Area Health Education Centers (AHECs) were developed by the Bureau of Health Professions to enhance access to quality healthcare, particularly primary and preventive care. They improve the supply and distribution of healthcare professionals through community and academic educational partnerships. Many of the AHECs are located in rural areas and serve to expose health professional students to rural health. For example, the Central Texas AHEC assists PA programs with placement of students in rural family medicine clinics. In some

instances, the organization arranges for student lodging and transportation as well as a per diem. The intent is to maximize the exposure of students to rural healthcare delivery.

Junior Commissioned Officer Student Extern Program

Students participating in JRCOSTEP work in federal agencies and programs as active duty commissioned corps officers. Typical assignments vary from 31 to 90 days during official school breaks. Applicants are accepted from a variety of fields, including environmental health, pharmacy, engineering, and nursing. Participants receive the basic pay and allowances of an ensign (pay grade 01) officer while in training.

RURAL HEALTH GLOBALLY

To provide a global perspective, this section presents an overview of the current status of rural healthcare in several countries. Each country is unique in its approach to addressing the problem of underserved populations.

Australia

The medical workforce shortage in Australia is significant countrywide but is particularly evident in rural and remote areas. One important document addressing this shortage is the *Report on the Audit of Health Workforce in Rural and Regional Australia*, published in 2008. This Australian Government Department of Health and Ageing report addressed shortages, compared the medical shortages in other countries with those in Australia, discussed the use of international medical graduates, and identified areas for improvement, which included the use of PAs.

As Australia thought about strategic ways to extend care with a limited cadre of doctors, the PA model emerged. The appeal is that the PA is under the supervision of a medical officer in a delegated practice model. Taking a cue from the United States and Canada—that they are trained by doctors in medical schools and can assume as much as 90% of the general practice visit safely—their skills may be particularly adapted to rural and remote settings where their team orientation to care can be highly leveraged.

A report to Parliament in 2008 contained an extensive review of the PA literature and was positive and endorsing of the PA concept, especially for rural areas. Additionally, a public health policy paper discussed specific roles that a PA could undertake within rural Australian society in such settings as hospitals, general practices, and indigenous health clinics.

Murray and Wronski (2006), two rural health observers, argue that there is compelling evidence that the "rural pipeline" (rural student recruitment and rurally based education and professional training) increased the rural workforce. The nexus between clinical education and training, a sustained healthcare workforce, clinical research, and quality and safety requires greater emphasis. The authors state that a "teaching health system" for nonmetropolitan Australia requires greater commitment to teaching as a core business, as well as provision of an infrastructure, including accommodation and access to the private sector. Because workforce flexibility is mostly well accepted in rural and remote areas, there is room for expanding the scope of clinical practice by nonmedical clinicians, such as PAs and NPs, in an independent codified manner with flexible local medical delegation (e.g., practice nurses, Aboriginal health workers, and therapists). The authors end with call to address the imbalance between subspecialist and generalist medical training. Improved training and recognition of Aboriginal health workers as well as continued investment in programs that will allow entry of indigenous people into other health professional programs, such as PA programs, remain policy priorities.

Lauftik (2014) describes the role and contributions of an American PA working in North Queensland, along with recommendations and insights for expanded implementation of the PA. This experience of a PA in Aboriginal care could serve as a model for other communities in bringing long-term stability and relationship-building to community care while improving the quality and efficiency of clinic management. The author suggests such partnerships will increase and improve training opportunities for health workers, medical students, and junior doctors.

Canada

Information on PAs in Canada in general and in rural areas specifically is beginning to emerge. From 1984 to 2008, the only development of PAs was by the Canadian Forces for use in the Canadian Forces Medical Group. However, because no PA legislation existed until Manitoba enacted an amendment under the Medical Act in 1999, these PAs were left without a place to go when they finished their military careers. Most either gave up healthcare work or sought employment in the civilian sector as health and safety officers in industry—sometimes in remote locations.

Manitoba and Alberta, two provinces with very remote and large indigenous populations, enacted PA legislation to address the shortages of medical care to rural communities. In 2012, the Ontario Ministry of Health and Longterm Care completed a demonstration project that recruited PAs from Canada and the United States to work in emergency departments, hospitals, and, particularly, community health centers. This impetus has allowed other provinces to consider PAs for their more rural and indigenous populations.

Great Britain

Although Great Britain is not known for its rural locations, at least 50 small towns are considered rural and difficult to service. These areas include parts of Scotland, and outlying islands.

An evaluation of US-trained PAs working in the National Health Service (NHS) in England and a similar project in Scotland delivered by NHS Education for Scotland (NES) identified a number of benefits with PA deployment (Woodin, McLeod, McManus, & Jelphs, 2005). American PAs have largely been replaced by English-educated PAs, and expanded deployment into rural areas is likely.

South Africa

The huge tracts of wilderness and distances between small towns and villages present challenges to the South African government. In clinics, whether they are in the outlying areas or in townships, the doctor-to-patient ratio is quite low. In addition, the number of professionals, including doctors, departing South Africa, is burdensome. To overcome this handicap, South Africa is looking for solutions. Implementing clinical associates (CAs) is one of the first steps in dealing with low doctor-to-population ratios, along with a PA program at the University of the Witwatersrand, Walter Sisulu University in the Eastern Cape, and the University of Pretoria. The intent is to train CAs for both urban and rural deployment.

The Netherlands

The Netherlands is a small country (about the size of Maryland) with a fairly dense population and little to identify as "rural." However, like other countries, it is experiencing a decline in physicians willing to work outside of metropolitan centers. These "shrink regions" are characterized by a decrease of younger population, declining facilities (shops, pharmacies, schools, sport clubs, medical services), and a lower average income compared with urbanized areas. It is in these regions that the Dutch are hoping PAs will help provide support.

FURTHER RESEARCH ON PHYSICIAN ASSISTANTS IN RURAL HEALTH

The literature about PAs in rural health is limited. A review of this literature reveals missing information and unanswered questions. The following are select research questions that might contribute to the successful deployment of PAs into rural health.

- **Case reports:** What is a unique rural health role for PAs? Writing about individual roles and settings using even 1 years' worth of data provides a foundation for others to build upon. A case report should describe the degree of isolation, how the organization functions, the community the organization serves, and the role of the PA in this setting.
- **Role delineation:** What is the role of the PA in a rural health setting? How is this

role shared between the PA and the supervising doctor?
- **Organizational research:** How does a RHC with a PA compare with a facility in an urban setting with a PA? Contrast and compare the practice setting, the population served, and the activity of each member of the team for each facility.
- **Economics:** How does a clinic in a rural setting staffed with a PA compare with a comparable clinic without a PA in terms of range of services?
- **Epidemiology:** What are the frequency of diagnoses, the characteristics of patients seen, and the incidences of diagnoses in the community when comparing rural PAs with urban PAs?
- **Quality of care:** How does the quality of care in a rural clinic staffed with a PA compare with similar clinics without a PA? Does the inclusion of a PA change the quality of care?
- **Procedures:** What are the procedures used and the skills needed for a family medicine PA in a rural setting?
- **Patient satisfaction:** Do patients have any different perceptions of PAs in rural settings versus those in urban settings?
- **Retention:** What are the social and economic factors that contribute to retention or attrition of PAs in rural locations?
- **Education:** Are there education strategies that can influence successful PA deployment to rural settings?

SUMMARY

The US rural healthcare system has changed dramatically since the early 1990s because of a general transformation of healthcare financing, the introduction of new technologies, and the clustering of health services into systems and networks. The result has been the expansion of PAs (and CAs) into rural health in unprecedented moves. Despite these changes, resources for rural healthcare systems remain relatively insufficient. Many rural communities continue to experience shortages of doctors, nurses, allied health professionals, and PAs. The percentage of rural hospitals under financial stress is much greater than that of urban hospitals. The healthcare conditions of selected rural areas compare unfavorably with the rest of the nation. Market and governmental policies have attempted to address some of these disparities by encouraging network development and changing the rules for Medicare and Medicaid payments to providers.

References

The following citations are key to supporting this chapter's content. You can find a complete list of citations for all chapters at www.fadavis.com/davisplus, keyword *Hooker*.

American Academy of Physician Assistants (AAPA). (2013). *2012 AAPA Physician Assistant Census Report*. Alexandria, VA: AAPA.

Baldwin, K. A., Sisk, R. J., Watts, P., McCubbin, J., Brockschmidt, B., & Marion, L. N. (1998). Acceptance of nurse practitioners and physician assistants in meeting the perceived needs of rural communities. *Public Health Nurse, 15*(6), 389–397.

Bergeron, J., Neuman, K., & Kinsey, J. (1999). Do advanced practice nurses and physician assistants benefit small rural hospitals? *Journal of Rural Health, 15*(2), 219–232.

Gamm, L. D., Hutchison, L. L., Dabney, B. J., & Dorsey, A. M. (Eds.). (2003). *Rural Healthy People 2010: A Companion Document to Healthy People 2010*. Volume 1. College Station, TX: The Texas A&M University System Health Science Center, School of Rural Public Health, Southwest Rural Research Center. Retrieved from http://www.srph.tamhsc.edu/centers/rhp2010/Volume1.pdf

Henning, G. F., Graybill, M., & George, J. (2008). Reason for visit: Is migrant healthcare that different? *Journal of Rural Health, 24*(2), 219–220.

Henry, L. R., & Hooker, R. S. (2014). Caring for the disadvantaged: The role of physician assistants. *Journal of the American Academy of Physician Assistants, 27*(1), 36–42.

Isberner, F. R., Lloyd, L., Simon, B., Joyce, M. S., & Craven, J. M. (2003). Utilization of physician assistants: Incentives and constraints for rural physicians. *Perspective on Physician Assistant Education, 14*(2), 69–73.

Jones, P. E. (2008). Doctor and physician assistant distribution in rural and remote Texas counties. *Australian Journal of Rural Health, 16*(2), 12.

Krein, S. L. (1997). The employment and use of nurse practitioners and physician assistants by rural hospitals. *Journal of Rural Health, 13*(1), 45–58.

Larson, E. H., Palazzo L., Berkowitz, B., Pirani, M. J., & Hart, L. G. (2003). The contribution of nurse practitioners and physician assistants to generalist care in Washington State. *Health Services Research, 38*(4), 1033–1050.

Lauftik, N. (2014). The physician assistant role in Aboriginal healthcare in Australia. *Journal of the American Academy of Physician Assistants, 27*(1), 32–35.

Marzucco, J., Hooker, R. S., Ballweg, R. M. (2013). A history of the Alaska physician assistant: 1970–1980. *Journal of the American Academy of Physician Assistants, 26*(12), 45–51.

Murray, R. B., & Wronski, I. (2006). When the tide goes out: Health workforce in rural, remote and indigenous communities. *Medical Journal of Australia, 185*(1), 37–38.

Woodin, J., Mcleod, H., McManus, R., & Jelphs, K. (2005). *Evaluation of US-trained PAs Working in the NHS in England. Final Report*. Birmingham, England: Health Services Management Centre, Department of Primary Care and General Practice, University of Birmingham.

CHAPTER 9

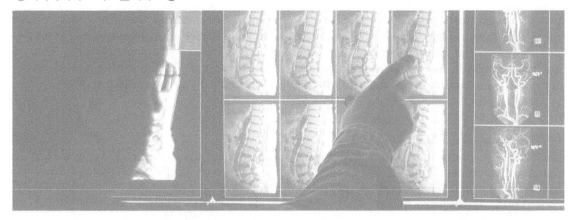

ECONOMIC ASSESSMENT OF PHYSICIAN ASSISTANTS

RODERICK S. HOOKER ■ JAMES F. CAWLEY ■ CHRISTINE M. EVERETT

"The introduction of physician assistants has been a responsible policy. Many other innovations mediated by medical practitioners have gained widespread acceptance with much less rigorous prior evaluation than was given physician assistants."

—Walter O. Spitzer, 1984

Are physician assistants (PAs) cost-effective? At the heart of this question is the matter of whether PAs are what they seem to be— a benefit to those they are intended to serve. Embedded in this opening question are accompanying questions, such as the following: Are PAs productive enough to be considered cost-effective for doctors? If they are cost-effective, do the benefits of employing PAs accrue to the employer, the patient, or society as a whole? What happens to the output of a physician's practice (or inpatient service or outpatient clinic) when a PA joins the clinical staff? Furthermore, what are the outcomes in terms of access to patient care services, level of quality of care, practice revenues, and productivity? Some of these questions have played out on the economic stage, and others

remain unanswered. This chapter is a summary of the literature on this topic.

Although the practice contributions of PAs are determined by multiple influences, several of which are difficult to measure, a number of clinical performance characteristics have been described in the health services research literature. Many of the findings, some of which are from studies performed decades ago, remain valid well into the new century.

Various studies over the past 50 years have shown that, within their spheres of practice competency, PAs provide lower cost healthcare that is comparable to that provided by physicians. Contemporary research has conclusively demonstrated that PAs are cost-effective in clinical practice, and substantial empirical and health services research evidence confirms the findings that they are cost-effective in almost all of the settings studied, with no perceptible differences in quality of care or patient safety. Probably more significant is that the popularity of PAs and their use in clinical settings, after a half-century, would be unlikely if they were not cost-effective.

Evidence indicates that the organizational setting is closely related to the productivity and cost benefits of PA use. The impact of PAs on access to healthcare services, quality of care, and physician and patient acceptance continues to be measured with positive results, although the precise degree of productivity and cost-effectiveness varies among settings and in roles performed. It is the downstream benefits of PA employment that are unclear because the vast majority of PA productivity studies have viewed PAs as substitutes rather than members of inter-disciplinary healthcare teams (Figure 9–1).

QUALITY OF CARE

PA utilization in medical practices has grown, partly as a result of practice efficiency and economic advantages and partly as a result of patient satisfaction with care. A number of healthcare services research studies conducted shortly after introducing a PA into practice concluded that PAs provide physician-equivalent levels of quality of patient care.

Patient satisfaction is a related but imperfect measure of healthcare-provider quality of care and is a partial determinant of the use of healthcare personnel. High level of patient acceptance of PA services has been a consistently observed finding in many of the healthcare services research reports published after PAs were introduced into clinical practice. These studies showed that the proportion of patients reporting acceptable to high levels of satisfaction with

FIGURE 9-1
Physician Assistants on the Medical Team

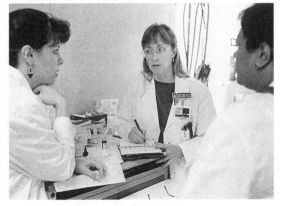

Courtesy of the American Academy of Physician Assistants

healthcare services delivered by PAs averaged between 80% and 90% among individuals not previously exposed to PA care. This figure subsequently rose more than 95% among patients surveyed after having received care from a PA (Henry & Hooker, 2014).

Public acceptance and familiarity with PA healthcare providers have grown substantially, particularly over the past decade. Data from a report based on findings from a random sample of 687 adults surveyed by telephone in the Kentucky Health Survey indicated that 1 in 4 (25%) had received medical advice or treatment from a PA within 2 years of being surveyed. More than 90% of these subjects reported satisfaction with the care they received. Recipients of care from PAs did not differ from recipients of care from physicians with respect to income, education, insurance status, self-assessment of health status, or rural versus urban location.

A 2005 study assessed the quality of care provided by PAs in primary care clinics of the Air Force, in which PAs deliver a considerable portion of primary care formerly provided by physicians. Quality of clinical care determinations were made on the basis of responses to predetermined diagnostic, therapeutic, and referral and disposition criteria. Therapeutic criteria included desirable actions on the part of the healthcare provider (e.g., prescribing the appropriate class of antibiotic for infectious otitis media at the first visit) and undesirable actions (e.g., prescribing an antibiotic for viral syndrome with gastroenteritis). On five of six such criteria, PAs performed as well as or better than physicians in identifying desirable therapeutic actions.

A more recent cross-sectional retrospective cohort study aimed to compare quality of care provided by PAs and nurse practitioners (NPs) with that provided by primary care physicians. To achieve this goal, the researchers reviewed the process and outcomes of care of Medicare beneficiaries with chronic obstructive pulmonary disorder (COPD) who had at least one acute hospitalization in 2010. They examined spirometry evaluation, administration of influenza and pneumococcal vaccines, use of COPD medications, and referral to a pulmonary specialist visit. Outcome measures were emergency department (ED) visit, number of hospitalizations, and 30-day readmission in 2010. In terms of process of care measures, PAs and NPs were more likely to prescribe short-acting bronchodilators, oxygen therapy, and consult a pulmonary specialist, but less likely to give influenza and pneumococcal vaccinations. Patients receiving care from PAs and NPs had lower rates of ED visits for COPD and had a higher follow-up rate with a pulmonary specialist within 30 days of hospitalization for COPD than those cared for by physicians (Agarwal et al., 2016).

PHYSICIAN ASSISTANT COST-EFFECTIVENESS

Most of the economic research on PAs has focused on cost-effectiveness of employment. Cost-effectiveness analysis is an economic technique to compare the positive and negative consequences of a specific resource allocation. The strategy is to measure the comparable benefit of a particular investment versus its cost. In healthcare, this technique is commonly applied to new medical technologies, diagnostic and laboratory tests, health facilities and delivery systems, and drug treatment and immunization programs. The application of cost-effectiveness analysis to the delivery of medical care services—and specifically to a provider of such services—is a complex endeavor. Accurately measuring the content of a medical encounter is difficult because of variations in such factors as severity of illness, types of treatment, patient preferences, extent of use of diagnostic tests, level of provider training, and the site and mode of care delivery. Add to these factors differences in the type of provider delivering a similar service and different styles of task delegation, and it becomes obvious that any efforts to determine cost-effectiveness tend to be methodologically difficult and quite expensive.

PAs provide medical care services that, to a large extent, overlap those services provided by physicians. Understanding what percentage of overlap exists constitutes the heart of the question for employers and health planners. Most studies suggest that PAs can substitute for (or complement) doctors in various ways. What is not clear is which services are included in these percentages and which are left out. The percentages vary considerably depending on practice setting and specialty, the degree of delegation of tasks by an individual physician to a PA, and the amount of supervision the PA requires or needs.

Given satisfactory quality and patient acceptance, the substitutability of PAs for physicians depends on the volume of services delegated and the degree to which the PA's productivity matches that of the doctor in performing the delegated services. The delegation and productivity numbers can be combined to produce a physician-PA substitution ratio. For example, if half of a physician's services are delegated to a PA (or the PA's productivity is half that of the physician), it will take one PA to substitute for half of a physician, and the substitution ratio will be 0.5 physician: 1 PA, or 0.5.

From the bulk of published studies that have evaluated PA performance, it is clear that most of the services performed by primary care physicians can be provided by PAs without consultation. The most rigorous of all PA economic studies showed that the conservative substitution ratio of traditional primary care medical office visits is 0.83, suggesting that it takes one PA to substitute for 83% of a physician in primary care ambulatory settings (Record et al., 1980). Other studies have found that the clinical productivity of PAs in family medicine and general internal medicine ranges between 75% and 100%.

In a state-level analysis in Utah, where PAs made up only 6.3% of the state's combined clinician (physician, PA, NP) workforce, PAs contributed approximately 7.2% of the patient care full-time equivalents in the state. The majority (73%) of Utah PAs worked at least 36 hours per week and spent a greater percentage of total hours working in patient care than physicians do. The rural PA workforce reported working a greater number of total hours and patient care hours compared with the overall statewide PA workforce (Pedersen et al., 2008).

If one accepts the old-school assumptions that PAs are at least three-fourths as productive as physicians and are capable of managing at least 83% of all primary care encounters, and if one recognizes that the mean salary of a PA is one-half that of a licensed primary care doctor, one can begin to appreciate the considerable cost-effectiveness that PAs bring to clinical practice. Unfortunately, these figures tend to become jumbled as a result of misunderstanding of the terms that economists use: *practice arrangements, delegation, supervision, consultation,* and *cost-effectiveness*. These terms, with explanations, are outlined in the following paragraphs.

Practice Arrangements

Practice arrangement refers to the organizational structure where a PA is employed. Studies have looked at estimates of PA productivity to try to determine the practice arrangements that best utilize the clinical services of PAs. Activity analyses used to develop a model of primary care practice organization and productivity consisted of listing the preponderance of tasks that fully describe most typical primary care practices. From this list, a model was developed that estimated that the introduction of a PA could increase medical practice

productivity from 49% to 74%; that is, a physician usually producing 100 office visits per week may increase that number to 150 to 175 visits per week simply by hiring a PA (a conservative assumption).

To estimate the savings in labor costs per primary care visit that might be realized from increased use of PAs and NPs in the primary care practices of a managed care organization, Roblin and colleagues (2004a; 2004b) analyzed 26 capitated primary care practices within a group model health maintenance organization (HMO). Data on approximately 2 million visits provided by 206 practitioners were extracted from computerized visit records. Payroll ledgers were the source of annual labor costs per practice. On average, PAs and NPs were the providers on record for one-third of adult medicine visits and one in five pediatric medicine visits. The likelihood of a PA or NP visit was significantly higher than average among patients presenting with minor acute illnesses, such as acute pharyngitis. In adult medicine, the likelihood of a PA or NP visit was lower than average among older patients (Figure 9–2). Practitioner labor costs per visit and total labor costs per visit were lower among practices with greater use of PAs or NPs,

FIGURE 9-2

Percent Reduction in Primary Care Visit Costs With Increased Integration of Physician Assistants/Nurse Practitioners Into Primary Care

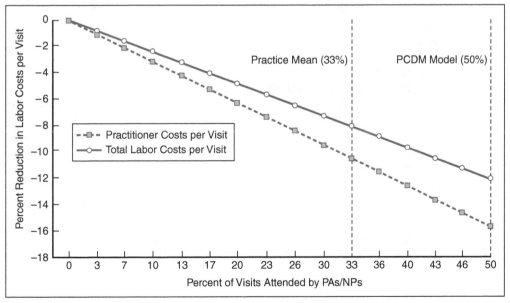

standardized for case mix. The authors concluded that primary care practices that used more PAs or NPs in care delivery realized lower practitioner labor costs per visit than practices that used fewer PAs or NPs (Roblin et al., 2011).

Delegation

Delegation is a legal term and an economic term. In this chapter, *delegation* refers to the percentage of primary care medical responsibilities that can be safely handled by a PA under optimal conditions (i.e., without supervision). The term *delegability* refers to the maximum level of delegation that can be achieved without threat to quality of care.

In one study, a multidisciplinary panel of health professionals developed a set of medical principles for determining the limits of PA substitutability, focusing on the patient's complaint and medical history. An outpatient utilization database was examined for a year of clinical experience to identify the office visits that would have been triaged to PAs had the panel's medical criteria been fully in effect. A number of conservative assumptions were used in undertaking this study. The theoretical construct was that the following would happen: significant illnesses such as cancer, renal failure, congestive heart failure, and similar progressive illnesses would be triaged away from PAs; all patients would be given a choice of seeing a physician or a PA at the time of the appointment; and no patient would be seen more than twice consecutively by a PA for the same diagnosis. PAs and physicians would be assigned the same number of appointments each day.

The research team found that the PA-appropriate medical office rate, or delegability, was 83% of the total in adult primary care during the study period (Record et al., 1981). As a result, the sentence "PAs can take care of 83% of all primary care visits" has become something of an industry standard in medical workforce research. Even though other studies have shown that the percentage of primary care diagnoses that PAs can assume is at least 90% in family or adult medicine, the 83% figure persists to this day.

Because of economy of scale, large medical practices seem to be more likely to use PAs and NPs. These organizations, which include health maintenance organizations (HMOs), the Department of Veterans Affairs, the military, and other vertically integrated systems, tend to experiment with new innovations in labor and technology. The other organizational trend in these settings is that doctors tend to delegate a larger percentage of medical services.

Van Rhee and colleagues (2002) compared a sample of patients admitted to an internal medicine service where cases were divided between PA and teaching services. A total of 16 PAs and 32 postgraduate residents (with 1–3 years of training) in internal medicine service were compared over a 180-month period in the mid-1990s (Table 9–1). Resource use was measured using direct costs expressed as relative value units. The results revealed that PAs used fewer ancillary services for pneumonia, stroke, and heart failure. One of the conclusions was that PAs might be more efficient than residents in providing some hospital services.

Dhuper and Choksi (2009) demonstrated that when PA hospitalists replaced medical resident house officers, patient satisfaction and quality of care between the two groups remained unchanged. The case mix of the two providers was the same and the mortality rate during this 2-year study was significantly lower than the preceding 2 years. The authors concluded that the implementation of PAs as hospitalists was relatively safe and effective.

Supervision

Supervision is a state-legislated term that has legal and economic implications. Competent supervision is a quality indicator of patient care. However, sometimes, restriction of delegated tasks can slow down productivity, such as interrupting a doctor to countersign all prescriptions. Loss of physician productivity can also occur if an employer's administrative tasks require every chart to be reviewed and countersigned. The amount of time devoted to supervision depends largely on the PA–physician relationship, yet little study has been devoted to this important function.

TABLE 9-1

Summary of Sampling Scheme, Comparing Physician Assistants to Internal Medicine Residents on a Random Assignment of Patients to Two Separate Wards: January 1994–July 1995

Diagnosis-Related Group	Initial Sample Size		Number (%) Expired		Length of Stay Outliers (%)		Sample Size (%) for Study	
	PA	Resident	PA	Resident	PA	Resident	PA	Resident
Cerebral vascular accident/stroke	87	139	7 (8.0)	16 (11.5)	13 (16.3)	17 (13.8)	67 (77.0)	106 (76.3)
Pneumonia	126	132	16 (12.7)	6 (4.5)	16 (14.5)	15 (11.9)	94 (74.6)	111 (84.1)
Acute myocardial infarction, discharged alive	38	39	0 (0)	0 (0)	1 (2.6)	2 (5.1)	37 (97.4)	37 (94.9)
Heart failure	170	171	11 (6.5)	7 (4.1)	29 (18.2)*	14 (8.5)	130 (76.5)	150 (87.7)
Gastrointestinal hemorrhage	91	118	2 (2.2)	0 (0)	8 (9.0)	8 (6.8)	81 (89.0)	110 (93.2)

*P < .05 according to chi-square test.

Data from Van Rhee, J., Ritchie, J., & Eward, A. M. (2002). Resource use by physician assistant services versus teaching services. *Journal of the American Academy of Physician Assistants, 15*(1), 33–38, 40, 42 passim.

Redesigning healthcare systems to deliver team-based care is important for improving patient care, especially care of chronically ill patients. Utilizing teams of PAs and NPs is one approach to the patient-centered medical home. In one large HMO that employed PAs and NPs, the supervising physician's patient load was purposely decreased by 10% per day. As a result, administrative time was inserted into the physician's schedule to compensate for supervising the PAs and NPs and reviewing medical records used by the PAs and NPs (Hooker & Freeborn, 1991). At that time, the supervision requirement was to see all charts, countersign the charts, and collaborate on patient care in a number of cases. Since then, however, most clinic schedules do not need to factor in collaborative time for the physician. When annual productivity in family medicine is examined from national studies the number of visits or the relative value units based on complexity of care for PAs is sometimes higher than that of NPs and physicians in family medicine offices (Essary et al., 2016).

In a cross-sectional analysis of administrative data from Veterans Health Administration (VHA) primary care encounters, patient encounter characteristics were compared across provider types (PA, NP, and physician). NPs and PAs attended to about 30% of all VHA general medical encounters, although these cases were slightly less complex than those seen by physicians. Interestingly, PAs attended a higher proportion of visits for the purpose of determining eligibility for benefits, suggesting some division of labor (Morgan et al., 2012).

In the same VHA setting, Moran and colleagues (2016) found PAs to be consistently more productive than NPs on an annual basis (Table 9–2). The importance of this study was the measurement of relative value units over full-time equivalents when clinically active. Administration, surgery, mental health, and nonclinical time was excluded from the analysis.

Consultation

Consultation is the PA's decision to request a physician's assistance in a specific medical office visit. It differs from delegation, which is the doctor's decision to assign to a PA some subset of the physician's service. The consultation can be a part of the total delegated medical office visits for which a PA is responsible.

The *consultation rate* is the number of consultations of any kind over the total number of visits assigned to the PA in a given time. Many circumstances determine a consultation rate, and consultations can take many forms, with varying time and cost results. For example, consultations involving signing a prescription, verifying a radiograph finding, or approving a proposed

TABLE 9-2
PA and NP Productivity by Practice Setting in all VHA settings, 2014

	Number of Providers	Sum of Weight (FTEs)	Mean Productivity	SD	P
PAs in nonrural settings	1,616	1,192	2,046	1,202	.0025
PAs in rural settings	180	132	2,349	1,510	
NPs in nonrural settings	3,825	2,842	1,904	1,083	.001
NPs in rural settings	338	255	2,042	1,061	
Total	5,959				
PAs in nonteaching roles	204	150	2,215	1,063	.0031
PAs in teaching roles	1,592	1,174	2,058	1,259	
NPs in nonteaching roles	514	381	2,102	1,022	<.0001
NPs in teaching roles	3,649	2,716	1,889	1,088	
PAs in Medical Center Complexity:					
1a	765	565	2,050	1,287	.0011
1b	251	186	1,915	1,199	
1c	343	251	2,171	1,206	
2	291	212	2,103	1,218	
3	146	109	2,214	1,150	
NPs Medical Center Complexity:					
1a	1,933	1,446	1,785	1,040	<.0001
1b	792	591	1,882	1,026	
1c	586	428	2,168	1,315	
2	407	303	2,030	1,019	
3	445	330	2,113	1,002	

FTE = full-time equivalent.
Data from Moran, E., Basa, E., Gao, J., Woodmansee, D., & Hooker, R. S. (2016). Factors associated with physician assistant and nurse practitioner productivity in the Veterans Health Administration. *Journal of the American Academy of Physician Assistants, 29*(7), 1–6.

medical management plan might take the PA's supervisor only a minute or two; however, in a more complicated case, the doctor might need to examine the patient and, as a result, the consultation takes more time (Figure 9–3).

The more time a physician spends consulting with a PA, the less time the physician has for his or her own tasks, thus decreasing the overall productivity of the PA–physician team. Another factor that influences consultation rate and duration is the PA's experience. Generally speaking, a newly graduated PA seeks more consultations from a physician than a PA who has been practicing primary care for 20 years (Figure 9–4).

Scope of practice (as defined by the particular state in which the PA works) can also influence consultation rates. One area of inefficiency is to be a PA employed in a state that limits PA prescribing and dispensing. In such a case, PAs have to consult with physicians on every patient who needs a prescription.

Consultation rates may be closely related to the level of delegation in a certain specialty. Specifically, the rate of consultation varies depending on whether the PA is being used as a substitute, working independently of the doctor, or being used as a complement, whereby the doctor may be using the PA as his or her personal assistant. In other circumstances, willingness to delegate a broad range of services to a PA may be based on the assumption that consultation will be infrequent or that the PA needs little supervision.

Other factors that affect consultation rates include the PA's relationship with the physician, the proximity to the collaborative physician (e.g., next door, down the hall, or upstairs), time, availability, and the patient mix. When a PA and a physician share an

FIGURE 9-3
Physician–Physician Assistant Consultation

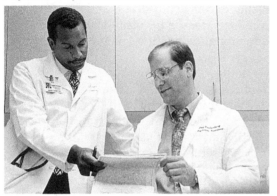

Courtesy of the American Academy of Physician Assistants

office, the rate is undoubtedly higher than when they are separated by distances and office layouts that inhibit formal and informal consultations. Because consultations are usually informal, little has been documented about PA consultation rates. Time-motion studies documenting every minute of a physician–PA relationship would need to be conducted over a prolonged time period to understand the importance of this labor shift.

Clinical Productivity

The first economists to study PA labor defined *productivity* this way:

> In theory, productivity is a simple concept: it measures changes in the total output that occur when small changes are made in one factor of production, with all other factors and circumstances held constant. Because these conditions can be met in the real world only rarely, productivity numbers are almost always rough estimates. Certainly that is the case with respect to [PAs]. (Record et al., 1981)

The findings on PA productivity reflect the changing policy concerns of the US healthcare system. Initially, emphasis relied on documenting increased access to solo practice services in rural areas. Later investigations focused on costs and delegation in organized healthcare settings.

An important contribution of health services research has been identifying the multifaceted effects of PAs on clinical productivity, meaning the overall output of a clinic or medical office when a PA is added to the medical staff. A common measure of productivity, one that can positively affect access to healthcare, is the number of patient visits provided in a

FIGURE 9-4
Percent of Physician Assistants by Time in Practice Who Spend Less Than 10% of Their Time Consulting With the Physician

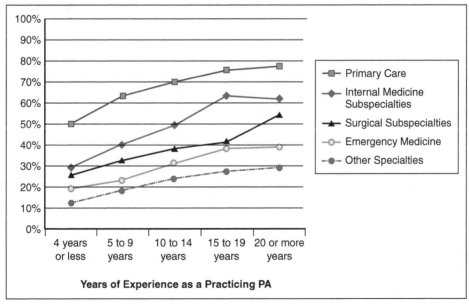

clinical setting. The next question is whether the productivity of PAs compares favorably with that of physicians.

In virtually every study on productivity, PAs compare favorably with physicians. In fact, evidence in some settings suggests that PAs see more patients per unit time than do physicians (Essary et al., 2016). When episodes of care are assessed, the cost of PA delivered care may be less costly than that of a physician (Hooker 1993). This may be the reduced labor cost or that the PA is using less resources, including return visits, differently than the doctor.

PA productivity can be compared with physician productivity in two other ways:

1. On the basis of tasks PAs are qualified to perform
2. On the full range of tasks performed by a physician

The comparison of the range of these tasks is sometimes known as the *functional delegation*. For most practices, depending on the degree of task delegation, practice case mix, the healthcare delivery system, the context in which the PA performs the clinical service, and institutional policy, the use of PAs results in higher clinical productivity rates.

Mathematical models have been developed to explore the most efficient contribution of healthcare personnel in different settings. The settings include private group practices, urban medical centers, military settings, managed healthcare settings, and tertiary care centers. Such models provide the documentation for the clinical productivity of PAs, with estimates ranging from 50% to 95% of physician productivity (where physician productivity equals 100%). These organizational and economic theories and carefully documented empirical approaches are similar in their assessment of PA clinical productivity. One study on the hourly, daily, and annual productivity of PAs, NPs, and physicians in the primary care departments of internal medicine, family practice, and pediatrics found that PAs see more patients than doctors do on an annual basis (29%). This difference is due in part to PAs being primarily clinic based, whereas physicians have hospital or administrative responsibilities that take them away from the medical office (Table 9–3). Patient visits to physicians and PAs tend to be similar in reason for visit in 90% of cases (the functional delegation level) but differ in illnesses associated with a hospitalization, such as acute cardiac events, cerebral accidents, and metastatic cancers (Hooker, 1993).

PA clinical productivity compares favorably with the productivity level of physicians, particularly in organized ambulatory care practice settings that use team approaches and structured division of medical care staffing. Although it seems likely that similar levels of PA clinical productivity exist for PAs working in other types of patient care settings, performance measures in newer practice areas, such as inpatient hospital settings, have not been performed.

One of the many variables difficult to control when comparing productivity of PAs in different settings is the population base. Many significant differences exist between groups of PAs depending on the work setting, type of specialty, and years of experience. However, interesting findings emerge when some of these data are aggregated.

Tables 9–4 and 9–5 present summary statistics on measures of outpatient productivity for

TABLE 9-3

Physician Assistant Clinical Productivity in an HMO Setting

Department	Patients per Hour	Patients per Day
FAMILY PRACTICE		
Physician	2.39	17.4
PAs	2.61	19.0
INTERNAL MEDICINE		
Physician	3.10	22.5
PAs	2.97	21.5
PEDIATRICS		
Physician	3.14	16.5
PAs	3.07	22.3

Data from Hooker, R. S. (1993). The roles of physician assistants and nurse practitioners in a managed care organization. In D. K. Clawson & M. Osterweis (Eds.), *The roles of physician assistants and nurse practitioners in primary care.* Washington, DC: The Association of Academic Health Centers.

TABLE 9-4
Outpatient Visits of Physician Assistants per Day by Work Setting, 2008

Specialty	No. of PAs in Practice	Mean Visits to a Typical PA per Week
Family/general medicine	20,554	88.8
General internal medicine	4,302	71.7
Emergency medicine	7,817	83.9
General pediatrics	1,891	94.2
General surgery	1,609	56.9
Internal medicine: cardiology	2,348	62.9
Other internal medicine subspecialities	5,310	59.9
Pediatric subspecialties	1,311	53.0
Surgery: orthopedics	5,776	69.7
Surgery: cardiovascular/thoracic	2,134	41.7
Neurosurgery	1,457	52.5
Other surgical subspecialities	4,606	60.6
Obstetrics/gynecology (women's health)	1,723	69.4
Occupational medicine	1,974	80.4
Dermatology	2,872	102.2
Other	8,118	65

Data from American Academy of Physician Assistants, Research Division, 2008. Based on PAs reporting outpatient visits but no inpatient or nursing home visits. Data collected on the 2008 AAPA member census.

TABLE 9-5
Mean and Standard Deviation of Outpatient Visits per Day by Years of Experience

Years of Experience	No. of Respondents	Mean	SD
Less than 1	139	18.6	7.2
1–3	821	20.8	8.8
4–6	505	21.9	10.1
7–9	341	21.2	8.5
10–12	410	21.6	8.6
13–15	371	22.5	10.2
16–18	343	22.8	10.5
More than 18	296	23.3	10.3
TOTAL	3,226	21.7	9.4

Data from American Academy of Physician Assistants, Research Division, 1996. Based on PAs reporting outpatient visits but no inpatient or nursing home visits. Data collected on the 1995 AAPA member census.

groups of PAs defined in terms of work setting, years of experience as a PA, and field of practice. All analyses used only data for PAs who reported being in full-time clinical practice and working for a single employer. Findings from this study include a statistically significant difference observed in the number of outpatients seen per day by work setting, with the largest differences reflected by PAs working in military and correctional treatment facilities. When data on years of experience are examined, PAs with more experience see more patients per day than PAs with less experience. Field of experience also seems to make a difference in terms of patients seen per day. The largest differences are found in emergency medicine, in which PAs report seeing 24.6 patients per day on average.

When the PA workweek was examined 10 years later, the vast majority of PAs self-reported working an average of 44 hours per week. On average, they saw the following number of patient visits per week: general pediatrics (97), family medicine (90), and emergency medicine (88) (AAPA, 2007).

The extent of PA productivity cannot be determined without reference to an array of interdependent variables, which, assuming that all of them can be identified, are difficult to evaluate. The classic conceptualization of how productivity should be measured—by observing what happens to total output when small homogeneous units of one input (in this case the

PA) are added while other inputs and the larger context are held constant—is difficult to measure in a big practice and virtually impossible in a small one.

EDUCATIONAL COSTS

The cost of PA education in the United States varies widely and is influenced by many variables: public versus private school, undergraduate versus graduate, duration, and type of institution (community college vs. academic health center). For example, in 2012, the full tuition for a PA education ranged from a mean of $35,839 (range $8,559 to $70,319) in a public funded university to $75,007 (range $42,125 to $137,291) in a private university (Cawley & Jones, 2013). In comparison to medical student educational costs, however, the overall expense of PA training is relatively low. The median education debt for medical school graduates in 2012 was $170,000, and 86% of graduates report having undergraduate education debt. Graduates from private medical schools are slightly less likely to have any debt but when they do have debt they typically have higher levels of debt than public medical school graduates. Controlling for type of school attended can be key to understanding some of the debt differences between groups of graduates. Debt levels for indebted medical school graduates and medical school cost of attendance have both increased faster than inflation over the past 20 years (Youngclaus & Fresne, 2013).

Student Costs

Student costs of a PA education include tuition and fees for the program as well as required expenses, such as medical equipment and textbooks. Also factored into student costs are the opportunity costs associated with pursuing PA education.

Tuition and Fees

A student can draw tuition from a number of sources, including personal income, family income, loans, and financial aid. Although a large number of PA students receive some type of financial aid, this aid is usually in the form of loans that must be repaid upon graduation.

To assess the economic burden that PA students assume when they begin the education process, Hooker and Warren (2001) showed how PA programs compared in terms of tuition. Drawing from the theory of human capital, the authors looked at individual decisions regarding education and training. Although educational decisions can be influenced by love of learning, desire for prestige, and various other preferences and emotions, human capital theorists find it useful to analyze schooling decision making as if it were part of a business plan. The optimal length of education, from this point of view, is the number of years of school needed until the marginal revenue (in the form of increased future income) of an additional year of schooling is exactly equal to the marginal cost.

The cost of tuition for a PA education ranges from $8,559 to $137,291 (Table 9–6) (Cawley & Jones, 2013). This more than 15-fold difference is found between public and private institutions, with state-supported programs being less expensive, on average, than private programs (duration ranging from 21–60 months). Although this difference does shrink when duration of education is held constant, the difference still demonstrates a remarkable market demand for PA education. It also represents a large differential in the expected economic return on the educational investment. Essary and colleagues (2014) found that PA programs rely significantly on student tuition as a source of revenue and that costs are rising substantially every year.

Additional Student Expenses

In 2008, PA programs were surveyed to determine what additional purchases they require students to make. Medical equipment, supplies, and textbooks were required by more than 90% of the programs (Figure 9–5). At the time of the survey, laptops were required by about one-third of the responding programs. Fewer than 20% of programs required their students to purchase medical software or assessment materials. Other major purchases by students are shown in Box 9–1.

Student Debt

The topic of student debt has become of increasing interest to economists and educators.

TABLE 9-6
Tuition and Expenses of US Physician Assistant Students, 2012

	Public Sponsorship	Private Sponsorship
Number of schools	58	110
Resident tuition range	$8,559–$70,319	$41,125–$137,291
Nonresident tuition range	$17,447–$117,547	$41,125–$137,291
Mean resident tuition	$35,839	$75,007
Mean nonresident tuition	$62,775	$75,283
Length range (months)	21–36	21–60
Average length	26.4	27.2
Class size range	18–105	18–98
Average class size	43.48	45.20
Average public program cohort, tuition generated (assuming all resident rates × mean class size)	$1,558,259	N/A
Average private program cohort, tuition generated (assuming nonresident rates × mean class size)	N/A	$3,402,785
Total tuition per matriculant cohort (assuming resident rates in 58 programs)	$90,379,013	N/A
Total tuition per matriculant cohort (assuming nonresident rates in 110 programs)	N/A	$374,306,330

Data modified from Cawley, J. F., & Jones, P. E. (2013). Institutional sponsorship, student debt, and specialty choice in physician assistant education. *Journal of Physician Assistant Education, 24*(4), 4–8.

FIGURE 9-5
Student Purchases Required by Physician Assistant Programs

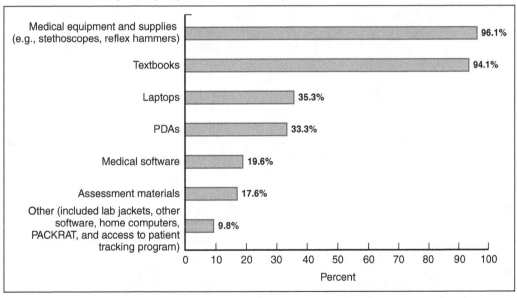

Data from *Physician Assistant Education Association (PAEA). (2008b)*. PA programs' purchasing power survey. *Alexandria, VA: PAEA.*

In one study on PA student debt, half of the respondents reported owing no pre-PA student loan debt, almost one-third reported owing an amount of $25,000 or less, and almost one-fifth reported owing more than $25,000. However, almost one-fourth of 2011 graduating PA students reported currently owing more than $100,000, slightly more than one-third reported owing between $50,001 and $100,000, slightly more than one-fourth reported owing an amount

BOX 9-1
Other Major Purchases by Physician Assistant Students

- PACKRAT
- Health insurance
- Malpractice insurance
- Transportation, parking, dues, etc.
- Housing at rotation sites
- Leasing fee for equipment/laboratory fees
- High-speed Internet access
- Course manuals
- Scrubs
- Advance cardiac life support certification
- Laboratory coats
- Infection control certification
- Basic life support certification
- Memberships
- Clearances
- Patient tracking program access

Data from Physician Assistant Education Association (PAEA). (2008b). *PA Programs' Purchasing Power Survey.* Alexandria, VA: PAEA.

of $50,000 or less, and approximately one-seventh reported owing no PA education loans (Moore et al., 2014).

Student debt is a contentious issue in American education systems because it contrasts sharply with many other socialized countries, where the cost of education is carried primarily by the state. For example, the 2.5 years of PA education in The Netherlands costs each student about €2,500, with the state paying the rest. Whether debt influences prospective PAs' decision to go to PA school or their employment selection later on has yet to be determined.

Opportunity Costs

What is the rational trade-off between continuing on to graduate school to become a PA or remaining in one's current career? Because the cost of becoming a PA includes more than just the cost of tuition, economic reasoning for such a decision needs to include many factors. When these factors are aggregated, the result is an *opportunity cost*. Opportunity cost decisions are made every day, although they are not always made consciously or articulated. The economist puts a monetary value on this behavior as a means to calculate the trade-offs an individual makes.

When economists refer to the *opportunity cost* of a resource, they are referring to the worth of the next highest valued alternative use of that resource. If, for example, a person spends time and money going to a movie, he or she cannot spend that time at home reading a book and technically cannot spend the money on something else. If the next best alternative to seeing the movie is reading the book, then the opportunity cost of seeing the movie is the money spent plus the pleasure you forgo by not reading the book. The opportunity cost of a PA education is the cost of a vocation foregone to obtain the education to embark on another career. It includes not only the tuition but also the earnings one would have if one remained a physical therapist or a paramedic instead of attending PA school.

In the only study on opportunity costs of PA education, Philpot (2005) examined the return to society by National Health Service Corps (NHSC) scholars who received training as PAs or NPs. By examining recipients of NHSC scholarships between 2003 and 2006, he was able to identify the payback potential between these two providers. The major findings were that (1) scholars repaid society's investment within 19 years after graduation, (2) PA scholars generated more tax revenue than NPs, (3) time to repayment was highly dependent on scholarship debt, and (4) NP students were required to forego an average of $5,216 more potential income than PAs during their training. The service period of NHSC scholars was not contingent on the amount of money invested in their scholarship award.

Doctoral degrees for PAs have become popular. One study analyzed the opportunity cost of a clinically active PA as a part-time student to obtain a doctorate in health sciences from Nova Southeastern University. This education was spread out over 4 years and involved travel to and from the university two times a year, tuition for online courses, and money for purchasing texts and other incidentals. In the aggregate, this PA was able to take vacations and extended weekends without having to take time off work at the VHA. The cost in 2008 dollars was $40,544 (Table 9–7).

This case illustrates some economic trade-offs required for obtaining a higher degree. The value of earnings over a lifetime varies according to whether the time forgone involves lost wages or lost leisure. Personal career satisfaction and status are social benefits of such an endeavor but are also elusive attributes not easily captured in social research. What does the investment of a terminal degree such as a technical doctorate (e.g., DHSc) bring to the individual? Perhaps salary increases, administrative roles, independent research, and prestige. How this investment in an additional degree is weighed over a lifetime will depend largely on where the individual starts and where at the end of his or her career the individual is situated.

State Funding of Higher Education

State or provincial (e.g., public) funding for higher education is related to the various policies the specific state or province is trying to promote. For example, in an effort to promote economic policies, states offer educational opportunities so that citizens will become educated, obtain higher paying jobs, and return something to the state in the form of higher taxable revenue. Although this approach is effective for undergraduate education, it is not necessarily the case with PA education. The debt incurred during PA education in terms of the opportunity costs (the income one foregoes and the debt one accumulates to obtain a higher paying degree) seems quite high for

TABLE 9-7
Clinical Physician Assistant Obtaining a Doctoral Degree Costs

Item	Cost
Tuition	$28,260
Books, fees, housing, car rental, incidentals, etc.	$12,284
TOTAL	$40,544

Data from Makinde, J. F., & Hooker, R. S. (2009). PA doctoral degree debt. ADVANCE for Physician Assistants, 17(3), 30–31.

many programs. Many PA students are embarking on a second career. The return rate for some of the high-end PA educational programs might never be realized if a well-paying job is abandoned to become a PA student. However, the potential benefit of state-supported education of PAs is that residents are then more likely to attend a state-supported school, thus remain in the state and offer a return to state taxpayers for their investment in higher education.

Institution Costs for Physician Assistant Programs

What are the costs associated with starting and sustaining a PA program? These questions are at the heart of educational economics and are part of *human investment*. The students and the institutions they attend are like firms—investing today for a return tomorrow. They are considered *investments in human capital*. Because these factors may be thought of as capital investments, the rate of return (educational costs) is viewed as an investment rather than the depletion of a resource.

Costs to Inaugurate a Physician Assistant Program

The cost to start up a PA program is expensive regardless of institution. Furthermore, costs are not easy to calculate because the analysis includes a number of variables and a number of unknowns. Some of the variables to consider are the following:

- Culture of the institution
- Type of institution (medical school or a health sciences–based institution)
- Funding of institution (private or public); private institutions have fewer rules and policies than do public institutions but have to fund internally; public institutions have more layers of administration and more policies and accountability but may be eligible for state or provincial funds for start-up and maintenance.
- Classroom and office space available
- Cost of faculty and supportive staff
- Cost of such facilities as clinical laboratories, simulations, and cadaver or autopsy laboratories

- Cost of a medical library
- Clinical education needs, such as clinical sites in the region and transportation and per diem cost for transportation, lodging, and meals for remote sites

To calculate start-up costs of a PA program, a PA program simulation was created. PA educational trends over 10 years (2011–2020) and program costs were analyzed. The costs were part of data collected on a public (state-sponsored) PA program. An *institutional cost model* was constructed. Built into the model was a set of assumptions of the program based on the experiences of the authors in consulting with new PA programs and the anticipated format of a new PA program that started up in the year 2010 (Table 9–8).

One of the assumptions built into this education model is the purchase of clinical sites for clinical experience. As of this writing the majority of American programs do not purchase clinical experiences, but programs outside of the United States do. A trend has emerged in which a small but growing number of PA programs compensate their preceptors between $250 and $1,000 per 40-hour week; others are likely to follow. In other systems the health authority (payor) compensates the preceptor.

Because of the many variables not accounted for, a cost of 2.5 million US (2014) dollars for the first 24 months of development before the first class entering the classroom might be expected. These are direct costs based on a public institution with a concentration in the health sciences.

Program Budgets and Expenses

In terms of the reported program budget, the cost of training an average PA student for 1 year of professional training can be roughly estimated by dividing the program budget by the total number of students enrolled. Thus, for the 2013 academic year, the cost for a typical program was approximately $15,820 to educate each student (mean budget of $1.2 million divided by an average enrollment of 87.5 students/program at 27 months per student).

The mean total annual budget of 178 PA educational programs in 2014 was $2,221,751. There were wide ranges of total budgets (10th percentile of $664,840 to 90th percentile of $4,147,783), depending on the size of the student body and the region of the country. The average cost per program to educate a PA student in 2014 was estimated to be $41,561 per year. The estimated cost per student is based on the number of students enrolled and the reported "program" budget. It should be noted, however, that these figures might exclude some costs, including:

- Overhead costs provided by the institution
- Faculty, other than "core" program faculty (e.g., basic science faculty) who are supported by their respective departments
- Preceptors responsible for the clinical training of PA students

The primary source of internal financial support for most programs is the sponsoring institution. Of the 23% programs that received federal grant awards during 2014, the average was $234,461 and accounted for 14% of the total budget. Over the past decade, when federal funding levels have remained constant at roughly $5 million a year, greater levels of internal support from sponsoring institutions have enabled programs to sustain operations and develop some measure of self-sufficiency. Other sources of support come from state grants (averaging $221,650 per program), research grants, program projects, hospital services, and practice plans (Cawley & Jones, 2013).

PA programs are periodically surveyed on their purchasing power and preferences. In 2008, a total of 139 program directors were surveyed; 53 responded (38%). According to the responses, PA programs spend an average of $32,488, primarily on the following five categories:

- Medical equipment and supplies
- Textbooks and other publications
- Nonmedical equipment, such as laptops, personal digital assistants (PDAs), and smart boards
- Software
- Other major purchases

TABLE 9-8
Institutional Start-Up Costs for a Physician Assistant Program: Year 0–Year 10

Year	2011	2012	2013	2014	2015	2016	2017	2018	2019	2020
Costs (renovation)	0	325,000	300,000	0	0	0	0	0	0	0
Budget (operating costs) 4% Inc.	1,200	307,110	1,062,517	1,105,017	1,149,217	1,195,185	1,242,992	1,292,711	1,344,419	1,398,195
Revenue (tuition) 8% Inc.	0	(750,000)*	0	718,000	1,640,400	1,771,632	1,913,362	2,066,431	2,231,745	2,410,284
Difference	(1,200)	(1,382,110)	(1,362,517)	(387,017)	491,183	576,447	670,370	773,720	887,326	1,012,089
Total spent to date	1,200	1,383,310	2,845,827	3,950,844	5,100,061	6,295,246	7,538,238	8,830,949	10,175,368	11,573,563
Total revenue to date				718,000	2,358,400	4,130,032	6,043,394	8,109,825	10,341,570	12,751,854

For the same categories, average student spending per program (for all students in the professional phase, a mean of 64) was $350,692. Table 9–9 shows details of spending patterns of these programs and their students.

Other purchases commonly reported by programs included simulators, training models, cadavers, office and classroom furniture, patient actors, and Physician Assistant Clinical Knowledge Rating and Assessment Tool (PACKRAT) standard examination fees. Technology, insurance, and consultation fees were mentioned as additional fees (Box 9–2).

Programs were asked about major purchases planned for the next 3 years. Nearly two-thirds of the responding programs were planning to purchase clinical training models, simulators, and other equipment in the next 3 years, and one-half of the programs reported having assessment materials in their 3-year purchasing plan. Figure 9–6 shows details of other planned purchases.

Efficiency of Physician Assistant Education

The theory side of educational economics asks whether PA education is efficient. As America increases its medical education system output to deliver more physicians, the efficiency of modern medical education comes into question. Does it require 7 or more years to adequately prepare physicians for a generalist role, particularly when PA education has shown that a similar task can be accomplished in far less time?

The notion of Eugene Stead that gave rise to the PA profession concept was that physician education was too long and that medical education was distorted in its mission. Medical education, then as now, is characterized by a reductionist approach, in which research and a singular biological focus crowds out teaching, caring for patients, and addressing broader public health issues. Critics have called for a fundamental redesign of the content of medical training by, for example, placing greater emphasis on the social, economic (reducing the length of training to 3 years), and political aspects of healthcare delivery and noting that "in academic hospitals, research quickly outstripped teaching in importance, and a 'publish or perish' culture emerged in American universities and medical schools." They go on to say: "Research productivity remains the metric by which faculty accomplishments are judged. Today's subordination of teaching to research, as well as the narrow gaze of American medical education on biologic matters, represents a long-standing tradition" (Cooke et al., 2006). Existing models that make the process shorter, more focused on the needs of society, and thus more efficient deserve greater consideration. These tenets comprise the heart of PA educational programs.

As of 2014, the majority of PAs graduate from a 2-year postbachelor education program, compared with a 7-year postbachelor program for internists, pediatricians, and family practice specialists. PAs receive much of their training on the job, having moved on with their lives and minimized their educational debt. In many practice

TABLE 9-9
Physician Assistant Program and Student Spending, 2008

	Medical Equipment and Supplies*	Textbooks and Other Publications	Nonmedical Equipment**	Software	Other Major Purchases
PROGRAM SPENDING					
Mean	$5,811	$3,202	$8,069	$2,998	$12,408
Median	$1,000	$1,000	$2,000	$2,500	$0
STUDENT SPENDING†					
Mean	$1,211	$2,408	$2,402	$70	$405
Median	$2,774	$5,503	$11,121	$130	$1,579

*E.g., stethoscopes, reflex hammers.
**E.g., laptops, PDAs, smart boards.
†Per student.
Data from Physician Assistant Education Association (PAEA). (2008b). PA programs' purchasing power survey. Alexandria, VA: PAEA.

BOX 9-2
Other Major Purchases by Physician Assistant Programs

- *Simulators, training models*
- Charting desks
- *Cadavers*
- Diagnostic laboratory setup (examination tables, paper and supplies, blood pressure monitors, x-ray readers, desks, lights)
- *PACKRAT/Standardized examination fee*
- Dry erase board
- *Office furniture*
- Wireless ports and electrical work to support laptops on student desks
- *Classroom furniture*
- Screens for projection
- Maintenance supplies
- Sonic foundry
- Casting supplies
- Audiovisual LED projector system
- Sutures
- Uniforms
- Needles
- Consultation for developing software for clinical rotations
- Linens
- Malpractice insurance
- Surgery tables
- Student fuel credit cards for travel to distant rural clinical training sites
- Surgery scrub sink
- Conference travel
- Surgery lights
- Storage cabinets
- Standardized patients and assessment/testing materials

Note. Items in italics had multiple entries.
Data from Physician Assistant Education Association (PAEA). (2008b). *PA Programs' Purchasing Power Survey.* Alexandria, VA: PAEA.

settings, PAs and their nursing counterparts, NPs, function semiautonomously. Kindman (2006) asks: "Two years or 7 years—what can allopathic and osteopathic medical education learn from that?"

PA education has shown us that it is possible to train healthcare providers who are competent to undertake most of the functions required of a generalist provider in a short time frame. Harvey Estes, Jr., a major shaper of the profession during

its first two decades, said, "The educational system producing physician assistants is more advanced, efficient, and cost-effective than that producing physicians" (Cawley, 2013).

Validation of this aspect of efficiency in education is seen in the choices that young people are making in terms of selecting healthcareers. Most faculty in PA education are familiar with the candidate who has the grade point average high enough to be admitted to medical school who chooses to enter PA training. These applicants have weighed the option related to the professional rewards and the length of training and have selected the PA profession. Estes and other contemporaries believed that medical educators must consider and incorporate the lessons learned from PA education and the profession itself (Cawley, 2013).

Comparing Physician Assistant and Medical Education Costs

Theoretic economic projections of the cost savings that could accrue under optimal conditions of use are considerable, perhaps as much as $4 to $5 billion a year for PAs alone. For physicians, the three education-cost components are:

- Medical school costs
- Graduate (resident) training costs
- Opportunity costs

The value of services to patients provided during medical training is often debated. There is a high cost of supervision and decreased productivity (at least in theory) because of this supervision, as well as staffing costs, inefficiencies in care, and overhead. Most economists tend to consider the value to society during the resident years (postgraduate years 1–3) as a net sum of zero in internal medicine and family medicine. More important, the opportunity cost (forgone years of independent practice) is large during this training period because "independent doctor" productivity is delayed until after the period of postgraduate training.

Because virtually no physician begins practice after medical school graduation, one must consider the cost of US medical training to be at least 7 years, based on 4 years of medical school and at least 3 years of postgraduate residency for most North American systems (although shorter in other countries). A PA chooses a different path

FIGURE 9-6
Major Physician Assistant Purchases Anticipated Over the Next 3 Years

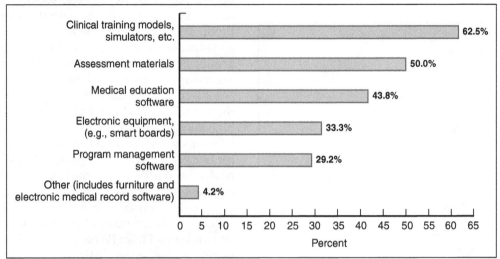

Data from *Physician Assistant Education Association (PAEA). (2008b).* PA programs' purchasing power survey. *Alexandria, VA: PAEA.*

of education that is approximately 2.5 years long. If the medical student had chosen to be a PA, practice income would be generated after 2.5 years of professional training. Using the PA salary rather than the potential income of a 4-year medical school plus 3-year postgraduate-trained physician, one can estimate the cost differential of physicians and PAs.

Both the PA and the medical student start approximately from the same place academically. The average PA student has a baccalaureate degree, as does the medical student. Most have the same type of background with varying combinations of academic course work in their undergraduate years. Given the overlapping training periods for doctors and PAs, the opportunity costs for these two can be calculated and compared.

In Figure 9–7, the PA and medical students are assumed to begin education after completion of 4 years of undergraduate study (most enter medical school and PA school with a baccalaureate degree acquired after 4 years). The PA becomes fully productive after 2 years of additional education, and the physician becomes a fully productive provider of care 5 years after the PA. Using the labor economic assumption that the PA's salary level is the value of a provider and that the PA salary is $100,000, the PA has delivered $500,000 ($100,000 × 5 years) worth of care

FIGURE 9-7
Cost Comparison of Physician Assistant and Physician Training Programs in 2014 Dollars

	PA student	MD student
Cost/year	$20,000	$40,000
Years of training	2.5	4
Total	$50,000	$160,000

before the physician begins practice. This figure is defined as the opportunity cost of additional medical education and training for the North American doctor. It is also the value of care that would have been delivered to society had the medical student chosen a PA training course.

Figure 9–7 also illustrates the opportunity cost of additional medical education and training. If direct training costs are assumed to be approximately $75,000 for a PA and $150,000 for a primary care allopathic physician, the difference between the physician and the PA in total training costs in 2014 may be calculated as $150,000 minus $75,000, plus the protracted training ($150,000 – $75,000 + $500,000). The differential is $575,000 per PA that society gains by having a PA trained instead of a physician. Put another way, the PA produces $575,000 worth of patient care before the physician begins practice.

If salary costs are used as a proxy for employment costs, the physician–PA differential is $50,000 (the differences between the average primary care salaries of $200,000 for physicians and $100,000 for PAs). This means the salary cost of a PA is 0.5 of a physician. If it requires 10% of a physician's time to supervise a PA, 10% of $200,000 should be added to the cost of employing a PA. The PA–doctor cost ratio as viewed by an employer would then become $100,000:$200,000, or 0.5.

COSTS OF PRACTICING PHYSICIAN ASSISTANTS

Cost implications of the use of PAs can be viewed from three perspectives. The first is that of the entrepreneurial doctor or medical

practice: Will revenue resulting from hiring a PA exceed the additional costs of compensating the provider? Second, if market conditions warrant, the focus is whether it is more desirable to hire a doctor or a PA. The third is the societal concern: How to deliver high-quality care at minimal cost? For many economists, the social economic view is all that counts, no matter where costs come from. In the end, all costs are ultimately borne by society.

Employment Costs of Physician Assistants

A number of direct and indirect costs must be considered when a PA is employed. These costs include salary, benefits, malpractice insurance, office space, equipment, support staff, supplies, and other direct and indirect expenses. Data on this subject are sparse, although there is little to suggest that costs other than compensation are different from those associated with employing a physician. Only one outcome study has been undertaken demonstrating that a PA uses no more laboratory and imaging orders and drugs for an episode of care than does a physician (Table 9–10; Hooker, 2002). Aside

TABLE 9-10
Multivariate Regression Cost Model Holding Different Valuables Constant While Examining for Differences Between Types of Providers

Provider	N	Total Cost	Visit Cost	Med Cost	Image Cost	Laboratory Cost
BRONCHITIS EPISODE COST						
Physician	1,336	$234.74	$133.63*	$96.42**	$3.31	$1.37
PA	411	$224.13	$92.23*	$125.74	$4.65	$1.50
TENDINITIS EPISODE COSTS						
Physician	264	$183.33**	$144.77*	$30.14	$7.50	$0.93
PA	90	$149.80**	$98.77*	$40.65	$9.53	$0.84
OTITIS MEDIA EPISODE COSTS						
Physician	6,264	$188.39*	$140.07*	$47.77	$0.0	$0.54
PA	2,008	$136.60*	$83.29*	$52.99	$0.0	$0.32
URINARY TRACT INFECTION EPISODE COSTS						
Physician	1,633	$262.17*	$142.73	$83.91	$17.67*	$17.86**
PA	878	$210.50*	$97.70*	$91.50	$5.80*	$15.48**
TOTAL	12,866					

*Significant at $P < .001$.
**Significant at $P < 0.01$.
Data from Hooker, R .S. (2002). A cost analysis of physician assistants in primary care. *Journal of the American Academy of Physician Assistants, 15*(11), 39–42, 45, 48 passim.

from anecdotal reports suggesting that malpractice insurance may be substantially less for a PA because the litigation rate is less than that for physicians, there seems to be little to suggest that PAs lose any of their cost-effectiveness by the way they practice medicine.

In contrast to other costs, the income differential for PAs and physicians is clearly quite large. Most PAs are employees and therefore are salaried, whereas self-employed physicians receive not only a stream of revenue for their own services but also entrepreneurial benefit from employing a revenue-generating provider.

PA Wages

Based on US Bureau of Labor Statistics published data in 2015, $98,180 was the mean annual wage

estimate for PAs employed in the offices of physicians in that year. The figure for a family medicine physician in the same year was approximately $215,650 (US Department of Labor, Bureau of Labor Statistics, 2013). Therefore, a family medicine PA earned approximately 0.45 of the salary of a physician in family medicine (Table 9–11). This ratio has fluctuated between 40% and 50% for 30 years. The ratio is higher when using American Medical Association (AMA) and AAPA data and lower when using Bureau of Labor Statistics data. Differences between the Bureau of Labor Statistics data and AAPA (or AMA) data may be due to bias selection; professional society members (such as doctors and PAs with high salaries) are more likely to join than those with low salaries.

TABLE 9-11
Physician Salary Data

Industry	Employment	Percent of Industry Employment	Hourly Mean Wage	Annual Mean Wage
Offices of physicians	48,140	2.03	$44.73	$93,040
General medical and surgical hospitals	18,380	0.35	$45.01	$93,630
Outpatient care centers	6,040	0.94	$45.35	$94,330
Federal executive branch (OES designation)	2,460	0.12	$40.27	$83,770
Employment services	1,910	0.06	$46.98	$97,720

INDUSTRIES WITH THE HIGHEST CONCENTRATION OF EMPLOYMENT IN THIS OCCUPATION

Industry	Employment	Percent of industry employment	Hourly mean wage	Annual mean wage
Offices of physicians	48,140	2.03	$44.73	$93,040
Outpatient care centers	6,040	0.94	$45.35	$94,330
General medical and surgical hospitals	18,380	0.35	$45.01	$93,630
Specialty (except psychiatric and substance abuse) hospitals	710	0.31	$48.11	$100,060
Offices of other health practitioners	1,150	0.16	$40.94	$85,160

TOP PAYING INDUSTRIES FOR THIS OCCUPATION

Industry	Employment	Percent of industry employment	Hourly mean wage	Annual mean wage
Specialty (except psychiatric and substance abuse) hospitals	710	0.31	$48.11	$100,060
Home health services	100	0.01	$47.23	$98,230
Office administrative services	120	0.03	$47.11	$98,000
Employment services	1,910	0.06	$46.98	$97,720
Outpatient care centers	6,040	0.94	$45.35	$94,330

OES = Occupational Employment Statistics.
Data from US Department of Labor, Bureau of Labor Statistics. (2013). "Occupational Employment and Wages, May 2013: 29-1071 Physician Assistants" [Online]. Retrieved from http://www.bls.gov/oes/current/oes291071.htm

More difficult to calculate are the benefits associated with each type of employment (doctor vs. PA). A doctor may be a partner of a medical group, have bonuses at the end of the year, have tax-deferred income with partnership shares, and have different time-off arrangements. PAs, on the other hand, tend to be salaried and not share-holding partners in the practice. As information emerges from various countries where salary and income are more standardized and can be more accurately accounted for, the differences may reveal a more reliable gauge of worth of a career.

Perquisites (Fringe Benefits)

Although the compensation package of a PA, which includes salary and benefits, may differ monetarily from that of a physician colleague in the same work organization, there are some parallels in the types of perquisites offered. The more consistent ones include health insurance, malpractice insurance, a retirement plan, allowances for journals and continuing education, and paid time off to take coursework or continuing medical education. Retirement benefits range between $4,500 and $4,800 for PAs compared with $14,225 for internists and $12,529 for family practitioners who do not deliver babies.

Financials are another fringe benefit that are folded into PA and doctor compensation. In 2006, 24% of PAs reported receiving a bonus based on their individual performance, with revenue generated being the most common yardstick. Extra pay was also received based on overtime, assistance on surgeries, administrative duties, and on-call availability and services. In all, 68% of PAs reported some form of additional pay besides their base salary (AAPA, 2016).

Compensation–Production Ratio

One of the better ways to examine the net value of a PA is the income generated to the employer in private practice. Compensation, which includes salary and benefits collectively, is usually examined. The most useful ratio is the amount of compensation the employer forgoes to retain the PA divided by the amount of revenue the PA returns to the employer. Basically, the smaller the ratio, the more economical the provider is to the practice. The Medical Group Management Association (MGMA) collects these data annually (Table 9–12). In 2010, the compensation–production ratio for PAs was 0.27. For comparison, the compensation-production ratio for family practice physicians was 0.57; for pediatricians, 0.49; for NPs, 0.42; and for psychologists, 0.79. These findings suggest that PAs are relatively more economical to employ because they return more revenue for their salary than do other providers.

TABLE 9-12

Compensation to Gross Charges Ratio for Physician Assistants and Other Types of Providers, 2010

Provider Type	Median	No. of Providers	Medical Practices
Overall for primary care PAs	0.341	440	124
Single specialty	0.208	69	36
Multispecialty	0.245	371	88
Family practice physician (without obstetrician)	0.527	1,621	232
Internal medicine physician	0.541	1,289	187
Pediatric physician	0.485	941	147
Nurse practitioner	0.470	258	74
Midwife (outpatient and inpatient)	0.424	61	25
Optometrist	0.447	84	32
Psychologist	0.655	89	34
Physical therapist	0.406	133	24

Data from Medical Group Management Association. (2010). *Physician Compensation and Production Survey: 2010 Report Based on 2009 Survey.* Englewood, CO: Medical Group Management Association.

Substitution Ratios

Substitution is the degree of labor one worker can assume for another. Primarily, the level of delegation and comparative productivity of physicians and PAs for the delegated services determine the physician–PA substitution ratio. A substitution ratio of 1.0 implies unity and is achieved when one PA completely substitutes for one doctor. PAs in rural and isolated clinics commonly function at very high levels, often replacing the physician who was previously occupying that role. These accounts are largely anecdotal, however, and little is known about the types and numbers of patients seen by physicians versus PAs in comparable settings. The best studies occur in large managed care settings in which some of the variables can be controlled and physicians and PAs work alongside each other, seeing similar patients at the same time and under the same circumstances.

Using a metropolitan medical center as a paradigm, one study constructed production functions that would best exploit the possibilities of substituting PAs for physicians. It was estimated that one PA could replace one-half of a full-time physician. From data developed in a national survey of physicians, Scheffler, Waitzman, and Hillman (1996) estimated that a 10% increase in the medical office visits output of a practice would require, on average, an increase of 3.5% in physician hours or 5.4% in PA hours. These percentages suggest a marginal substitution ratio of 0.63, compared with the overall 0.50 ratio.

Record and Schweitzer (1981a, 1981b) estimated that if enough PAs were hired to perform all of the services for which physicians in the Department of Internal Medicine at Kaiser Permanente considered them competent, and if the PA and physician workweeks were equal, the substitution ratio would be 0.76. However, Hooker (1993) using more developed data in the same institution showed that the ratio was 0.90, considerably higher than theorized.

Most of the contemporary estimates of substitution ratios in primary care fall in the range of 0.75 to 0.95, suggesting it would take, on average, approximately one PA to substitute for three-fourths of a family physician. For managers, this suggests that four PAs could replace

three physicians conservatively. What is not accounted for is the efficiency that develops with division of labor, economy of scale, and increased throughputs decreases the patient waiting times and improves patient satisfaction. The Essary et al study (2016) showed that annual productivity of PAs at times exceeded that of physicians when the same setting was held constant.

Resource-Based Relative Value Scale

The Resource-Based Relative Value Scale (RVS) is widely used to measure healthcare provider productivity and to set payment standards, although its limitation is in its assessment of "preservice" and "postservice" work and other potentially non–revenue-generating healthcare services, or service-valued activity (SVA). A time and motion study assessed PA/NP productivity in hospital and outpatient settings. Using personal digital assistants (PDAs), 19 PA/NPs identified their location and activity each time the PDA randomly prompted them to input their activity. The data from the providers in multiple inpatient and outpatient settings was separated into revenue-generating services (RGSs) and SVAs. The inpatient PA/NPs spent 62% of their time on RGSs and 35% on SVAs. Providers in the outpatient settings spent 59% of their time on RGSs and 38% on SVAs. This novel information gathering system can be used to accurately document productivity, determine clinical practice patterns, and improve deployment strategies of healthcare providers (Ogunfiditimi et al., 2013).

Controlling the overall cost of medical care requires controlling the number of physician visits. Nurse practitioners and physician assistants (NP/PAs) may function as lower-cost substitutes for physicians or they may complement physician services. The association between NP/PA and physician visits when they are not working as primary care providers (PCPs) has not been thoroughly studied. A sample of 400 family medicine patients drawn from a Mayo Clinic multisite practice was studied using multiple logistic regression analysis. NPs/PAs did not function as PCPs during the study period. Patients were defined as outliers if they visited physicians more than five times in a year. Patients who visited NP/PAs in non-retail clinics were significantly more likely to be physician visit outliers. Visits to NP/PAs in retail clinics were not related to physician visits. The authors concluded that NP/PA visits in standard medical office settings *complement* physician visits when the NP/PAs were not working as PCPs in this large multisite practice. Healthcare reform proposals relying on increased use of NP/PAs may be more cost-efficient if NP/PAs are located in retail settings or function as PCPs (Rohrer et al., 2013).

Both the Essary et al study (2015) and the Moran et al study (2016) showed that when RVUs were tabulated the annual productivity of PAs and NPs were closely aligned with physicians in the same settings.

REIMBURSEMENT

There are four major ways a physician is reimbursed for his or her labor: fee for service, fee per case, per capita, and salary. As employees of doctors, PAs must be cost-effective to allow the reimbursement rate to adequately compensate for their labors and the cost to the physician employer for his or her risk in employing the PA. Reimbursement of PAs can occur depending on various scenarios. The three major methods of reimbursing PAs for services in the United States are Medicare, Medicaid, and third-party reimbursement from private insurance companies (Box 9–3).

BOX 9-3
Payment for PA services

Payment for provider services in the United States can occur in the following ways:

■ Private insurance (which includes the federal TriCare for military dependents)
■ Medicare/Medicaid:
  ■ Medicare + Medicaid
  ■ Medicare + private insurance
■ Worker's compensation
■ Self-pay/out-of-pocket payment
■ No charge/charity care (*pro bono*)

Medicare Coverage for Physician Assistants

Since 1998, Medicare pays the PAs' employers for medical services provided by PAs in all settings at 85% of the physician's fee schedule (Table 9–13). This payment includes work performed in hospitals (inpatient, outpatient, and emergency departments); nursing facilities; homes; and offices and clinics as well as first assisting with surgery. Assignment of fees is mandatory, and state law determines supervision and scope of practice. Hospitals that bill Medicare Part B for services provided by PAs may not at the same time include PA salaries in the hospital's cost reports.

Outpatient services provided in offices and clinics may still be billed under Medicare's "incident-to" provisions if Medicare's restrictive billing guidelines are met. This form of billing allows payment at 100% of the fee schedule if (1) the physician is physically on site when the PA provides care, (2) the physician treats all new Medicare patients (PAs may provide the subsequent care), and (3) established Medicare patients with new medical problems are personally treated by the physician (PAs may provide the subsequent care).

According to the Balanced Budget Act, PAs (using the 85% reimbursement benefit) may be W-2 employees, leased employees, or independent contractors. The employer still bills Medicare for the services provided by the PA, no matter the employment arrangement. All PAs who treat Medicare patients must have a national plan and provider number (NPI). In 2002, the Centers for Medicare and Medicaid Services issued new instructions that permitted PAs to have an ownership interest in an approved corporate entity (e.g., professional medical corporation) that bills the Medicare program if that corporation qualifies as a provider or supplier of Medicare services. The new policy also removed a provision that prohibited ambulatory surgical centers from employing PAs.

Medicaid Coverage

All 50 states, the federal district, and most US territories cover medical services provided by PAs under their state-based Medicaid programs.

TABLE 9-13
Medicare Policy for Physician Assistants

Setting	Supervision Requirement	Reimbursement Rate	Services
Office/clinic when physician is not on site	State law	85% of physician's fee schedule	All services a PA is legally authorized to provide that would have been covered if provided personally by a physician
Office/clinic when physician is on site	Physician must be in the suite of offices	100% of physician's fee schedule*	Same as above
Home visit/house call	State law	85% of physician's fee schedule	Same as above
Skilled nursing facility and nursing facility	State law	85% of physician's fee schedule	Same as above
Office or home visit if rural Health Professional Shortage Area	State law	85% of physician's fee schedule	Same as above
Hospital	State law	85% of physician's fee schedule	Same as above
First assisting at surgery in all settings	State law	85% of physician's first assist fee schedule**	Same as above
Federally certified rural health clinics	State law	85% of physician's fee schedule	Same as above
HMO†	State law	85% of physician's fee schedule	Same as above

HMO = health maintenance organization.
*Using carrier guidelines for "incident to" services.
**For example, 85% × 16% = 13.6% of surgeon's fee.
†Some Medicare/HMO risk contracts may exclude nonphysician providers.

The rate of reimbursement, which is paid to the employing practice and not directly to the PA, is either the same as or slightly lower than that paid to physicians.

Private Insurance

There are more than 100 health insurance companies in the United States. Private insurers generally cover medical services provided by PAs when they are included as part of the physician's bill or as part of a global fee for surgery.

Although insurance companies have discretion regarding the rate at which they reimburse a PA for services, the standard rate that emerged after the Balanced Budget Act of 1997 is at 85% of the prevailing rate for a doctor in the same setting. Over the past two decades, a number of actions by state insurance regulators and a few litigations against companies such as Blue Cross of Georgia in the early 2000s resulted

in most companies honoring the medical services of PAs and NPs.

ISSUES REGARDING THE EFFECTIVENESS OF PHYSICIAN ASSISTANTS

How cost-effective is a PA? The answer is contained in the difference between the physician–PA substitution ratio (0.75) and the PA–physician compensation ratio (0.45). The meaning of these two numbers is that a PA can substitute for *at least* 75% (conservatively) of primary care physician's range of services. This service is undertaken at approximately 45% of the physician's salary. If the physician's time to see patients is reduced because of supervision, then the ratio is 50%. The social cost figures are even more impressive because the PA–physician ratio, including training costs, is smaller than the employment cost ratio. Finally, the employment of a primary care PA is fairly economical because the compensation–production ratio at 27% is more efficient than that of most other types of providers (including family medicine doctors at 53% and NPs at 38%).

Table 9–14 summarizes the economic exercises in this chapter. These figures, however, must be viewed with caution because they are based on the "best studies" (those studies considered the most rigorous in investigation) or the average of different studies, using fairly conservative figures.

Prescribing Authority

All states, the District of Columbia, and four of the five territories authorize prescribing privileges for PAs; most allow some prescribing of controlled substances. Prescribing authority generally applies to the outpatient or ambulatory setting. Medications for patients in hospitals are considered medical orders and usually fall under the purview of institutional medical staff bylaws. States typically place certain stipulations on PA prescribing activities. These may include:

- Requiring a physician cosignature for a PA prescription
- Limiting the drugs that a PA may prescribe (e.g., those listed in a specific formulary)
- Excluding selected schedules of drugs, usually schedule II agents (i.e., those defined by the Controlled Substances Act as having the potential for abuse)

- Prescribing using drug treatment protocols
- Limiting the quantities of certain drugs that PAs may prescribe

National trends in PA and NP prescribing research found, on average, doctors, PAs, and NPs wrote prescriptions for 60% to 70% of their visits. The mean number of prescriptions was 1.3 to 1.5 per visit depending on the provider. PAs were more likely to prescribe a controlled substance than were physicians and NPs (19.5%, 12.4%, and 10.9%, respectively). Overall, PAs and NPs prescribe in a manner similar to doctors (Hooker & Cipher, 2005).

Prescribing Behavior

Although all 50 states permit PAs to prescribe, a full understanding of the implications of this policy is yet to be determined. In 2008, the AAPA Research Division estimated that PAs practicing in family medicine and general internal medicine wrote 1.5 prescriptions, whereas those in emergency medicine wrote 1.4. These three specialties wrote the most prescriptions (AAPA, 2008).

JOB SATISFACTION OF PHYSICIAN ASSISTANTS

Job satisfaction is not usually thought of as an economic issue. However, a high rate of turnover of professional personnel in a clinic is disruptive to patient care and organizational stability as well as to the individual clinician. When employment

TABLE 9–14
Cost-Effectiveness of Primary Care Physician Assistants*

Issue Examined	Range	Average or Best Study
Delegation	0.40:1.0	0.83
Supervision	0.10:0.60	0.10
Physician–PA substitution ratio	0.40:1.0	0.75
PA–physician cost ratio (salary)	0.40:0.50	0.43
PA–physician cost ratio (with supervision)		0.52
Compensation–production ratio	0.25:0.52	0.38
Societal cost training a PA (compared with a physician)		0.20
Average number of outpatients seen	18:35	21.7
PA–physician cost–benefit ratio	Unknown	Unknown

*Based on a review of the literature, using conservative estimates, and extrapolating to 2005 costs.

attrition occurs, productivity and the efficiency of the healthcare service are negatively affected.

Research on PAs and job satisfaction is fairly extensive. PAs seem to be reasonably satisfied with their work experience and practice conditions. They express an overall level of satisfaction that compares favorably to that of other professionals, including lawyers, accountants, and engineers, and PAs report less stress and lower turnover rates than nurses and many other health personnel (Hooker et al., 2015).

The major determinants of job satisfaction among PAs seem to be the professional and personal support provided by the supervising physician, the amount of responsibility for patient care, income, and opportunities for career advancement. Two studies suggest the strongest correlates of both job performance and job satisfaction are the degree of physician supervisory support and amount of responsibility for patient care (Freeborn et al. 2002). Inadequate financial compensation and control over income are other reported sources of dissatisfaction. Acceptance by patients and by other healthcare workers has not been found to be a significant problem (Hooker et al., 2015).

Clinical responsibility and professional autonomy among PAs is highly correlated with the level of job satisfaction, the extent of professional and personal support provided by the supervising physicians, and the opportunities for career advancement. The majority of studies addressing the job/career satisfaction of PAs reveal that they are largely satisfied in their professional roles and are quite happy with their career choice—a set of findings that is a bit surprising in view of the status of PAs as dependent practitioners.

Holmes and Fasser (1993) reported findings of occupational stress and professional retention in a survey conducted of 1,360 randomly selected practicing PAs responding to a mailed questionnaire. The typical respondent was male (53%), white (88%), and age 37 years (mean) and devoted most work time to patient care activities. Job satisfaction was high overall, and it was correlated positively with independence, challenge, and job security. Issues of salary, perceived opportunities for advancement, and the management style of the employer were associated with the highest levels of job dissatisfaction and role stress.

In one of the few career satisfaction studies involving health professionals that have similar levels of responsibility, PAs in an HMO were compared with others in the same setting: NPs, optometrists, mental health workers, and chemical dependency counselors. PAs expressed the most satisfaction with the amount of responsibility given, support from coworkers, job security, working hours, supervision, and task variety. They were less satisfied with workload, control over the pace of work, and opportunities for advancement. Chemical dependency counselors expressed the highest levels of satisfaction across various dimensions of work; optometrists expressed the lowest level of satisfaction (Figure 9–8). NPs also tended to be satisfied with most aspects of practice in this setting. In a number of instances, they were more satisfied than the PAs. Most PAs were also satisfied with pay and fringe benefits (Freeborn & Hooker, 1995).

These findings, along with those of other studies, suggest that institutions, group practices, and HMOs are favorable settings for PAs. The organization of care in an HMO model may be consistent with how the PA views himself or herself as a member of a team.

As of 2013, the annual annulment (death, disability, retirement) rate for PAs in the United States was estimated at 2.9%. This estimate is considered very low for any occupation. How long PAs remain in their careers as clinicians remains for further analysis. Clear evidence exists that PA employment results in the production of more revenue than the costs of that employment in almost all settings (Coombs et al., 2013).

FURTHER RESEARCH ON PHYSICIAN ASSISTANT ECONOMICS

The literature about the economics of PA education and employment is sparse. It is also somewhat outdated in the sense that national productivity has not been evaluated. Because

FIGURE 9-8
Comparison of Job Satisfaction Between Nonphysician Providers

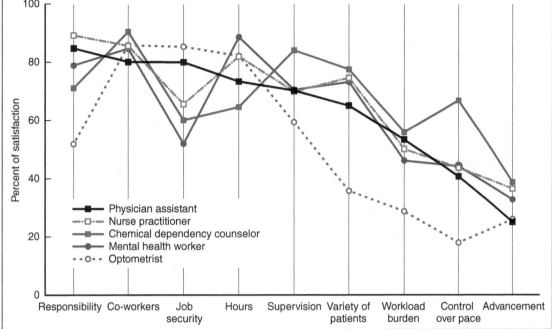

Data from *Freeborn, D. K., & Hooker, R. S. (1995). Satisfaction of physician assistants and other nonphysician providers in a managed care setting.* Public Health Reports (Washington, D.C. 1974), 110(6), 714–719.

this literature reveals large areas missing and many questions unanswered, a brief list of suggested economic questions and areas for future research are presented follows.

- **Case reports:** How does the PA's clinical role compare with that of a doctor in the same role? A case report of two or more clinicians provides an opportunity to see how a PA can be used in common situations. Diagnostic codes, procedure codes, patient characteristics, and revenue generated should be compared.
- **Cost benefit:** What is the cost benefit of a PA to an organization? Do PAs negate any of their cost-effectiveness by managing patients differently? What are some of the differences between clinics with and without PAs?
- **Cost utility:** What is the cost utility of a PA, and does the chronic disease management of a patient by a PA have any different utility than with a doctor?

- **Team use:** Does the incorporation of a PA on a team of doctors and nurses change the productivity and output? Does a doctor–PA team improve care compared with a doctor–doctor team?
- **Economy of scale:** Is there some optimal level when the addition of one more PA to an organization changes the output?
- **Education:** What is the opportunity cost of a PA education? How does this differ by type of institution and by size of PA program? What are the differences between public and private tuition PA programs? Do these differences in cost of education have any predictive value on the role the PA selects?
- **Rate of return:** What is the rate of return to a PA education for the individual, institution, and society?
- **Cost of PA programs:** What is the cost of starting a PA program and maintaining a PA program? What is the cost per student

per month, and is this changing compared with inflation?

- **Patient benefit from PA education:** What does a patient receive in turn for being a patient attended by a PA in training?
- **Role satisfaction:** Are PAs satisfied with their roles? Are some PA roles more satisfying than others?
- **Productivity over time:** What is the lifetime productivity of a PA under given circumstances?

Furthermore, additional studies examining levels of PA clinical performance characteristics are needed because the content of clinical care (the specific medical tasks) delivered by PAs differs within various clinical settings. Comparing the number, content, and patient outcomes of clinical services of PAs with those of physicians would be useful.

SUMMARY

Knowledge about performance and the potential contribution of PAs continues to be a significant source of scrutiny by health services researchers. Virtually all studies demonstrate an advantage to systems, whether they are large or small, when a PA is added to the staff. Clearly a large portion of primary care services can be safely delegated to PAs. In settings where PAs provide these services, they perform at levels of productivity that compare favorably with physicians. When the difference between substitution ratios and cost ratios are compared (even when the ratios are conservatively estimated) the differences are so large as to ensure cost savings for employers. Prepaid group practice studies and research from other large institutions suggest that physician comfort levels and practice styles in delegating medical tasks to the PAs with whom they work have a significant influence on PA use and effectiveness in clinical practices. In studies of performance and patterns of utilization of PAs and NPs, scholars have noted a marked difference in the observed versus normative rates of delegation of medical tasks by HMO physicians when working with both PAs and NPs.

Measures of the clinical practice activities and professional characteristics of various healthcare providers continue to be observed in inpatient and outpatient settings. Results suggest that PAs and NPs are underused in many healthcare systems. The factor most critical in determining the effective use of PAs is the medical task delegation style of the supervising physicians. Staffing efficiency in many organizations could be increased if physicians were more aware of the clinical roles and practice capabilities of these PAs and were better equipped to delegate tasks appropriately.

The societal cost benefits of PAs in the form of education suggest that a great deal is gained when PAs are trained because they provide care at substantial savings for 5 years longer than physicians. Many of the barriers in the form of restrictive legislation and reimbursement policies that at one time interfered with full use of PAs have largely been removed.

Finally, the cost advantages of employing PAs rather than physicians remain strong after 4 decades of observation. The cost difference between the income of doctors in primary care and PAs in primary care has been hovering around 50% salary ratio since the early 1990s. However, this employment investment could diminish if the gap between physician and PA earnings significantly narrows.

References

The following citations are key to supporting this chapter's content. You can find a complete list of citations for all chapters at www. fadavis.com/davisplus, keyword *Hooker*.

Agarwal, A., Zhang, W., Kuo, Y., & Sharma, G. (2016). Process and outcome measures among COPD patients with a hospitalization cared for by an advance practice provider or primary care physician. *PLoS ONE, 11*(2), e0148522.

American Academy of PAs. (2016). *2016 AAPA Salary Report.* Alexandria, VA: Author.

Cawley, J. F. (2013). A conversation with E. Harvey Estes, Jr., M.D. *Journal of Physician Assistant Education, 24*(2), 22–24.

Cawley, J. F., & Jones, P. E. (2013). Institutional sponsorship, student debt, and specialty choice in physician assistant education. *Journal of Physician Assistant Education, 24*(4), 4–8.

Cooke, M., Irby, D. M., Sullivan, W., & Ludmerer, K. (2006). American medical education 100 years after the Flexner report. *New England Journal of Medicine, 355*(13), 1339–1344.

Coombs, J. M., Hooker, R. S., & Brunisholz, K. D. (2013). What do we know about retired physician assistants? A preliminary study. *Journal of the American Academy of Physician Assistants, 26*(3), 44–48.

Dhuper, S., & Choksi, S. (2009). Replacing an academic internal medicine residency program with a physician assistant-hospitalist model: A comparative analysis study. *American Journal of Medical Quality, 23*(2), 132–139.

Essary, A. C., Green, E. P., & Gans, D. N. (2016). Compensation and production in family medicine by practice ownership. *Health Services Research and Managerial Epidemiology, 1,* 3.

Essary, A., Wallace, L., & Asprey, D. (2014). The relationship between physician assistant program costs and student tuition and fees. *Journal of Physician Assistant Education, 25*(1), 29–32.

Freeborn, D. K., & Hooker, R. S. (1995). Satisfaction of physician assistants and other nonphysician providers in a managed care setting. *Public Health Reports (Washington, D.C. 1974), 110*(6), 714–719.

Freeborn, D. K., Hooker, R. S., & Pope, C. R. (2002). Satisfaction and well-being of primary care providers in managed care. *Evaluation & The Health Professions, 25*(2), 239–254.

Henry, L. R., & Hooker, R. S. (2014). Caring for the disadvantaged: The role of physician assistants. *Journal of the American Academy of Physician Assistants, 27*(1), 36–42.

Holmes, S. E., & Fasser, C. E. (1993). Occupational stress among physician assistants. *Journal of the American Academy of Physician Assistants, 6*(3), 172–178.

Hooker, R. S. (1993). The roles of physician assistants and nurse practitioners in a managed care organization. In D. K. Clawson & M. Osterweis (Eds.), *The Roles of Physician Assistants and Nurse Practitioners in Primary Care.* Washington, DC: The Association of Academic Health Centers.

Hooker, R. S. (2002). A cost analysis of physician assistants in primary care. *Journal of the American Academy of Physician Assistants, 15*(11), 39–48.

Hooker, R. S., & Cipher, D. J. (2005). Physician assistant and nurse practitioner prescribing: 1997–2002. *Journal of Rural Health, 21*(4), 355–360.

Hooker, R. S., & Freeborn, D. K. (1991). Use of physician assistants in a managed healthcare system. *Public Health Reports (Washington, DC: 1974), 106*(1), 90–94.

Hooker, R. S., Kuilman, L., & Everett, C. M. (2015). Physician assistant job satisfaction: A narrative review of empirical research. *Journal of Physician Assistant Education, 26*(4), 176–186.

Hooker, R. S., & Warren, J. (2001). Comparison of physician assistant programs by tuition costs. *Perspective on Physician Assistant Education, 12,* 87–91.

Kindman, L. A. (2006). Medical education after the Flexner report. *New England Journal of Medicine, 356*(1), 90.

Moore, M., Coffman, M., Cawley, J. F., Crowley, D., Bazemore, A., Cheng, N., Fox, S., & Klink, K. (2014). *The impact of debt load on physician assistants.* Washington, DC: Robert Graham Center.

Moran EA, Basa E, Gao J, Woodmansee D, Lamenoff PL, Hooker RS. PA and NP productivity in the Veterans Health Administration. *Journal of the American Academy of Physician Assistants.* 2016; 29(7): 1-7 on-line.

Morgan, P. A., Abbott, D. H., McNeil, R. B., & Fisher, D. A. (2012). Characteristics of primary care office visits to nurse practitioners, physician assistants and physicians in United States Veterans Health Administration facilities, 2005 to 2010: A retrospective cross-sectional analysis. *Human Resources for Health, 10*(1), 42.

Ogunfiditimi, F., Takis, L., Paige, V. J., Wyman, J. F., & Marlow, E. (2013). Assessing the productivity of advanced practice providers using a time and motion study. *Journal of Healthcare Management, 58*(3), 173–185.

Pedersen, D. M., Chappell, B., Elison, G., & Bunnell, R. (2008). The productivity of PAs, APRNs, and physicians in Utah. *Journal of the American Academy of Physician Assistants, 21*(1), 42–47.

Philpot, R. J. (2005). *Financial returns to society by National Health Service corps scholars who receive training as physician assistants and nurse practitioners.* Unpublished doctoral dissertation, University of Florida.

Record, J. C., Blomquist, R. H., McCabe, M. A., McCally, M., & Berger, B. D. (1981). Delegation in adult primary care: The generalizability of HMO data. *Springer Series on Healthcare and Society, 6,* 68–83.

Record, J. C., McCally, M., Schweitzer, S. O., Blomquist, R. M., & Berger, B. D. (1980). New health professions after a decade and a half: Delegation, productivity and costs in primary care. *Journal of Health Politics, Policy & Law, 5*(3), 470–497.

Record, J. C., & Schweitzer, S. O. (1981a). Staffing primary care in 1990: Effects of national health insurance on staffing and costs. *Springer Series on Healthcare and Society, 6,* 115–127.

Record, J. C., & Schweitzer, S. O. (1981b). Staffing primary care in 1990—Potential effects on staffing and costs: Estimates from the model. *Springer Series on Healthcare and Society, 6,* 87–114.

Roblin, D. W., Howard, D. H., Becker, E. R., Adams, E. K., & Roberts, M. H. (2004a). Use of midlevel practitioners to achieve labor cost savings in the primary care practice of an MCO. *Health Services Research, 39*(3), 607–626.

Roblin, D. W., Becker, E. R., Adams, E. K., Howard, D. H., & Roberts, M. H. (2004b). Patient satisfaction with primary care: Does type of practitioner matter? *Medical Care, 42*(6), 579–590.

Roblin, D. W., Howard, D. H., Ren, J., & Becker, E. R. (2011). An evaluation of the influence of primary care team functioning on the health of Medicare beneficiaries. *Medical Care Research and Review, 68*(2), 177–201.

Rohrer, J. E., Angstman, K. B., Garrison, G. M., Pecina, J. L., & Maxson, J. A. (2013). Nurse practitioners and physician assistants are complements to family medicine physicians. *Population Health Management, 16*(4), 242–245.

Scheffler, R. M., Waitzman, N. J., & Hillman, J. M. (1996). The productivity of physician assistants and nurse practitioners and health work force policy in the era of managed healthcare. *Journal of Allied Health, 25*(3), 207–217.

US Department of Labor, Bureau of Labor Statistics. (2013). Occupational Employment and Wages, May 2013: 29-1071 Physician Assistants. Retrieved from http://www.bls.gov/oes/current/oes291071.htm

Van Rhee, J., Ritchie, J., & Eward, A. M. (2002). Resource use by physician assistant services versus teaching services. *Journal of the American Academy of Physician Assistants, 15*(1) 33–38, 40, 42 passim.

Youngclaus, J., & Fresne, J. A. (2013). *Physician education debt and the cost to attend medical school: 2012 update.* Washington, DC: Association of American Medical Colleges.

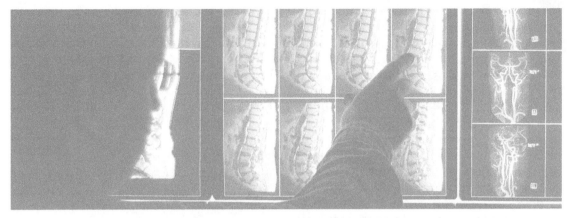

CHAPTER 10

LEGAL ASPECTS OF PHYSICIAN ASSISTANT PRACTICE

JAMES F. CAWLEY ■ CHRISTINE M. EVERETT ■ RODERICK S. HOOKER

"Law and order are the medicine of the body politic and when the body politic gets sick, medicine must be administered."
—*B. R. Ambedkar, Indian economist and social reformer*

In 1965, Dr. Eugene A. Stead, Jr., Chair of the Department of Medicine, founded Duke University's Physician Assistant Program. The Duke program was the first in the US to formally train this professional group in general medicine. However, upon graduating from the program in 1967, the only legal framework to authorize physician assistant (PA) practice was a 1966 opinion from the Attorney General of North Carolina, which provided that the performance of delegated, physician-supervised activities by a PA did not violate state law. By 1974, 37 states had passed legislation to authorize practice by these new practitioners. Within 4 decades, a series of laws developed to govern the PA practice, including a network of statutes and regulations in the states, the District of Columbia, the United States Territories, and federal systems. In general, states are far from achieving uniformity in

their laws, and PA legislation is no exception. In less than 50 years, PA regulation originated through considerable legal activism, largely on the part of state and national PA organizations, with considerations of appropriate medical scope of practice, concern for public safety, and assurance of professional conduct. This chapter reviews the key legal concepts and principles that pertain to PAs and their practice of medicine.

LEGAL BASIS FOR PHYSICIAN ASSISTANT PRACTICE

Supervision and Delegation

PAs were created in response to a changing healthcare system. As a result, the US legal system has needed to address the PA phenomenon. One of the primary aspects of using PAs is supervision. State, provincial, and federal systems have put into place regulatory and contractual arrangements in which a medical doctor is obligated to properly supervise a PA. Lack of proper supervision not only results in potential tort liability of the practice but may also affect reimbursement for services provided. In 2000,

Mississippi became the 50th state to formally authorize PA practice, and in 2007, Indiana became the 50th state to grant PAs prescriptive authority. Upon enactment of legislation to authorize PA practice in Mississippi, the medical board immediately adopted regulations to authorize PA prescribing.

A major defining characteristic of PA scope of practice is physician delegation. Unlike some health personnel who have unique skills, such as physical therapists and occupational therapists, PAs have a general skill set similar to that of physicians. They perform acts of medical diagnosis and treatment that comprise the legal definition of medical practice. The scope of services that PAs are trained to perform is broad, ranging from routine examinations and diagnostic maneuvers to prescribing medications, performing minor surgical procedures, and assisting at surgery. For PAs to apply their skills in clinical practice, states require that PAs practice with a physician or group of physicians and are delegated specific tasks. Procedures performed by PAs can be explicit or implicit in scope of practice, depending on state law, the reviewing medical board, and the arrangement between the supervising doctor and the PA.

Credentialing and Privileging

Credentialing and privileging are the processes used by licensed healthcare facilities to authorize licensed PAs, physicians, and others to practice in the institution. *Credentialing* is the process used to evaluate the qualifications and practice history of an applicant for medical staff privileges. The intent of credentialing is to safeguard the public and the institution. This process involves a review of the PA's education and training, including postgraduate studies, continuing medical education, certification, and state licensure. Additionally, a thorough background check, including any past disciplinary actions or malpractice claims, may also be sourced. The credentialing process typically takes place as the individual seeks hospital privileges.

Once a PA is credentialed by a hospital or licensed facility, he or she is authorized to engage in a specific scope of practice through a process known as *privileging*. The standards of The Joint Commission (a major hospital accrediting agency) require hospitals to credential and privilege PAs in a manner similar to that of physicians. After privileges are granted, the PA is permitted to see patients, assist in surgery, or perform other specific duties delegated by the supervising physician.

The *Whittaker* Case

What is the legal basis for the expansion of PA activity? For example, does a state's medical practice act or PA practice act permit a PA to insert a pacemaker in a patient suffering severe bradycardia? For most jurisdictions, legal authorities have not had to deal with the underlying issues associated with these questions. In a few states, however, the answers have begun to emerge from court decisions, opinions of attorneys general, and legislative enactment. As a practical matter, delegation of health service functions is predominantly governed by prevailing custom and practice. In the few relevant court decisions, however, it has been held that professional custom is no defense for a contravention of licensure laws.

One case in particular is important to illustrate, not only because of the court's handling of elements of licensure, custom, and supervision in deciding the delegation question, but because of its influence on the development of the PA profession. The case *People v. Whittaker* (No. 35307, Justice Court of Redding Judicial District, Shasta County, Calif. [December 1966]) involved the right of a neurosurgeon to use a trained surgical assistant to assist in brain surgery. For various reasons, the case became a pivotal event affecting the fledgling PA profession.

Roger G. Whittaker was a former Navy corpsman and engineering technology student at the University of California. He had attended the Navy's Hospital Corps School and Operating Technician School. A Vietnam veteran, he was attending college with veterans' benefits and took a job as an assistant with neurosurgeon George C. Stevenson. Stevenson was the only practicing neurosurgeon within 275 miles of Redding, California. Whittaker and Stevenson were reported to the California State Board of Medical Examiners.

Whittaker was charged with practicing medicine without a license because he operated a cranial drill and Giegle saw, positioned by the surgeon, to bore holes and excise skull flaps during neurosurgical operations. The surgeon was charged with aiding and abetting an unlicensed person to practice medicine. Despite the testimony of the chairman of the board of Redding Memorial Hospital that said the defendant was a "better neurosurgical assistant than I am," Whittaker was found guilty in one of three cases before the jury, and his employer was found guilty of having aided and abetted him. However, Whittaker and Stevenson were found not guilty on the other two charges because the jury felt that their services were beneficial. The court imposed nominal penalties. Both received suspended sentences of 30 days in jail; Whittaker was fined $50, and his employer $200. A jury impaneled before a justice of the Peace Court found both parties guilty of the charge in which the surgeon had sufficient time to call another physician to assist him but did not try to do so. As a standard for judging the physician's use of an unlicensed trained assistant, working under direct supervision, the following instruction was given to the jury:

> In determining whether acts in this case, if any, performed under the direct supervision and control of a duly licensed physician, were legal or illegal, you may consider evidence of custom and usage of the medical practice in California as shown by the evidence in this case.

The *Whittaker* judgment was successfully appealed because of its importance as a test of the right of a physician or surgeon to use an extra pair of hands under conditions not constituting a medical emergency. This particular case was significant for its allowance of prevailing "custom and usage of the medical practice" in the state to determine the propriety of a physician's delegation and supervision of patently medical, but essentially mechanical, functions.

An interesting footnote to this case is that Dr. Eugene Stead, the founder of the PA program at Duke University, was called to serve as an expert witness. Stead testified that Whittaker provided a much-needed medical service and put forth the concept of the delegation of medical tasks to assistants. In the course of the legal proceedings, Stead had the opportunity to meet Whittaker and told him about the new educational program that had been inaugurated at Duke (Carter & Thompson, 2008). Whittaker became a member of the third PA class at Duke and, later, president of the American Academy of Physician Assistants (AAPA) (Figure 10–1).

The key issue in the licensure of PAs is the scope of functions that may be delegated to them and the educational and certification qualifications to permit such delegation safely. A shortage of PAs and other skilled healthcare personnel, new scientific and technological developments, and new methods of organizing health services have made the question of delegation all the more important. Across the states, licensure laws are being amended to authorize broader scope of functions for qualified PAs.

Medical Boards

Medical boards are charged with administering systems to monitor provider behavior, ensure public safety, and provide appropriate medical regulation. As such, most jurisdictions license and regulate PAs through the state medical board. However, 11 states have regulatory bodies strictly for PAs. Nearly all of the states where PAs are regulated by the medical board have PA committees. All states require two basic criteria for licensure: graduation from a

FIGURE 10-1
Roger Whittaker, PA-C (left), Passing the AAPA Presidential Gavel to Daniel Fox, PA-C, 1977

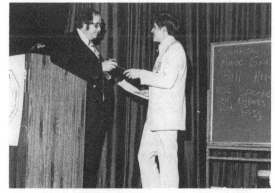

Courtesy of the American Academy of Physician Assistants.

PA program accredited by the Accreditation Review Commission on Education for the Physician Assistant (ARC-PA) and passage of the Physician Assistant National Certification Examination (PANCE), administered by the National Commission on Certification of Physician Assistants (NCCPA). The NCCPA's PANCE examination functions as the de facto licensing examination for PAs.

Most medical boards require continuing medical education (CME) as a condition of license renewal. CME credits can be earned in lecturer-learner format at conferences and seminars or online. However, a wide range of alternatives for earning CME credits has emerged in recent years. For instance, they may also be earned though journal-based activities, such as completing a set of questions derived from a specific journal article. Performance improvement and self-assessment are newer types of processes that can be part of the CME requirements. Most medical and osteopathic licensing boards condition license renewal on a specific number of earned CME credits. The same is true for most PA licensing boards.

The Federation of State Medical Boards (FSMB) is a national organization that represents the nation's 70 medical and osteopathic boards. It assesses policy documents on topics that range from credentialing to disciplinary alert services. The organization has a section on PA regulation in its *Essentials of a Modern Medical and Osteopathic Practice Act* ("*Essentials*"). Among other goals, the *Essentials* are developed "to encourage the development and use of consistent standards, language, definitions and tools by boards responsible for physician and physician assistant regulation." In alignment with the policies of the AAPA, the American College of Physicians, and other organizations, the *Essentials* call for PA scope of practice to include those medical services that are within the PA's training and expertise, that are delegated by a physician, and that form a component of the physician's scope of practice.

The ultimate objective of the FSMB is to promote excellence in medical practice and protect the health and welfare of society by ensuring fair and accurate monitoring of quality of care. To meet this goal, the FSMB collects third-party disclosures on provider behavior and brings that information to the public's attention. The information must be guided by unbiased and accurate state-based information on medical provider mishaps.

LIABILITY

In general, each state-licensed practitioner is directly liable for his or her own actions in tort and negligence; therefore, physicians, nurses, PAs, and others are independently liable for their malpractice. Licensed practitioners are also separately liable to their individual licensing and registration boards for any professional misconduct. Hospitals and physician professional groups may also be responsible for the malpractice of any employed licensed practitioner that occurs within the scope of employment (Davis, Walker, Radix, Cawley, & Hooker, 2015).

Liability of Physicians Who Supervise PAs

One of the most discussed topics regarding employment of a PA is the set of legal doctrines that binds the doctor to the action of the PA. Doctrines are principles of government and tend to have a legal connotation. Legal doctrines commonly used to assess a physician's liability for mistakes of a PA include:

- *Respondeat superior* (from the Latin "let the master answer"), in which the employer is considered responsible for the actions of the employee
- *Negligent supervision,* in which an employer is held responsible for failing to reasonably monitor and control an employee's actions
- *Negligent hiring,* in which an employer can be considered negligent if it had awareness of an employee's past misconduct or if an employee had an easily discoverable record of misconduct that went unnoticed
- *"Captain-of-the-ship" doctrine,* in which a physician is considered liable for the negligent acts of other employees
- *"Borrowed-servant rule,"* in which an employing physician is considered liable for the actions of a (borrowed servant) PA

because the physician is considered the person in control of the PA's actions

Since the mid-1980s, statutory regulations have emerged from various jurisdictions suggesting a legislative trend to reduce and limit the liability of physicians who supervise PAs. Generally, the standard of care applicable to PAs is the same as the standard of care for a physician. The tendency is for the elements of each cause of action to reflect the mistakes of PAs and not to hold supervising physicians liable (Gore, 2000).

However, physicians striving to reduce liability from PAs working under them should focus on three main areas: (1) selection, (2) supervision, and (3) standard of conduct. PAs appear to learn most from the habits of the physicians who supervise them, irrespective of whether the habits are good or bad.

The American Medical Association (AMA) recognized these concepts when its 1995 House of Delegates adopted the following guidelines for physician/PA practice (AMA, 2001):

- The physician is responsible for managing the healthcare of patients in all practice settings.
- Healthcare services delivered by physicians and PAs must be within the scope of each practitioner's authorized practice as defined by state law.
- The physician is ultimately responsible for coordinating and managing the care of patients and, with the appropriate input of the PA, ensuring the quality of healthcare provided to patients.
- The physician is responsible for the supervision of the PA in all settings.
- The role of PAs in the delivery of care should be defined through mutually agreed-on guidelines that are developed by the physician and the PA and based on the physician's delegatory style.
- The physician must be available for consultation with the PA at all times either in person or through telecommunication systems or other means.
- The extent of the involvement by the PA in the assessment and implementation of treatment should depend on the complexity and acuity of the patient's condition and the training and experience and preparation of the PA as adjudged by the physician.
- Patients should be made clearly aware at all times whether they are being cared for by a physician or a PA.
- The physician and PA together should review all delegated patient services on a regular basis, as well as the mutually agreed-on guidelines for practice.
- The physician is responsible for clarifying and familiarizing the PA with his or her supervising methods and style of delegating patient care.

Physician Assistant Liability

Although the physician employer is ultimately responsible for the activities of the PA, the PA is not immune from liability. With regard to liability, PAs are usually held to the same standards as physicians or the communities in which they work.

Agency

In the eyes of the law, the PA serves as the agent of the physician. *Agency* refers to a legal relationship in which one party (the agent—the PA) is authorized to represent another (the principal—the physician) in dealings with third parties (patients). Agents owe their principals three duties: loyalty, obedience as to reasonable directions, and care (which includes the duty to notify).

Agency authority may be contractual, apparent, or inherent:

- When *contractual,* the scope of authority is clearly communicated to the agent.
- When *apparent,* the authority is communicated to the third party.
- Under *inherent,* the principal is liable even when the agent acts in violation of the principal's orders or exceeds the scope of authority.

Authority also may either be *expressed,* in which the orders from the principal are clearly defined, or *implied,* in which authority is based on a reasonable belief by the agent. The circumstances under which the authority is granted may result from contract, custom, or circumstance, or it may be judicially defined in the event that litigation occurs.

Under the theory of *apparent agency*, a principal (an employing physician or hospital) "holds out" an agent (a PA) to the community as one who possesses certain authority, inducing the formation of a belief on the part of the third party that the agent may provide certain services. Principals that employ PAs have a legal duty to their prospective patients to ensure that the PAs in their service provide non-negligent care. This is referred to as *vicarious liability*.

Agency, or more precisely, apparent agency, assumes that caregivers do not misrepresent themselves. Plaintiffs have claimed that they assumed a provider was a physician simply because the provider wore a stethoscope and lab coat. Therefore, most state PA practice laws require PAs to clearly identify themselves as PAs. For example, statutes in Texas, Maryland, and other states—in addition to imposing legal responsibility on the employing physician for the PA's acts or omissions—expressly require a PA to wear a name tag identifying himself or herself as a PA while engaging in professional activities. The distinction between the PA and the physician must always be clear and obvious to patients, and the PA must never be misrepresented to patients as a medical student, student in training, or any other inaccurate typing. One area that has resulted in misperception is addressing a PA who holds a doctorate as "doctor." Misrepresenting the status of a PA or failing to disclose that status has resulted in administrative sanctions and can form liability under the theory of misrepresentation.

MALPRACTICE

In addition to being responsible for licensing services, medical boards are responsible for administering systems to monitor provider behavior, ensure public safety, and provide appropriate medical discipline. Each state board has investigative units responsible for the identification of medical misconduct.

Examples of medical misconduct include (but are not limited to):

- Practicing fraudulently
- Practicing with gross incompetence or gross negligence
- Practicing while impaired by alcohol, drugs, physical disability, or mental disability
- Being convicted of a crime
- Filing a false report
- Guaranteeing that treatment will result in a cure
- Refusing to provide services because of race, creed, color, or ethnicity
- Performing services not authorized by the patient
- Harassing, abusing, or intimidating a patient
- Ordering excessive tests
- Abandoning or neglecting a patient in need of immediate care

Although malpractice insurance data are not readily available, some evidence since 2010 indicates that the increases in the number of malpractice claims, size of awards, and malpractice insurance rates that physicians have experienced have not been the experience of PAs. Still, PAs are not immune from malpractice claims. As the number of PAs in practice increases, the number of reported cases of malpractice lawsuits involving allegations of negligence by PAs also increases. Legal precedents have been set.

Negligence

A claimant who brings a medical negligence action against any healthcare provider must prove that four elements existed in the situation in question: duty, breach of duty, proximate cause, and damages.

Duty

A claimant first must show that the healthcare provider had a *duty* to provide medical care. For example, in all states but Vermont, healthcare providers are not required to stop and render care in a roadside emergency (Vt. Stat. Ann. tit. 12 519). Therefore, they cannot be found negligent for failure to provide care in such a situation. On the other hand, some courts have ruled that a physician on call in an emergency department has a duty to render medical assistance to any emergency patient whether or not the person is eligible for treatment at that facility (*Guerrero v. Copper Queen Hospital,* 537 P2d 1329). In most circumstances, the duty to treat is activated when medical treatment is begun and continues until the patient has recovered from the condition or has released the healthcare provider from the continuing duty to treat.

Breach of Duty

Breach of duty is predicated on provision of the standard of care of a reasonably prudent physician practicing under the same or similar circumstances. This is an objective standard, and an expert witness in a medical negligence trial is not asked what he or she personally would have done in the situation. Rather, the determination of breach of duty is based on what an average, reasonably prudent healthcare provider in the community would have done. Of the four requisite elements in negligence cases, breach of duty is the most difficult to prove.

Proximate Cause

In addition to the duty to treat and a breach of that duty, negligence involves proving that the breach of duty was the cause of the claimant's injury. For example, a healthcare provider may have been negligent in a case of wrongful death. However, if the healthcare provider can show that the patient would have died regardless of the treatment rendered, the negligence cannot be held to be the *proximate cause* of death.

Damages

The fourth criterion for a negligence suit is that a claimant must have sustained some form of *damage.* For example, medication errors frequently are made in hospitals; too much, too little, or the wrong type of medication is given, or a medication is administered to the wrong person. Although many of these errors can be blamed on negligence, the vast majority of them result in little or no damage. One reason

is the cost of bringing a case to trial or settlement: medical negligence suits routinely cost more than $20,000 to prosecute, and an experienced malpractice attorney is unlikely to accept any case with estimated damages less than $50,000.

Standard of Care

In a medical negligence action involving a physician, standard of care may seem straightforward. Duty is breached only when the physician has not performed as a reasonable and prudent physician would have performed under the same or similar circumstances. But to what standard of care should a PA or other healthcare professional be held: to that of a reasonably prudent PA or that of a reasonably prudent physician? Two federal court opinions involving a technician and a PA illustrate the confusion in this area.

In the case of *Haire v. United States* (No. 75-55-ORL-CIV-R, 1976), the mother of a 23-month-old girl took her child to a pediatric clinic at a military treatment facility in Florida. A medical technician saw the child. The technician had worked as a medic in Vietnam for 2 years and had received in-service training, which primarily involved observing the supervising pediatrician, before being assigned to the clinic. The medical technician examined the child and recorded that she had a runny nose as a result of an upper respiratory infection. He prescribed a decongestant and discharged her. Over the next 10 days, the child's appetite diminished, and her runny nose persisted. On the 10th day, her temperature was noticeably elevated. The next day, her mother brought her back to the clinic, and the medical technician saw the child again. He examined the child's ears and throat and listened to her chest. He then told the mother that the patient's tonsils were causing her distress and discharged the child without referring her to a physician. The next day, the patient's mother noted "twitching" of her daughter's hands and a temperature of 103°F. She rushed the child to a local emergency department, where a physician performed a lumbar puncture and diagnosed *Haemophilus influenzae* meningitis. Despite the rapid institution of appropriate treatment, the child died 3 days later.

The child's family sued the medical center, claiming that the "physician extender" failed to diagnose or test for meningitis and that the child should have been referred to a physician on her second clinic visit. At the trial, a board-certified pediatrician testified on behalf of the family that if a pediatrician had seen the child on the second visit, the physician would have suspected meningitis and conducted ophthalmic and neurological examinations to confirm the diagnosis. The court held the technician to the standard of care of a board-certified pediatrician, and because he had not performed the neurological and ophthalmic examinations that a board-certified pediatrician would have performed, the court found him negligent. In 1976, the parents were awarded $15,000 each for emotional suffering.

In the case of *Polischeck v. United States* (535 F Supp 1261 [ED Pa. 1982]), another federal court took a different approach. A 44-year-old woman experienced a headache associated with nausea, vomiting, and fever. She complained to her husband of pressure behind her eyes and the feeling that the "top of her head was blowing off." The next day she went to the emergency department of a government medical center and was evaluated by a PA. Her temperature was 100.4°F and her blood pressure was 144/90 mm Hg. The PA questioned the patient about her illness and recorded that she had experienced "sudden onset of headache 4 days ago with malaise, nausea, and ocular myalgia." A brief neurological examination revealed photophobia but no nuchal rigidity. A complete blood count demonstrated a slightly elevated white blood cell count. The PA diagnosed flu syndrome, prescribed an analgesic/anxiolytic/muscle relaxant, and instructed the patient to return to the emergency department if her symptoms became worse. This medical center allowed PAs to use their discretion in deciding whether to consult a physician and did not require supervising physicians to review the charts of patients seen by PAs, so the patient was not seen by a physician, and her chart was not reviewed or countersigned by a physician.

Two days later, on a Friday, the patient returned to the emergency department when her condition had not improved. The same PA saw her and referred her to the emergency department physician. A physician examined the patient, diagnosed "headaches, etiology unknown," and advised the patient to go to the internal medicine clinic the following Monday if her headaches persisted, or sooner if they became worse. That evening, the patient's husband could not rouse her. He took her back to the emergency department, where the same physician examined her and diagnosed intracerebral hemorrhage. Because the medical center was not equipped to handle this type of patient, she was transferred to another hospital, where an arteriogram demonstrated a large subdural hematoma and a right posterior communicating artery aneurysm. A frontoparietal craniotomy was performed. However, the patient never regained consciousness, and she died 3 days later.

The patient's husband filed suit in federal court, claiming that the medical center was negligent in not having his wife seen by a physician on her first visit. He also claimed that the physician was negligent in treating the patient on her second visit. At the trial, a licensed physician had reviewed the plaintiff's brief. The expert medical witness testified that the standard of care in the community required that patients not be discharged from emergency departments until they had been seen by (or at least their charts had been reviewed by) a physician. However, the court reasoned that the PA himself was not negligent in failing to diagnose the patient's subarachnoid hemorrhage on her first visit. Indeed, it hardly seems reasonable to expect a person with only 2 years of general medical training to be able to recognize a medical condition when it is presented in a patient possessing only some of the condition's textbook symptoms.

The court held the PA to the same standard of care as other PAs in the community with similar training, and, compared with these peers, he was found not negligent. However, the court found the medical center negligent for failure either to have the patient seen or to have her records reviewed by a physician on her first visit, as was standard in the community.

These two decisions disagree about the standard of practice that a PA must meet. Decisions in other cases involving healthcare extenders may be helpful in clarifying this issue:

- *Thompson v. Brent* (245 S2d 751 [La. 1971]): In removing a cast from a patient's leg with a Stryker saw, a nurse accidentally cut the patient's leg, leaving a scar. The court held her to the standard of care of a physician and ruled that she was negligent.
- *Barber v. Reinking* (411 P2d 861 [Wash. 1966]): A practical nurse administered an injection that caused injury to a patient. In that state, only registered nurses were authorized by law to administer injections. The court held the practical nurse to the standard of care of a registered nurse and ruled that she had been negligent.

Evidence of Standard of Care

How is the standard of care proved in a medical negligence suit? In addition to hiring an expert witness, the plaintiff's attorneys are likely to subpoena all hospital or clinic manuals, regulations, and protocols referring to PAs. These usually are admissible evidence of the applicable standard of care. A PA's failure to follow a hospital's protocol or other applicable regulation offers strong, although not necessarily conclusive, evidence that the standard of care was not met. Violation of a state law regarding the duties of PAs is also strong evidence of a breach of the standard of care.

In addition to hospital or clinic protocols and regulations, the courts may consult guidelines issued by professional organizations, including standards used by The Joint Commission. Therefore, PAs must also be aware of the guidelines issued by these organizations.

NATIONAL PRACTITIONER DATA BANK

Are PAs safe to employ? Can they provide competent care? For 5 decades, policymakers and opponents of PAs have questioned whether the introduction of PAs is in society's best interest. The question that arises most often is whether PAs increase liability. Unlike doctors, nurses, dentists, and some other health professionals, PAs have a relatively short history, and their scrutiny for quality of care has not been as lengthy because they were first legislated under the 1966 Allied Health Professions Act (PL-751) and legislation was fully extended to all 50 states only in 2000 (with, as noted earlier, Mississippi being the last state to do so). Because this scrutiny of PAs has been relatively brief, a full assessment of their safety has not been undertaken. With that said, some attempts have been made to address the question of safety, including the National Practitioner Data Bank (NPDB).

The NPDB is a federal electronic data repository that contains information about licensed healthcare providers in the United States, including records of all state board actions and malpractice actions (Box 10-1). Introduced in 1987 by the Medicare and Medicaid Patient and Program Protection Act and implemented in 1990 by the US Department of Health and Human Services, the NPDB was designed to protect patients from incompetent healthcare providers by restricting the ability of unfit practitioners to simply move from state to state and continue practicing. The NPDB was originally designed to record data on physician and dentists, but in 2007, the Health Resources and Services Administration proposed to add other

BOX 10-1
Information Tracked by the National Practitioner Data Bank

- Total number of malpractice payments
- Average amount of malpractice payments
- Average years of practice
- Total number of adverse events/actions
- State medical board licensing actions
- Clinical privileges actions
- Professional society membership actions
- Practitioner exclusions from Medicare and Medicaid programs
- US Drug Enforcement Administration actions
- Year of adverse action
- Basis of action
- State of license

practitioners, including PAs and nurse practitioners, to the NPDB. The overall goals of the NPDB are to improve healthcare quality, promote patient safety, and prevent fraud and abuse.

All healthcare practitioners applying for privileges to a hospital or medical center must provide in-depth personal and professional background information, which is submitted to the NPDB for clearance. Through this clearance process, from 1990 through 2015, the NPDB produced information on more than 414,000 reported board actions, malpractice payments, and Medicare/Medicaid exclusions that involved 18 different types of providers.

Analysis of data from the NPDB can provide valuable comparisons of the rates of adverse outcomes, fraud, misappropriations of professional role, malpractice, and other variables for different healthcare providers. Between 2004 and 2015, 364,893 providers were registered with the NPDB. During this same period, the NPDB recorded 154,621 medical malpractice payments and 392,100 adverse action reports. The per capita malpractice payments ranged from 9.9 to 16.6 for every 1,000 active physicians, 1.40 to 2.35 for every 1,000 for PAs, and 1.09 to 1.43 for every 1,000 nurse practitioners (NPs). In other words, 11.4% of physicians, 3.3 % of PAs, and 1.3% of NPs made malpractice payments during the specified period. Median physician payments were 1.56 to 2.31 times higher than those of PAs and NPs. Malpractice allegations associated with diagnosis varied by provider type, with physicians having significantly fewer reports (31.8%) than PAs (52.8%) and NPs (40.6%). Declining trends in malpractice awards and adverse actions may be the result of policy enactments designed to decrease liability issues in American medicine. The malpractice analyses of PAs and NPs were less than 0.01% of the total payment made during that period (Table 10–1).

The median malpractice payments by year for the study period for all three providers, adjusted to 2014 dollars, are displayed in Table 10–2. Physician median malpractice total payments were significantly greater than those of PAs and NPs for each year of data (each $P < .001$). When the slopes of the CPI adjusted median malpractice payments were calculated, the adjusted median physician malpractice award demonstrated a significant decrease ($r^2 = .74$, $P < .001$) across the 10-year period. PA and NP payments fluctuated by year, but the CPI adjusted trend for malpractice awards were not significant.

Figure 10–2 graphically compares adverse action risk ratios among three providers. It reveals significant downward trends in the risk

TABLE 10-1
Comparison of Malpractice Counts and Rates Among Providers

	Number of Providers			Malpractice Counts			Rate per 1,000 Providers		
Year	Physicians	PAs	NPs	Physicians	PAs	NPs	Physicians	PAs	NPs
2005	842,384	63,350	88,532	13,992	110	125	16.61	1.74	1.41
2006	854,045	62,960	92,266	12,475	113	104	14.61	1.79	1.13
2007	868,171	67,160	96,000	11,459	94	118	13.2	1.4	1.23
2008	882,297	71,950	100,000	11,001	115	133	12.47	1.6	1.33
2009	896,249	76,900	104,000	10,715	131	147	11.96	1.7	1.41
2010	910,201	81,420	112,000	10,158	139	122	11.16	1.71	1.09
2011	921,050	83,540	118,400	9,743	196	144	10.58	2.35	1.22
2012	931,898	83,640	125,600	9,362	163	179	10.05	1.95	1.43
2013	947,304	88,110	136,800	9,656	164	180	10.19	1.86	1.32
2014	960,419	91,670	153,600	9,477	190	190	9.87	2.07	1.24

Data from the National Practitioner Data Bank.

TABLE 10-2
Malpractice Allegation Groups for Physicians, PAs, and NPs

Malpractice Allegation	Physicians		PAs		NPs		Total	
Diagnosis related	34,360	31.8%	747	52.8%	586	40.6%	35,693	32.2%
Surgery related	28,745	26.6%	56	4.0%	26	1.8%	28,827	26.0%
Treatment related	21,135	19.6%	377	26.6%	465	32.2%	21,977	19.8%
Obstetrics related	8,194	7.6%	10	0.7%	53	3.7%	8,257	7.4%
Medication related	5,606	5.2%	132	9.3%	184	12.8%	5,922	5.3%
Monitoring related	3,329	3.1%	36	2.5%	69	4.8%	3,434	3.1%
Anesthesia related	2,925	2.7%	6	0.4%	16	1.1%	2,947	2.7%
Other miscellaneous	2,490	2.3%	39	2.8%	21	1.5%	2,550	2.3%
Equipment/Product related	639	0.6%	7	0.5%	4	0.3%	650	0.6%
Behavioral health related	410	0.4%	3	0.2%	16	1.1%	429	0.4%
IV and blood products related	205	0.2%	2	0.1%	2	0.1%	209	0.2%

Data from the National Practitioner Data Bank.

ratio of adverse action records of physicians compared with those of PAs and NPs. The risk ratios of PAs to NPs show a moderate upward trend in adverse actions records across the 10-year period (Brock et al., 2016).

Although the NPDB has some shortcomings in its collection methodology because arbitration might not be recorded, its data should not be discounted completely for these nuances because the criteria for data bank entry essentially affect all providers equally. Analysis of the existing NPDB data supports perceptions that PAs pose a low risk of malpractice liability to the public in general and to employing practices in particular. Even taking into account the agency that exists between

FIGURE 10-2
Comparison of Provider Adverse Action Risk Ratios

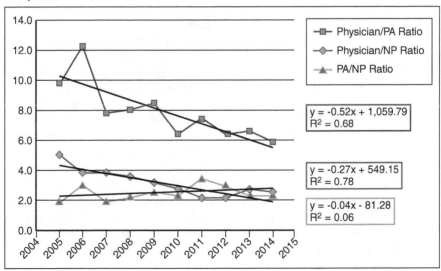

PAs and physicians, physicians are still implicated in a far greater percentage of malpractice suits and claims than PAs are. Overall, the data offer some reassurance that the delegated responsibility of patient care from the physicians to PAs is relatively safe.

Building on the NPDB data findings, one study found that a great level of physician supervision or involvement does not guard against malpractice claims. Overall, the study determined that PA–physician teams were much less likely to face malpractice claims and suits than physicians practicing without PAs (Hyams et al., 1996). One postulated reason for observed differences in PA and physician malpractice rates is that PAs employ certain communication skills in patient encounters that limit their liability (Brock, 1998). Another possible explanation is that PAs limit their liability by avoiding risky encounters with patients and procedures with high liability profiles, such as births and anesthesia. However, further research on the causes of the difference between PA and physician malpractice rates and the types of visits managed by different providers is warranted.

TORT REFORM

Tort reform refers to measures that would modify the current medical liability system to limit the number of legal claims and amounts awarded in cases prosecuted by personal injury lawyers that are perceived to unfairly burden insurance policyholders with high premiums. At times, tort reform has become a politicized matter with medical groups, particularly the AMA, labeling tort reform a "crisis" issue. The AMA has spent considerable sums lobbying for legislation favorable to their hoped-for objectives to change the present medical malpractice liability law.

Proposed Changes to Tort Law

Tort law is traditionally a matter of state "common law" and legislation. A number of states have addressed this issue in the past by passing various types of measures that modify the tort liability and resolution system. In some states, legislation has passed attempting to deal with alleged abuses of the tort system by placing caps on the amount of money that juries can award for "pain and suffering." Bills of this sort cap awards for noneconomic damages at a certain level (e.g., $250,000) and place limits on attorneys' fees and other damages that plaintiffs can collect in medical malpractice suits.

Some proposals go beyond simply applying liability caps to physicians and hospitals and extend such limits on liability to any entity providing healthcare products or services. Under such legislation, civil suits against drug makers, insurance companies, and medical device manufacturers would be subject to the same caps on noneconomic and punitive damages as suits against physicians.

Federal versus State Purview

One issue surrounding tort reform is the question of the necessity for a federal remedy to the matter of medical malpractice liability, as has been proposed in the past decade. Is this approach the most appropriate way to deal with an issue that is primarily in the purview of the states because they license and regulate the practice of medicine? Most would agree that the overall goals for the reform of medical malpractice liability include limiting overall health system costs, adequately compensating the victims of medical mistakes, and providing incentives for health providers and facilities to avoid errors. Many believe that more needs to be done within the medical care system to reduce the number of errors. States commonly deal with these matters and may be in a better position to solve them than a federally imposed ruling.

Tort reform has been front and center in a number of states where legislatures have struggled with the competing interests of medical professionals and trial lawyers. For example, in 2004, Maryland's medical malpractice carrier announced that premiums would rise by 33%. This led to considerable wrangling between the governor and the legislature, who differed on remedies to deal with the malpractice issue. After considerable polarization of the issue, the final legislative solution—in addition to limitations of awards on noneconomic damages—was for the state to essentially levy a health maintenance organization (HMO) user's fee to subsidize physician malpractice insurance premiums. Several years later, a large amount of this subsidization was shown not to be used by the state's malpractice carrier and was subsequently refunded to the state treasury. In confrontations of this sort, consumers seem to be caught in the crossfire.

The Debate Over Tort Reform

Tort reform adherents advocate the idea of capping malpractice awards, and this notion has found some degree of legislative acceptance. Caps exist in 16 states and have been in place in California since 1975. Typically, such laws limit awards that a plaintiff may receive for pain and suffering at $250,000 to $500,000. However, there is no conclusive evidence that caps save much money. One study of verdicts in 22 states concluded that caps have no effect on the size of the overall compensation awarded by juries and that what seemed to influence outcomes were factors such as the severity of injury, the requirement for medical expert screening of cases, and the election experiences of the judge (Studdert, 2004). Another reason that caps may not work to limit overall compensation awarded to plaintiffs is that lawyers can shift the damage awards to categories of compensation that are not capped.

One perceived change resulting from these caps has been reluctance on the part of lawyers to take medical malpractice cases, thus reducing the opportunity for victims of medical negligence to have access to the court system. Some argue that such caps are futile and unfairly penalize less fortunate groups, such as the poor and the elderly, who have less economic capacity than the average citizen.

On the other side of the argument are growing data that show there is no such thing as an "epidemic" of medical malpractice. Reviews of existing evidence of the rates of serious injuries and malpractice suits cite data from research studies done over the past 30 years in Utah, Colorado, and California. Findings show that rates have not risen steeply in the past 10 years, remaining between 6 and 25 serious injuries from medical malpractice for every lawsuit

filed. In the states for which the best recent information is available—Texas, Florida, and Mississippi—reports show that the rate of claims has been steady or even declined in relation to population and economic growth over the past 15 years (Baker, 2005).

In the overall picture of health policy, the cost of medical malpractice is small—less than 1% of total healthcare costs. The automobile liability and workers' compensation businesses total amounts are higher than medical malpractice, and overall numbers and premium rates in these areas are proportionately higher than the premiums paid by physicians.

A view commonly held by advocates of tort reform is that the tort system is responsible for rising medical insurance premiums. However, Baker (2005) identified cyclical economics of the insurance industry and states that tort reform has little impact on malpractice insurance premiums; he also posed that little connection exists between the rates and amounts of medical malpractice awards and insurance premiums. The combination of the stock market bubble bursting in 2001—coupled with a downturn in interest rates and the September 11, 2001, attacks—led insurance companies to be at the bottom of the cycle. The result was that premiums rose steeply thereafter, not only in the medical malpractice area but also in the entire property and casualty insurance business.

Implications of Tort Reform for the PA Profession

For the PA profession, the tort reform issue presents some difficult choices. On one hand, there is seemingly natural temptation to side with physicians on this issue because most PAs are employees of physician practices. In addition, PAs are sometimes the targets of lawsuits when physicians and healthcare facilities are sued and share their frustrations with the current system. On the other hand, PAs view themselves as advocates for their patients and espouse the values of the rights of citizens to seek appropriate redress of alleged medical negligence.

The AAPA developed a policy statement on this issue that was approved by the 2004

AAPA House of Delegates. This position holds that:

> It is critical to assure that any medical liability insurance reform in the United States treats patients fairly…tort reform alone is not the answer. Caps on noneconomic damages may perhaps be appropriate if they are part of comprehensive medical liability insurance reform whose impact is borne equitably by attorneys, insurers, providers, and patients.

On the matter of liability caps, the AAPA believes that "a $250,000 cap on noneconomic damages paid for medical malpractice is too low and that fair and comprehensive reform of the medical liability insurance system is needed. Appropriate goals of a fair medical liability insurance system include compensating injured patients, deterring poor quality medical care, and assuring affordable medical liability insurance."

A Modern Physician Assistant Practice Act

State laws vary widely in the level of physician oversight required for PAs to practice medicine in America. Within 50 states and six additional US jurisdictions, the range of policies is broad.

Puerto Rico permits no PAs to practice. On the other end of the spectrum, Alaska has a unique law that permits PA autonomy but requires a collaborative arrangement with a physician (the collaborating physician need only be within contact). Some states grant PAs authority to diagnose, treat, and prescribe medications to patients with limited supervision; however, states such as Alabama grant licensure only when the supervising physician is in the same building. Still other systems such as the Department of Veterans Affairs, Department of Defense, and the US Coast Guard authorize PAs to practice independently.

The AAPA, in 2015, revised model legislation for the states to adopt. This model ranks states by level according to six criteria (Table 10–3). The model legislation put forth by the AAPA has not been analyzed to see whether there is some utility to a high level of permissiveness or strictness. Stated differently, does the maximum amount of the AAPA model legislation have some benefit to society? One question is whether the enactment of model legislation correlates with deployment of PAs that in turn permit greater healthcare access for citizens?

TABLE 10-3
Key Elements of a Modern PA Practice Act

State	Licensure as Regulatory Term	Full Rx	Scope Determined at Practice Site	Adaptable Supervision Requirements (No Mile Limit, No On-Site)	No chart Co-Sig	No Ratio Restriction
Alabama	√					
Alaska	√	√	√		√	√
Arizona	√	√	√	√	√	
Arkansas	√		√		√	√
California	√	√	√	√		
Colorado	√	√	√			
Connecticut	√	√	√	√	√	
Delaware	√	√	√		√	
District of Columbia	√	√		√	√	
Florida	√				√	
Georgia	√			√		
Hawaii	√		√	√		
Idaho	√	√	√		√	
Illinois	√	√	√	√	√	

TABLE 10-3
Key Elements of a Modern PA Practice Act—cont'd

State	Licensure as Regulatory Term	Full Rx	Scope Determined at Practice Site	Adaptable Supervision Requirements (No Mile Limit, No On-Site)	No chart Co-Sig	No Ratio Restriction
Indiana	√	√	√	√		
Iowa	√					
Kansas	√	√	√			
Kentucky	√					
Louisiana	√		√			
Maine	√		√	√	√	√
Maryland	√	√		√	√	
Massachusetts	√	√	√	√		√
Michigan	√	√	√	√	√	
Minnesota	√	√	√	√	√	
Mississippi	√	√				
Missouri	√		√			
Montana	√	√	√			√
Nebraska	√	√	√			
Nevada	√	√	√			
New Hampshire	√	√	√	√		
New Jersey	√	√				
New Mexico	√	√	√		√	√
New York	√	√	√	√	√	
North Carolina	√	√	√		√	√
North Dakota	√	√	√	√	√	√
Ohio		√			√	
Oklahoma	√					
Oregon	√	√	√	√		
Pennsylvania	√	√				
Rhode Island	√	√	√	√	√	√
South Carolina	√	√				
South Dakota	√	√	√	√	√	
Tennessee	√	√	√			√
Texas	√	√	√	√		
Utah	√	√	√	√		
Vermont	√	√	√		√	√
Virginia	√	√				
Washington	√	√		√		
West Virginia	√					
Wisconsin	√	√			√	
Wyoming	√	√	√	√	√	

FURTHER RESEARCH ON LEGAL ISSUES

Although liability is one of the excuses that practices use for not employing PAs, little research has been conducted to assess PA safety and efficacy. A number of questions arise regarding the legal considerations of PA employment that afford opportunities for further research:

- **Liability:** Does the inclusion of a PA in a medical practice reduce or increase liability exposure? What is the rate of liability per 10,000 visits in family medicine comparing a PA, an NP, and a physician? How do these rates compare across medical specialties, such as orthopedics and urology?
- **Supervision liability:** When does physician supervision become an issue in liability involving a PA and when is the PA alone held accountable for his or her actions without involving the physician?
- **Adverse events:** What changes and trends are occurring in adverse events regarding PAs? What is the rate of various disciplinary issues brought before state boards of

medical examiners by state, population, and type of provider?

- **Case studies:** In what type of cases are PAs found liable or incompetent, convicted of fraud, or exonerated for skill and duty?
- **State comparisons:** How do the various states compare in their laws of liability?

SUMMARY

Although the scope of practice granted by state laws governing PAs varies somewhat, there is more convergence than difference. Quality care research generally supports a broad scope of practice for PAs. Studies document high patient acceptance, quality, productivity, access, and skill for PA-provided care. PAs provide access to care in all fields of medicine and their availability to meet the demands of more complex patient types means their adaptability to the standards of quality of care is an important part of meeting workforce needs. The knowledge that PAs do not increase a medical practice's liability has enabled PAs to broaden their role.

References

The following citations are key to supporting this chapter's content. You can find a complete list of citations for all chapters at www.fadavis.com/davisplus, keyword *Hooker*.

American Academy of Physician Assistants. (2006b). *Physician assistants: State laws and regulations* (10th ed.). Alexandria, VA: Author.
American Academy of Physician Assistants. *AAPA model state legislation for PAs*. https://www.aapa.org/WorkArea/DownloadAsset.aspx?id=548
American Medical Association. (2001). *Guidelines for physician/physician assistant practice*. Chicago, IL: Policy Compendium.
Baker, T. (2005). *The medical malpractice myth*. Chicago, IL: The University of Chicago Press.
Banja, J. (2005). *Medical errors and medical narcissism*. Boston, MA: Jones & Bartlett.
Brock, D. M., Nicholson, J. G., & Hooker, R. S. (2016). Physician assistant and nurse practitioner malpractice trends. *Medical Care Research and Review*, 1077558716659022.
Carter, R., & Thompson, A. (2008). People v Whittaker: The trial and its aftermath in

California. *The Journal of Physician Assistant Education, 19*(2), 44–51.
Cawley, J. F., Rohrs, R., & Hooker, R. S. (1998). Physician assistants and malpractice risk: Findings from the National Practitioner Data Bank. *Federal Bulletin, 85*(4), 242–247.
Davis, A., Radix, S. M., Cawley, J. F., & Hooker, R. S. (2015). Access and innovation in a time of rapid change: Physician assistant scope of practice. *Annals Health L., 24*, 286.
Gore, C. L. (2000). A physician's liability for mistakes of a physician assistant. *Journal of Legal Medicine, 21*, 125–142.
Hyams, A. L., Shapiro, D. W., & Brennan, T. A. (1996). Medical practice guidelines in malpractice litigation: An early retrospective. *Journal of Health Politics, Policy and Law, 21*(2), 289–313.
Studdert, D. M., Yang, Y. T., & Mello, M. M. (2004). Are damages caps regressive? A study of malpractice jury verdicts in California. *Health Affairs, 23*(4), 54–67.

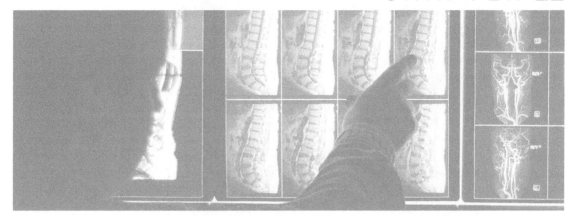

CHAPTER 11

PROFESSIONAL AND WORKFORCE ISSUES

RODERICK S. HOOKER ■ JAMES F. CAWLEY ■ CHRISTINE M. EVERETT

"The reward for work well done is the opportunity to do more."

—*Jonas Salk*

Issues related to the professional practice of medicine as a physician assistant (PA) and the practice dynamics associated with the workforce tend to shape policy and governance. Factors that may affect the culture and environment of PA practice are job satisfaction, scope of practice, supervising physician relationship, compensation, and role delineation. Although these professional and workforce issues are viewed as peripheral to the clinical practice of medicine, they have a clear influence on the behavior of PAs.

Professional issues may be organizationally based or political in nature, and many issues tend to fall on one side or the other when viewed by physicians. The topics discussed in this chapter are issues about the PA profession. They are part and parcel of changes in healthcare delivery and the way in which PAs fit into the greater health workforce. As new patterns of service delivery evolve, the boundaries between and within some professions begin to blur.

Healthcare workforce issues—defined as the interaction among the various health professions as they relate to supply and demand, professional territory, and compensation in the medical marketplace—have become increasingly important for policymakers and providers alike. A key characteristic that has made PAs valuable in the healthcare workforce is their adaptability. PAs, like pluripotent stem cells, begin with all the basic ingredients for development. Both are able to grow and change to meet the environment where they come to rest. The healthcare environment continues to be the greatest influence on the end product of PAs.

PROFESSIONAL ISSUES

Throughout their history, PAs have faced such professional issues as enabling legislation, prescriptive authority, and insurance reimbursement. By encountering and overcoming or evolving past each issue, the PA profession has grown into what it is today. However, PAs continue to be confronted with issues related to their professional growth. In this decade, the issues that have been more or less prominent include the changing name of the profession, autonomy, doctoral degrees, postgraduate training, and the ever-changing relationships with other healthcare professionals.

Physician Assistant Name Change

As discussed in earlier chapters, the appropriate name for a professional group that stands alongside physicians providing medical services has a long and controversial history. PAs did not determine the title by which they would be known. Instead, educators, physicians, regulators, and advocates of the concept made the first suggestions for a name. Early on, a wide range of names was attached to the graduates of training programs, including *physician assistant, physician associate, health associate, Medex,* and many others. *Physician assistant* evolved to become the dominant title and has gained a considerable degree of acceptance and penetration into the laws, literature, and culture of American medicine.

Thus, after more than 50 years, the term *physician assistant* has become embedded as the name of the profession. In some countries the name is protected; in others, it is not protected and as such can be adopted by a variety of health workers. As the PA role has evolved and expanded, certain parties continue to express concern regarding the name. For some in the profession, the term *physician assistant* is no longer appropriate. The definition of a PA is one who practices medicine with physician supervision; the scope of medical services and the level of care that PAs provide go far beyond assisting physicians. PAs are now licensed in almost all U.S. jurisdictions, have prescription privileges throughout, are able to order tests under their own names, and dispense care without reporting each case to a supervising physician. Given this scope of practice, selected individuals and groups assert that the term *assistant* does not accurately represent what PAs do. Specifically, they argue that the term *assistant* is demeaning and inconsistent with the level of responsibility and autonomy involved in the role. Others argue that *assistant* implies that PAs are mere helpers or auxiliary personnel who facilitate the work of their superior or function in a subordinate position. Moreover, inclusion of the word *assistant* leads people to draw parallels with medical assistants, clinical assistants, and nurses' aides. To those in the profession, the confusion of a PA with a medical assistant is insulting and demeaning. It fails to reflect PAs' substantial clinical and didactic education and the fact that many PAs have earned graduate degrees. Furthermore, it is not representative of the substantial responsibility PAs discharge in delivering clinical care.

Intellectually, many agree with change proponents that *physician assistant* is an undesirable name for the profession and agree that *physician associate* would be a far better and more accurate designation. In 2014, the United Kingdom replaced the title of *physician assistant* with *physician associate,* a change that seems to have resonated both with the medical establishment as well as PA clinicians. The same name change is being advanced as a possibility in India and Australia. In the Netherlands, it is a protected name used only by graduates of an approved program. In The Kingdom of Saudi Arabia, it is "associate physician," and in South Africa, it is "clinical associate."

Changing the name of the PA profession in the United States presents substantial challenges. It would be a monumental task that would require the amendment of the statutes of virtually all states and legislative jurisdictions, plus all federal and state regulations pertaining to PAs. Employers and such payers as insurance companies would need to accept such a name change. Accomplishing this task could take a lot of years and millions of dollars. Years would pass, during which many different individuals would reap the benefits achieved by the PA profession by assuming the older name and calling themselves PAs.

From a practical standpoint, the drain of resources, the amount of work required, and the risk that would accompany an effort to change the name has yet to be justified. Moreover, the PA profession has already made an enormous investment in educating the public, other health professions, and patients about the true meaning of the PA title and the vital roles that PAs play in the delivery of medical care services. A public opinion poll conducted by the American Academy of Physician Assistants (AAPA) in 2008 revealed that two-thirds of all Americans were familiar with (had heard of) a PA and one-third had received medical care from a PA. In many respects, the PA profession has finally become an American institution. Still, as discontent over the name remains, this issue is likely to reemerge at various times and for various reasons.

Autonomy

Among various clinicians and PA leaders, PA autonomy is another topic that resurfaces from time to time. This self-sufficiency is not so much a push as a pull. *Autonomy* in this regard refers to the ability to apply for a license in a jurisdiction as a PA, be employed with a physician or group of physicians, and be held accountable for one's activities and actions without involving a physician. Supervision under this purview of PA practice would occur on an individual basis (by a physician) or on an organizational basis (by a corporation). However, the AAPA is not currently pushing for such a change, and there is no concerted effort to make sure a change at this time on any other front. What is pulling is economic and labor history—the inevitable evolution of a profession, the tendency to be self-sufficient and self-governing. The trend of dependent roles to evolve to positions of independent licensure is embedded within many occupations, such as psychology, optometry, physical therapy, podiatry, audiology, midwifery, and nurse anesthetists, to name a few.

As the PA profession has developed and matured, some PAs have questioned the necessity of the PA–physician relationship. The U.S. nurse practitioner (NP) profession is in full quest of total practice independence, similar to the status held by many other health professions. In light of these trends, some healthcare workforce observers believe that PA autonomy is "inevitable" and that PAs will seek a separate autonomous practice stance relative to physicians. The evolution of legislation and regulation since the 1970s has been remarkable. In this short span, all states and most jurisdictions now enable PAs to function, write prescriptions, and

be reimbursed for their services. Many states permit this role to be semiautonomous and remote. The federal government, the largest single employer of PAs, has decided that autonomy is appropriate for the military, the Coast Guard, and the Veterans Health Administration. It is the outcome of care that guides this policy—if PAs were not safe, they would not be employed. Any discussion of autonomy must first be viewed through the lens of patient safety. For nearly 50 years, the PA profession has established an impressive patient safety record that is documented in quality-of-care studies, malpractice reports, sanction reports, and reports of adverse actions and, according to these documents, fairs better than that of physicians. A growing number of studies have shown that PAs embedded in practices with doctors provide excellent care, with quality indices indistinguishable from physician practice. PAs are far less likely to be the subject of malpractice suits, and patient satisfaction surveys remain consistently high.

The issue of PA autonomy is not a domestic one: The Netherlands PA independent license has emerged as well, as a directive from the government. This accomplishment stems from the Dutch strongly held belief about the nature of professional independence. Such permanent autonomy may be inevitable if history is to repeat itself and patient safety is not compromised (Hooker 2015).

Still, some believe that the analogy between PAs and other types of health professions in terms of the pursuit of autonomous practice is not valid. Unlike other clinicians, such as podiatrists and optometrists, PAs do not typically have explicit limits on their scope of practice. These professions may be "independent" in that they do not practice collaboratively with physicians, but they actually have far greater legal limits on their practices than PAs do.

One form of practice autonomy is the concept of "negotiated performance autonomy," the idea that PAs grow in their scope of practice with increasing levels of autonomy as they demonstrate increasing skills and knowledge. This approach appears to be effective. After a few years in practice, PAs enjoy considerable autonomy within a practice along with the advantage of having a built-in consultant. This arrangement allows PAs to grow in their profession without having to seek further credentials or licenses to increase their scope of practice. It is what gives PAs the flexibility to change specialties over their lifetimes.

Theoretically, relinquishing an employee-like relationship with doctors may necessitate changes in the way PAs are trained. Typically, PA programs offer no more than a few weeks of training in most medical or surgical specialties, which is certainly not comparable to the years of specialty training taken by physicians. For PAs to practice autonomously, they would either require longer training or choose an area of specialty training (as NPs do) upon entry to the PA program.

The counterargument to autonomy is that success of the PA profession and acceptance by patients and doctors owes much to its close practice relationship with physicians. Patients appear to be less concerned about seeing a provider who has less training when they know that the physicians whom they know and trust have trained and are available to consult with PAs (Dill et al., 2013). For some, the politics of severing the well-developed relationship PAs have with physicians are unappealing. Others argue that organized medicine has not reciprocated PA loyalty and that a declaration of independence would not improve this relationship. The argument goes that PAs benefit from the public trust in physicians, and endorsement of physicians on both the policy level and the clinical level substantially benefits PAs. In the end, these patient perceptions of PAs might have more of an effect on the autonomy of PA practice than any formal legislation.

Doctoral Degrees

Clinical doctoral degrees have become commonplace in health professions education. The trend in American higher education for institutions to develop professional or clinical doctoral degrees has led to the establishment of entry-level doctoral degrees in a number of health professions, including physical therapy (i.e., DPT), audiology (i.e., AuD), and advanced practice nursing (i.e., Doctorate of Nursing Practice, or DNP) among others. Educational institutions have strong financial incentives to make available professional doctorates due to a number of reasons, one being the increased tuition revenue associated with doctoral study. This trend has led to speculation that clinical doctorates specific to PAs are an inevitable progression, similar to the patterns observed in other health professions. The AAPA recognizes the prerogative of individual PAs to pursue advanced training and encourages graduates to pursue advanced education and professional development. As of 2016, at least two U.S. PA programs have decided to award an optional clinical doctorate to their students. Given the continued strength of the PA program applicant pool and the growth and desirability of the PA profession, it is possible that more academic institutions will consider the option of doctoral programs for PAs (Box 11–1).

Some health professions who have moved to the doctorate cite the following reason: a desire for increased autonomy, improved professional respect, a unique body of knowledge on which to base doctoral studies, and the need to stay competitive with other practitioners. Those who advocate for a doctorate associated with PA concentration of studies are concerned that without it, PAs will soon become marginalized among healthcare providers. For example, nurse practitioner programs have moved to a DNP as the entry-level degree. In many instances, though, the transition to doctoral studies has originated from academic and association leaders within the profession and not a push from its practitioners. The success of the PA profession is in part due to its competency-based educational model that does not depend on specific academic degrees for licensure. Unfortunately, the concept of competency-based education is not well understood by regulatory agencies and credentialing bodies, who may place greater importance on the degree. If practicing PAs do not feel a DPA is necessary to provide the highest level of care, academic and association leaders should not push the doctorate as a means to bring more money into programs or "keep up" with other practitioners. Other health professions that have moved in

BOX 11-1
Types of PA Doctoral Degrees

There are three configurations of doctoral degrees either intended or potentially intended for PAs: nonclinical doctorates, postgraduate PA-specific clinical doctorates, and entry-level PA-specific clinical doctorates.

NONCLINICAL DOCTORATES
A nonclinical doctorate is the "traditional" academic (or research-based) doctorate that PAs may seek to achieve tenure, to advance in an institutional or corporate setting, or for personal edification. Degrees commonly awarded to PAs in this category include doctor of education (EdD), doctor of philosophy (PhD), and doctor of public health (DrPH). Wake Forest University has an MMS-PhD PA program focused on research that falls into this category. The doctor of health science (DHSc) programs at Nova Southeastern University and A.T. Still University is another example.

POSTGRADUATE PA-SPECIFIC CLINICAL DOCTORATES
PA-specific doctoral degrees are awarded upon completion of an intensive PA postgraduate residency program. The one existing PA-specific doctoral programs is the Army's postgraduate training program in orthopedics and emergency medicine at Baylor University that awards a Doctor of Science Physician Assistant (DSc) degree. Another potential type of PA-specific postgraduate degree is one that would award a doctoral degree based in part on the coursework that a PA obtains in a master's degree PA program, so-called degree completion programs.

ENTRY-LEVEL PA-SPECIFIC CLINICAL DOCTORATES
This type of doctoral degree is awarded upon completion of an entry-level PA program similar to physical therapy's doctoral degree. The development of such a curriculum represents a significant change in the nature of a PA. Announced in 2015, Lynchburg College students who enroll in the physician assistants' doctoral program spend 27 months earning a master's degree and then begin a 9-month program, consisting of courses and a clinical fellowship, before obtaining their doctoral degree.

---

the direction of the clinical doctorate have their own unique body of knowledge on which to base further studies. PAs, on the other hand, lack a unique knowledge base because PA education is based on the same medical model used to train physicians. Without a unique body of knowledge for PA training, a doctoral degree granted to PAs would likely be a professional degree similar to the present day MD, DO, and MBBS degrees.

One option for PAs who seek professional doctorate degrees is the PA to MD/DO bridge program. This option bridges the PA profession to physician training and ultimately licensure and practice as a physician. It allows PA seeking more autonomy or professional recognition to earn a doctorate in medicine. Some argue that this transition is a natural next step for PAs who want to pursue additional education because it moves them into a model that already exists instead of having to create a new model for the PA with a technical or professional doctorate. The added benefit is keeping a uniform standard for the awarding of doctorate degrees because there has been concern about the lack of standards that exist for the clinical doctorates awarded.

The relationship between PAs and physicians in healthcare is one argument for rejecting the DPA. The PA profession was developed as part of a team-based approach to healthcare led by a physician where all PAs are required to practice under the supervision of a physician. Generally, PAs have a large scope of practice and are fairly autonomous, but ultimately, the eyes of the law and supervising physicians determine their scope and degree of autonomy. It may be possible for PAs to obtain a DPA and still work within a physician-led healthcare team; however, it seems likely that with a doctorate, PAs may push for more autonomy. This is where a PA to MD/DO bridge program would be beneficial. For PAs, however, a core component of the profession is working as part of a physician-led team. The opposing argument continues with the notion that the PA–physician collaboration may also be undermined with any conflict that could potentially arise from both parties being considered "doctors." If physicians feel that PAs are imposing on their occupation, the relationship is likely to be negatively affected.

Concerns about PA-specific doctoral degrees abound. There is a lack of any demonstrated or apparent benefit to the profession or to the public. Outside of the Army model, there is no evidence that a doctoral-prepared PA, whether entry-level or postgraduate, would differ in any way from a PA who is not doctoral-prepared in terms of clinical acumen, professional responsibility, or salary. Examinations of the experiences in other professions undergoing transformation from a master's to doctoral entry-level preparation (e.g., physical therapy) reveal no detectable differences in salary or level of clinical capabilities. Although no evidence has yet emerged, it appears that the cost of doctoral-level training increased among many professions without demonstrable benefit to practitioners, the public, or the healthcare system.

Postgraduate Training

Postgraduate education is an avenue of additional formal training that a few PAs opt for. It is not a cornerstone of PA education but an add-on to the American PA movement. Strong opinions come down on both sides of the notion of PAs spending additional time in training. One of the main observations is that less than 1% of all PAs who have ever graduated from a PA education program, approximately 110,000, have entered into PA postgraduate training. The other 99% have obtained employment in highly specialized roles from neurosurgery to rheumatology and have done so with on-the-job training. Only 50 of the 10,000 or so PAs in orthopedics have been fellowship trained.

The argument for postgraduate education is that the PA of the new century needs to be more specialized. Technology, expectations, and trends dictate this requirement, and medical educators have called for a shift in PA education. A rationale for this opinion is that PA education is too short to learn the intricacies of modern medicine. Concentrated experience in a specialized setting is apprentice development at its best, with scholarly activity and tertiary medicine intertwined.

The argument against postgraduate education is that 5 decades of experience in deploying PAs trained in general medicine says a lot. PAs appear to be quick to learn and adaptable to a broad spectrum of medical services. The evidence of PA residencies' producing something more than a cadre of house officers is limited. At best, the residencies generate approximately 100 graduates annually, less than 1% of the U.S. physician assistant graduation rate. Takers are few, the growth is stagnant, and more than one-third of the programs have folded. But to what degree does this extra education benefit the individual, society, or the training institution? Protracted training for 12 to 24 months results in the added burden of opportunity costs and delays career entry and repayment of education debts. Deferring a PA from working in a semiautonomous setting for that period of time means fewer patients are seen, those seen are done so inefficiently, and the lifetime employment span is shortened by the training years.

Most arguments tend to be based on the logical consequence of the premise. The premises for and against PA residencies appear inadequately laid out. More than 4 decades of experience have generated little more than strongly held opinions because postgraduate PA programs have not produced evidence of their value. For more detailed information on this topic, see Chapter 4, "Physician Assistant Education."

Relationship with Nurse Practitioners

The origins of PAs and NPs are similar in time, concept, and federal policies. Although the ideologies of the two professions might remain distinct to some, enough analysis exists to suggest that NP service in the United States and elsewhere is remarkably similar to the service provided by PAs. Approximately one-third of U.S. PAs and somewhere over two-thirds of NPs work in primary care (Hooker et al., 2016). *Primary care* in this case is defined as family practice, general internal medicine, pediatrics, and obstetrics and gynecology. NPs are five times more likely to be in pediatrics, geriatrics, or women's health than PAs are (Hooker et al., 2016). However, when other subspecialties are included, such as urgent care, corrections medicine, and occupation and environmental medicine, the percent of PAs in primary care approaches half (Table 11–1).

TABLE 11-1
Comparison of PA and NP Characteristics: 2013

Characteristic	Category	PA	NP	Source
Estimated licensed (2013)		84,000	171,000	Hooker, 2014; AANP, 2014
Estimated employed (2013)[a]		88,110[a]	113,370	BLS, 2014
Per capita (2013)	(100,000)	26.8	31.2	
Gender (%)	Female (%)	75.0	92.3	Hooker, 2014;
	Male (%)	25.0	7.7	AANP, 2015
Age (2013)	Years (median)	38	49	NCCPA, 2014; AANP, 2015
Race/Ethnicity (%)	Black/African American (non-Hispanic)	8.0	4.4	HRSA, 2014; AANP, 2015
	Asian (non-Hispanic)	7.2	3.7	
	Native Hawaiian/Other Pacific Islander (non-Hispanic)	NR (b)	NR (b)	
	Native American/Alaska Native (non-Hispanic)	0.3	NR (c)(b)	
	White/European (non-Hispanic)	63.4	86.5	
	Hispanic or Latino	10.8	3.7	
	Multiple / Other Race (non-Hispanic)	2.9	1.6	

NR = not reported or not fully represented.
[a]Numbers between licensed and employed differ because of two methods for counting. A BLS employer of a PA may include one licensed PA with two employers. The Hooker and Muchow analysis only counted one PA regardless of whether two licenses were held.
[b]Number withheld due to lack of stability.
[c]Number merged with multiple other/other race (non-Hispanic).

Despite their divergent training (and sometimes acrimonious debate), PAs and NPs are commonly thought of as similar types of healthcare providers, especially from a human resources standpoint. In a number of clinical settings, such as managed care health systems and ambulatory clinics, the roles of PAs and NPs are regarded as interchangeable, and open positions are advertised as being able to be filled by either provider (Morgan et al., 2016). Not surprisingly given this fact, PAs and NPs are also paid similarly in the same settings (Figure 11–1). Major research reports and policy analyses that have examined both of these health professions consider PAs and NPs to be equivalent when used in ambulatory practice roles. Even on the clinical level, PAs and NPs have similar views about their roles.

The differences are that NPs can practice either independently or collaboratively—that is, with limited supervision by doctors—in a growing number of states. In most states, they can prescribe medications with some level of authority, although some states do prohibit them from prescribing narcotics. Such restrictions are changing as much for NPs as for PAs.

The relationship between PAs and NPs depends on the perspective. Educators might not comingle, but clinicians at the patient-interaction level do to a large degree. No formal relationship exists between PAs and NPs on an organizational level; however, NPs commonly attend PA-type educational meetings and conferences, such as PAs in oncology conferences and PAs in family medicine conferences. NPs argue that they are filling an

FIGURE 11-1

Comparison of PA and NP Wages by Employer

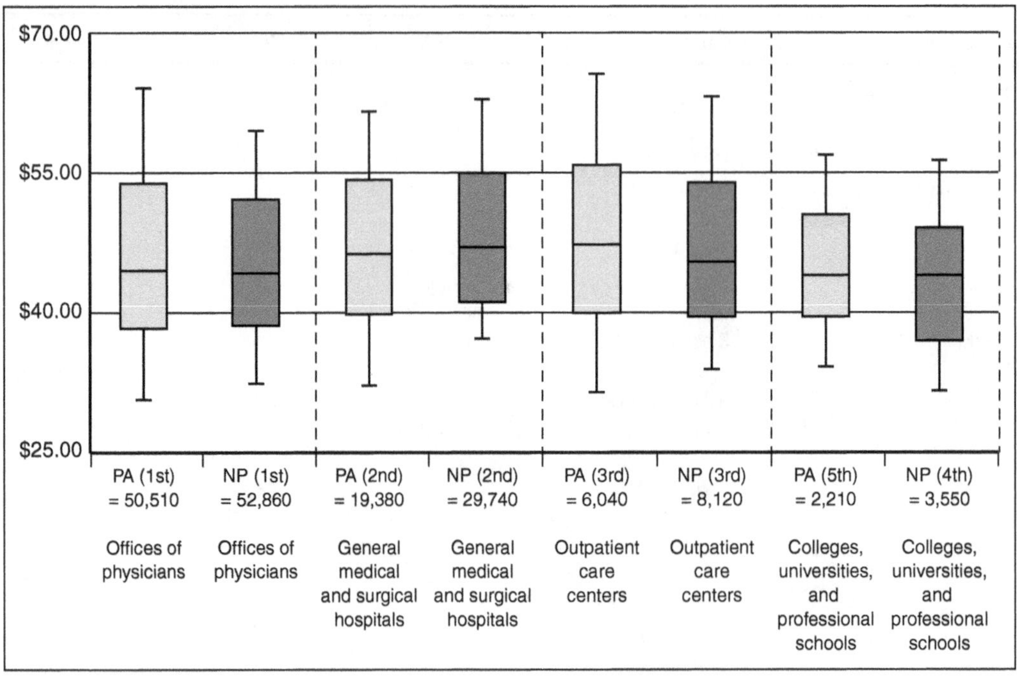

PA (1st) = 50,510	NP (1st) = 52,860	PA (2nd) = 19,380	NP (2nd) = 29,740	PA (3rd) = 6,040	NP (3rd) = 8,120	PA (5th) = 2,210	NP (4th) = 3,550
Offices of physicians	Offices of physicians	General medical and surgical hospitals	General medical and surgical hospitals	Outpatient care centers	Outpatient care centers	Colleges, universities, and professional schools	Colleges, universities, and professional schools

acute workforce need in primary care by providing services in areas that physicians are neglecting or avoid. To say so without mention of the considerable overlap with PAs may be a bit parochial. Doing so also ignores the observation that nonprimary care comprises about two-thirds of health delivery systems in the United States. Just the burden of chronic disease alone is a needed role substantially attended to by both PAs and NPs (Hooker et al., 2013).

A relevant claim of NPs is that they can provide the full range of medical care diagnostic and therapeutic services required for primary care. One notable study, conducted by NPs, asserted that NP outcomes in care of patients with certain conditions were equivalent to those of family physicians in primary care practice (Mundinger et al., 2000). Although the study found that patient outcomes were equivalent for diabetes (a finding corroborated by other studies as well [e.g., Morgan et al., 2012]), generalizing this finding across the full spectrum of primary care medical problems needs further investigation.

In the end, there seem to be more similarities between PAs and NPs than differences. They are deployed in similar surroundings, work in both primary care and nonprimary care, work with the disadvantaged at increasing rates, and seem satisfied with their roles.

WORKFORCE ISSUES

A key characteristic that has made PAs valued in the U.S. healthcare workforce is their adaptability to a wide range of work environments and roles. The role plasticity of PAs is their capability to work with physicians in almost any clinical practice setting. Over time, they have been able to adjust to the changing demands in the healthcare system and fill niches in the medical workforce—and physicians appear to appreciate this capability. After a period in which PAs were somewhat invisible on the healthcare workforce policy scene, influential leaders in medicine have recently taken note of their current roles and potential.

The Changing Healthcare Workforce

Healthcare workforce issues—the interplay among the various health professions as they relate to supply and demand in the medical marketplace—have become increasingly important in the discussion of who will address the growing need for access to care. A shortage of physicians has led to some expansion of medical school enrollment and output. The prevailing wisdom in healthcare workforce policy circles is that medical schools must expand their capacity to meet the anticipated demand for physician services expected in the next 10 to 20 years (Phillips et al., 2014). This projected demand is based on the assumptions of an expanding and aging population, decreased physician productivity, more disenfranchised becoming insured, and an increasing gross domestic product that correlates with medical care demand.

The expansion of medical education to meet anticipated demand brings direct challenges to the PA profession and to PA education, suggesting that changes are needed in the profession's educational direction, structure, and output. One belief is that PAs and NPs are likely to assume a greater role in medical care. In part, this view holds that the physician workforce will not be able to meet the anticipated future demand for medical care services and that PAs will assume new responsibilities for patient care that involves technical procedures, such as robotic surgery and interventional radiology. This view has led to suggestions to lengthen the period of PA education, which averages 26 months in the United States, and 24 to 36 months in other countries. Given the increasing complexities of modern medicine and the difficulties faced by primary care providers in patient management, it is easy to understand how individuals outside of the PA profession may feel that 2 years is a relatively short time in which to prepare for encountering the wide range of clinical problems faced by modern clinicians.

Various advocates for the expansion of the healthcare workforce believe the United States is facing a substantial physician shortage and that U.S. workforce policy should call for an increase in the output of medical school graduates, NPs, and PAs. In speaking about PAs and NPs, a growing consensus is that both disciplines have expanded their training capacity and may have a supply of practitioners that will meet future demand.

Leaders in medicine are essentially saying that they are counting on PAs to pick up a proportion of the workforce demand and that raising the output of educational programs should be considered (Cooper, 2013). In an attempt to determine the dimensions of program expansion, surveys have been conducted but little has been done in terms of policy direction with the information in response to calls for a greater supply of PA graduates. This raises the question of who determines PA educational policy: Is it the professional organizations, or is it left to individual institutions? In most countries it is the state that underwrites university-based education and as such controls the purse for such undertakings.

Recent history suggests that it is market forces in higher education, rather than a concerted effort by the professions' organizations, that tends to set the course of PA education. This was certainly the case in the second phase of PA program expansion in the late 1990s, when the number of US programs more than doubled. In this instance, the professions' organizations refrained from taking any public positions on program expansion. Generally, since its development, the Physician Assistant Education Association has traditionally shied away from taking official positions on workforce policy issues. In view of the recent challenges presented to PA education by prominent leaders in medicine, it may be time for a more assertive organizational approach to addressing PA workforce policy issues to shape the direction for the profession.

Federal Involvement in Workforce Issues

For decades, the federal government has been extensively involved in helping to shape workforce policy in the United States. The federal role in healthcare workforce policy was prominent and included the funding of workforce study groups, such as the Graduate Medical Education National Advisory Committee and the Council on Graduate Medical Education, as well as programs that offered direct support to schools for training health professionals. However, the federal government is less involved in healthcare workforce activities.

The expansion of US medical education in the second decade is occurring more as a private-sector activity than it was with the traditional federal subsidy it enjoyed for almost a century. PA programs are expanding their enrollment a private-sector activity as well (Cawley & Jones, 2013). What this trend means is uncertain. Federal support of healthcare workforce training typically took into consideration perceived problematic areas that affected society and the health sector, such as insufficient numbers of providers in primary care and in rural and underserved areas and imbalances in racial and ethnic composition. Consequently, in recent years, the federal training grants for PA education have integrated these identified priorities as preferences. In doing so, they have selected proposals for grant support that has attainable goals consistent with these priorities.

FURTHER RESEARCH ON PROFESSIONAL AND WORKFORCE ISSUES

The literature about PA professional and workforce issues is limited. For the most part, the research on the PA labor force is underdeveloped and poorly promulgated. Increasing evidence identifies PAs as team players (see Chapter 12, "Physician Assistants on Multidisciplinary Teams"). To date, researchers have not identified the relationships between the professional and workforce issues facing PAs and such factors as demographics, age, intellectual curiosity, family, patient perceptions, personality profiles, and specialty and supervisory roles that PAs occupy. This breach leads to the following suggestions for areas of further research related PA professional and workforce issues:

- **Professionalism:** What are issues for PAs in the 21st century with regard to professionalism?

- **PAs and NPs:** What is the overlap in skills and roles between PAs and NPs? How will this affect the changing workforce by 2025?
- **Economics:** Do PAs and NPs substitute one for the other? Are some skills unique to one practice and not the other?
- **Prescribing:** What are the trends in the pharmaceutical industry regarding targeting PAs and NPs? How do those trends differ from those seen with doctors? Does such targeting enhance or diminish the stature of PAs?
- **Healthcare workforce policy:** Will private sector expansion in the workforce address issues of shortages? Can Americans attain the workforce needed without federal policy direction or subsidies?
- **Global PA movement:** What political and professional issues do PAs in other countries face? Are these issues universal ones that PAs in all countries face or are they unique to only one country?

These topics are not meant to be inclusive but are merely suggested ideas for further research.

SUMMARY

Professional issues for PAs vary depending on the era, prior accomplishments, experience, and policy climates. Some current issues include autonomy, doctoral degrees, nomenclature of the profession, postgraduate training, and NP and PA relationships. Although some of these issues are uniquely specific to PAs, many are shared in common with other health professionals.

Similarly, workforce issues have become increasingly influenced by PAs. As the total number of PAs in the workforce increases, the PA profession appears to have reached a critical mass that has caused national organizations and individual investigators to increasingly include PAs when examining the national healthcare workforce. The PA profession would benefit from additional original research on many workforce-related questions to be prepared to assist policymakers in developing programs to address the nation's needs for healthcare providers.

References

The following citations are key to supporting this chapter's content. You can find a complete list of citations for all chapters at www.fadavis.com/davisplus, keyword *Hooker*.

AANP. (2014). 2012 NP Sample Survey (NPSS). American Association of Nurse Practitioners. Austin, TX

AANP. (2015). 2013-14 National NP Practice Site Census. American Association of Nurse Practitioners. Austin, TX.

BLS [Bureau of Labor Statistics]: OES: http://www.bls.gov/oes/tables.htm. BLS code: 29-1071 Physician Assistants; BLS code: 29-1171 Nurse Practitioner

Cawley, J. F., & Jones, P. E. (2013). Institutional sponsorship, student debt, and specialty choice in physician assistant education. *Journal of Physician Assistant Education, 24*(4), 4–8.

Cooper, R. A. (2013). Unraveling the physician supply dilemma. *Journal of the American Medical Association, 310*(18), 1931–1932.

Dill, M. J., Pankow, S., Erikson, C., & Shipman, S. (2013). Survey shows consumers open to a greater role for physician assistants and nurse practitioners. *Health Affairs, 32*(6), 1135–1142.

Hooker, R. S., Benitez, J. A., Coplan, B. H., & Dehn, R. W. (2013). Ambulatory and chronic disease care by physician assistants and nurse practitioners. *Journal of Ambulatory Care Management, 36*(4), 293–301.

Hooker, R. S., Brock, D. M., & Cook, M. L. (2016). Characteristics of nurse practitioners and physician assistants in the United States. *Journal of the American Association of Nurse Practitioners, 28*(1), 39–46.

Hooker RS. (2015). Is physician assistant autonomy inevitable? *Journal of the American Academy of Physician Assistants. 28*(1): 18–19.

Hooker, R. S., & Muchow, A. N. (2014). The 2013 census of licensed physician assistants. *Journal of the American Academy of Physician Assistants, 27*(7), 35–39.

HRSA. (2014). U.S. Department of Health and Human Services, Health Resources and Services Administration, National Center for Health Workforce Analysis. Sex, Race, and Ethnic Diversity of U.S. Health Occupations: Technical Documentation, Rockville, Maryland: Author.

Morgan, P. A., Abbott, D. H., McNeil, R. B., & Fisher, D. A. (2012). Characteristics of primary care office visits to nurse practitioners, physician assistants and physicians in the United States Veterans Health Administration facilities, 2005 to 2010: A retrospective cross-sectional analysis. *Human Resources for Health, 10*, 42. Retrieved from http://www.human-resources-health.com/content/10/1/42

Morgan, P., Everett, C. M., & Huminick, K. (2016, February 4). Scarcity of primary care positions may divert physician assistants into specialty practice. *Medical Care Research and Review.* Advance online publication.

Mundinger, M. O., Kane, R. L., Lenz, E. R., Totten, A. M., Tsai, W. Y., Cleary, P. D, et al. (2000). Primary care outcomes in patients treated by nurse practitioners or physicians: A randomized trial. *Journal of the American Medical Association, 283*(1), 59–68.

NCCPA. (2014). National Commission on the Certification of Physician Assistants. 2013 Statistical Profile of Certified Physician Assistants. Johns Creek, Georgia.

Phillips, R. L., Jr., Bazemore, A. M., & Peterson, L. E. (2014). Effectiveness over efficiency: Underestimating the primary care physician shortage. *Medical Care, 52*(2), 97–98.

CHAPTER 12

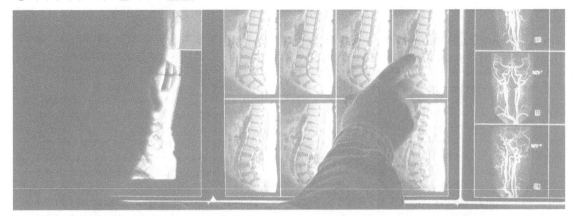

PHYSICIAN ASSISTANTS ON MULTIDISCIPLINARY TEAMS

CHRISTINE M. EVERETT ■ RODERICK S. HOOKER ■ JAMES F. CAWLEY

"A boat doesn't go forward if each one is rowing their own way."

— *Swahili proverb*

Across the world, many systems are looking for ways to improve access to healthcare. Not just the access but to improve and the quality and efficiency of the care they deliver. Since the inception of the profession, physician assistants (PAs) have worked within the context of teams. This chapter provides an introduction to the concepts associated with teams and roles as well as team effectiveness. Moreover, it explores the application of these concepts to healthcare teams. Defining the PA's role within the healthcare team is a critical aspect of this dynamic.

OVERVIEW OF THE TEAM CONCEPT

The major challenges facing our healthcare system have encouraged utilization of team-based approaches to system redesign. The US Population is approximately 320 million, and 2015 is the first year healthcare spending reached $10,000 per person (3.2 trillion dollars). This spending accounts for more than 17% of the gross domestic product (GDP) and is nearly twice the average spent in countries with similar economies (Organisation for Economic Co-operation and Development [OECD], 2013). Despite the significant investment in healthcare, the quality of care experienced by US citizens is far from ideal. Access to healthcare is reduced for the poor, the uninsured, and those living in rural areas. Those who are able to access healthcare often visit multiple healthcare providers in a year but are still not routinely receiving guideline-recommended care (Pham et al., 2007). With the aging of the population, increasing complexity and fragmentation of care, and projected physician shortages, the solutions to these issues require significant system changes. One frequently recommended approach to dealing with these forces is team-based care delivery.

Teams Defined

The idea of healthcare professionals working together is not a new idea; it is the predominant organizational structure in healthcare

(Figure 12–1). Less than one-third of physicians work in solo practice, and almost 50% of physicians' offices include PAs, nurse practitioners (NPs), or certified nurse-midwives (Hing & Hsio, 2015). However, only within the past decade has the focus on teams emerged. What distinguishes a group of healthcare professionals who are "together and working" from a team that is "working together" (Morgan et al., 1993)? The term *team* has an abundance of definitions. At their essence, the definitions state that a *team* is a group of two or more individuals with defined roles who work interdependently toward a common goal (Bosch et al., 2009). It is important to note that it is possible for individuals with defined roles to work together and not be a team. For example, a family physician and a specialist physician such as a psychiatrist may have patients in common. Both professionals have defined roles, and the work of one may even be dependent on the work of the other. However, if both do not explicitly coordinate their efforts to meet a shared objective, they are not functioning as a team. The absence of working together toward a shared objective is not uncommon in the US healthcare system. Often, the information needed to share an objective is unclear. One study reported that 68% of specialists responding to a survey regarding physician referral processes reported that they did not receive information from primary care providers before a referral visit (Gandhi et al., 2000). Another study that evaluated referrals found that referring physicians made the purpose of the visit explicit in only 76% of cases (McPhee, 1984). Similarly, coordination is often lacking. Consulting specialty physicians communicated their findings in only 55% of consultations (McPhee et al., 1984).

In reality, groups and teams fall on a continuum (Saltman et al., 2005) (Figure 12–2). At one extreme are people in groups, who interact minimally but work in a group setting. Examples of this approach have historically been used in primary care group practices. At the other extreme are highly structured teams with well-defined, interdependent roles, such as surgical teams. Unfortunately, no agreement exists regarding the cutoff between *group* and *team*. Additionally, there is still much debate as to which factors are critical in determining where health professionals working together may fall on this continuum. Although interdependence and common goal are considered essential factors, other factors (such as length of time the team will work together, reason for forming, decision-making, and communication) can also influence where a group falls on the team continuum.

FIGURE 12-1
Distribution of Physicians Employed in Physician-Owned Groups by Practice Size, 2001

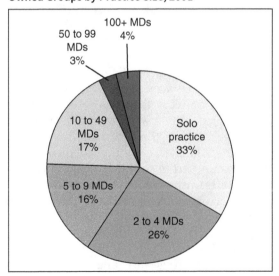

Source: Gauthier, A., Schoembaum, S. C., & Weinbaum, I. (2006). Toward a high performance health system for the United States. New York: The Commonwealth Fund. Data source: Kane, C. (2004). The practice arrangements of patient care physicians (Physician Marketplace Report No. 2004-02). Chicago, IL: American Medical Association.

FIGURE 12-2
The Group-Team Continuum

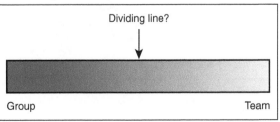

To Team or Not to Team?
That Is the Question

In healthcare, professionals work together due to the nature of the needs of patients. In other words, no individual professional provides 100% of the care for an individual patient. However, under what circumstances is it best to behave like individuals working in a group versus forming a team? Due to the positive connotation of the word *team*, many people would say that it is always best to form a team. Like all things, however, teams come with disadvantages as well as advantages (Table 12–1). If a group contains professionals with diverse professional backgrounds, knowledge, and skills, then a team can provide multiple advantages. First, the variety of skills available provides the potential for cross-training, which can allow the workers more flexibility in roles. It also allows for the potential to combine multiple approaches to create unique approaches to patient care and solutions to problems. Social support is another added benefit of teams, particularly in situations with difficult decision-making, such as is the case in emergency departments and palliative care.

Despite the advantages working in teams also has potential disadvantages. For example, not everyone may wish to be part of a team, which can be a significant challenge to overcome. Teamwork also requires additional time for such activities as communication and coordination, which could reduce the efficiency of the group. This can be the case when professional backgrounds are diverse, as variety in perspectives can often make decision-making challenging. Even teams with cohesive views have risks. Decision-making in these circumstances could become less creative due to "group think"—a phenomenon that occurs when people want to avoid conflict. Determining whether a team is an appropriate work design for a clinical practice requires consideration of whether the potential advantages are worth the disadvantages. Unfortunately, there is little evidence to support when teams, and what type or model of team, are best for any given circumstance in healthcare (Saltman et al., 2005).

MODELS OF TEAM CARE

Since the Institute of Medicine report *Crossing the Quality Chasm* recommended developing healthcare delivery teams as an approach to improving quality, a wide array of teams have been described in the literature (Institute of Medicine, 2001). All cases involve inclusion of professionals from multiple disciplines. For example, teams in intensive care units may include doctors from several specialties as well as nurses. Surgical teams that include surgeons, PAs, and nurses have also been described. The team models used in primary care are numerous and range from a small "teamlet," consisting of a single doctor and nurse, to large teams with doctors, PAs, NPs, pharmacists, and social workers.

Although the types of professionals and specialties involved in a team may vary significantly,

TABLE 12-1
Advantages and Disadvantages of Teams

Advantages	Disadvantages
■ Mutual learning opportunities ■ Workforce flexibility with cross-training ■ Opportunity for synergistic combinations of ideas and abilities ■ Social support for difficult tasks and situations ■ Beneficial for interdependent tasks ■ Increased communication and information exchange ■ Potential to stimulate performance and attendance due to commitment to team	■ Potential to involve individuals who are incompatible with teamwork ■ Additional need to select worker to fit team as well as job ■ Potential for some members to experience less motivating jobs ■ Increased competition and conflict between teams ■ Time required for coordination, socializing, and consensus-building ■ Inhibition of creativity; possibility of group-think ■ Less powerful evaluation and rewards; may result in social loafing or free-riding

Adapted from Campion, M. A., Papper, E. M., & Medsker, G. J. (1996). Relations between work team characteristics and effectiveness: A replication and extension. *Personnel Psychology, 49,* 429–452.

these models of team care can be categorized according to their approach to hierarchy and collaboration. *Multidisciplinary teams* are the most hierarchical. Each member contributes a discipline-specific skill set, and collaboration is defined by the communication between supervisor and subordinate(s). An example would be a primary care teamlet model that includes a doctor and a medical assistant. A team becomes *interdisciplinary* when its members are considered to be on the same level of the hierarchy, with collaboration between colleagues. An example would be a cancer treatment team that involves surgical and medical oncologists. Finally, a team could take a *transdisciplinary* approach, which extends the focus on collaboration. This type of team generally involves overlapping roles and cross-disciplinary education. It is also the only model that explicitly includes patients on the team. An example might be a primary care team with a doctor, a PA, an NP, and the patient. Theoretically, a PA could be involved in any of the three team models. It is important to note that despite their separate definitions, many people are not aware of the distinctions among these types of teams and use the terms *multidisciplinary* and *interdisciplinary* interchangeably.

TEAM EFFECTIVENESS

With so many options for healthcare teams, how does one decide which is best for a given clinical situation? Although this information might not yet be available, enough is known about teams to describe which characteristics influence team effectiveness. The literature contains many models of team effectiveness from a variety of disciplines. However, at their essence, most of them have a common set of relationships: team design (i.e., structure) affects work processes (i.e., team work and work of the team) and outcomes (Figure 12–3).

Team Structure

Team structure can be roughly divided into two categories: team context and the team itself (Lemieux-Charles & McGuire, 2006). *Team context* is the milieu in which the team works. Many contextual factors can potentially influence the

FIGURE 12-3
Teams Effectiveness Models

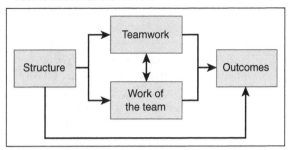

effectiveness of a team. For example, studies have demonstrated that organizational cultures that enhance team orientation have a positive impact on healthcare team outcomes (Lemieux-Charles & McGuire, 2006). Larger regulatory factors, including scope of practice laws and reimbursement policies, could also potentially affect team effectiveness; however, research evaluating these relationships is limited. Other structural issues that are characteristics of the team itself also influence team effectiveness (Lemieux-Charles & McGuire, 2006). Many of these characteristics are factors related to the tasks the team has to perform. Features of the care or the setting can influence outcomes. For example, one can imagine that work related to geriatric patients in long-term care facilities would be quite different from that of emergency departments in rural settings. Other important structural features are characteristics of team composition. Examples include the size of the team, diversity of its membership, and length of time the members have been performing as a team. Research on healthcare teams particularly suggests that these factors can have mixed effects on team outcomes (Bosch et al., 2009; Lemieux-Charles & McGuire, 2006). For example, diversity of membership seems to improve professional performance but may or may not improve patient outcomes. These structural components can have an impact on effectiveness directly or indirectly through team processes.

Team processes are the ways in which teams work. They include two major categories: teamwork and work of the team. The teamwork processes are the processes that most people think of when they think of the word *team*. They include leadership, communication, conflict resolution, and collaboration. Although significant work remains to be done in this area, evidence suggests that these factors are more likely to influence staff satisfaction than are patient outcomes (Lemieux-Charles & McGuire, 2006). The factors related to the ways in which healthcare providers perform healthcare duties on a team are also important. They are frequently the focus of studies that concentrate on healthcare quality. An illustrative example is the work done by Pronovost and colleagues (2006), who significantly reduced bloodstream infections in intensive care units through the implementation of a checklist for catheter insertion. These two groups of processes—teamwork and work of the team—can have an impact on each other as well as the team's effectiveness.

Outcomes and Team Effectiveness

Team effectiveness can be defined by outcomes at the patient, team, or organizational level (Lemieux-Charles & McGuire, 2006). Important patient outcomes could include quality of care, functional status, and patient satisfaction. Team outcomes that have been considered include perceived team effectiveness and team member satisfaction. Finally, organizational outcomes include provider turnover and costs. Most studies on teams do not evaluate the full range of important patient, team, and organizational outcomes. However, different team structures result in different patterns of outcomes. For example, in primary care teams with PAs or NPs as usual providers, the quality of care delivered has been found to be similar to that of doctors, but patients were more likely to use the emergency department (Everett et al., 2013). As a result, designing a team approach to care delivery will likely require that organizations prioritize their goals and ensure that the team structure reflects those goals.

PAs and Teams

The PA profession prides itself on its focus on teamwork. A leader in the profession recently captured this pride when he said, "PAs did teams before teams were cool" (J. Cawley, personal communication, September 2013). In fact, this issue is a frequent point of challenge. There are important distinctions between groups and teams—can one say that PAs really work on teams or that PAs are legally required to work on teams (at least in the United States). Because of the regulation of PA practice, the minimum requirements for a team are met. In the U.S. a PA must work under the supervision of a doctor. This means that at least two people are working together. It also creates the condition for interdependence and shared goals. Presumably, a physician would not work with a PA unless a need to fill a gap in patient care existed. A PA cannot practice without working with a doctor. Their shared goal is the treatment of a common group of patients. Finally, the laws also specify roles for each person in the group, at least those related to leadership.

ROLES

Role Theory

Roles are the defining features of organizations. It is the interaction between roles that affects an organization's ability to meet its goals (Katz & Kahn, 1966). A role is recognized as a relational concept that is defined in terms of other positions, is task oriented (i.e., oriented toward the work performed), and is hierarchical (Fig. 12-4). The expectations for any role within an organization are influenced by the individuals in related positions (role senders), such as supervisors and coworkers. This idea of organizational role is useful for understanding that general patterns of behavior define roles.

PAs and Roles

In healthcare, clinical roles can be defined by the division of patient care between members of the team. Sibbald et al. (2006) discuss healthcare provider patient care roles in terms of skill mix, or task profiles. They contend that the roles of healthcare professionals are continuously revised in response to contextual or outside pressures, including patient perceptions

FIGURE 12-4
Organizational Role Theory

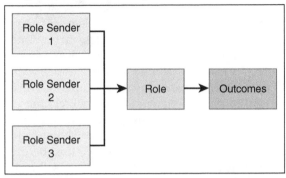

Based on Katz, D., & Kahn, R. L. (1966). The social psychology of organizations. New York: John Wiley & Sons.

and expectations, policy and payment systems changes, professional regulation and training, and professional attitudes. Role revision related to defined tasks that were previously the domain of physicians falls under two categories: supplement/complement and substitute. Clinicians such as PAs that "provide additional services that are intended to complement or extend those provided by physicians" are *supplements or complements* for physicians. However, clinicians that "provide the same services as physicians" act as *substitutes*. For example, in primary care, a PA who acts as a usual provider (i.e., has his or her own panel of patients and provides the full range of care delivered in primary care settings) is a substitute. A PA who assists in hip replacement surgery is a complement.

This distinction between *substitute* and *supplement/complement* provides a useful and broad generalization for PAs according to their similarity of function to that of physicians. However, it does not provide enough specificity to fully capture the distinct roles of PAs. Specifically, it does not identify the key factors or domains that are considered when determining *how* to divide patient care services within the PA–physician dyad. For example, because of the heterogeneity of patient care tasks, the broad range of patients served in primary care, and the longitudinal nature of the patient–provider relationship, factors that can

determine PA roles in primary care include the following:

■ Type of services provided
■ Complexity of patients served (i.e., the number and type of diseases for each patient)
■ Level of involvement of a PA in the care of a patient

While the necessary conceptual work to understand teams in other specialties has not yet occured, the factors that are important for other specialties are likely different. It is possible that the nature of emergency medicine may make urgency of the issue a more important factor than patient complexity. In medical specialties, severity of the disease may be more pertinent. There are other factors that influence PA roles, such as level of interdependence with the partnering doctor. Research is needed to identify and define the important factors involved in PA role definition in each medical and surgical specialty if the impact of PA roles on access, quality, and cost of care is to be understood.

FURTHER RESEARCH ON TEAMS AND ROLES

The work on team roles is in its infancy and there is much to learn. Here is a brief listing of some of the areas requiring further exploration:

■ **Regulatory and organizational contexts:** How do laws and organizational policies influence team and role designs?
■ **Team structure:** How does the PA clinical role influence team and organizational outcomes? How does length of time on the team influence teamwork?
■ **Team processes:** How does the PA role affect key teamwork processes, such as leadership, communication, and coordination? How does the PA role influence the work of the team?
■ **Outcomes:** Does the PA role or other team design features affect team member satisfaction? Does team design affect patient access or organizational costs?

SUMMARY

The idea of healthcare professionals working together is not new; it is the predominant organizational structure in healthcare. However, what distinguishes a group of healthcare professionals who are "together and working" from a team that is "working together" is the presence of two or more individuals with defined roles who work interdependently toward a common goal. Multiple models for team care exist and can be categorized according to their approach to hierarchy and collaboration. The regulatory requirement for PAs to work in collaboration with physicians sets the stage for meeting the minimum definition of a team. Team effectiveness is a function of the structure and processes of that team. An important structural element of any team is role definition. PA roles vary within and between specialties. PA roles can be broadly categorized into two categories: complement and substitute. Preliminary work identifying the important factors included in role definition for primary care PAs has been completed. However, similar work needs to be completed for all other specialties before identification of team designs that will lead to the best outcomes for patients, providers, and organizations can occur.

References

The following citations are key to supporting this chapter's content. You can find a complete list of citations for all chapters at www. fadavis.com/davisplus, keyword *Hooker*.

Bosch, M., Faber, M. J., Cruijsberg, J., Voerman, G. E., Leatherman, S., Grol, R. P.,...Wensing, M. (2009). Review article: Effectiveness of patient care teams and the role of clinical expertise and coordination. *Medical Care Research and Review, 66*(Suppl. 6), 5S–35S.

Everett, C. M., Thorpe, C., Palta, M., Carayon, P., Bartels, C., & Smith, M.A. (2013). Physician assistants and nurse practitioners perform effective roles on teams caring for Medicare patients with diabetes. *Health Affairs, 32*(11), 1942–1948.

Gandhi, T. K., Sittig, D. F., Franklin, M., Sussman, A. J., Fairchild, D. G., & Bates, D. W. (2000). Communication breakdown in the outpatient referral process. *Journal of General Internal Medicine, 15*(9), 626–631.

Hing, E., & Hsiao, C. J. (2015). In which states are physician assistants or nurse practitioners more likely to work in primary care? *Journal of the American Academy of Physician Assistants, 28*(9), 46-53.

Institute of Medicine. (2001). *Crossing the quality chasm: A new health system for the 21st century.* Washington, DC: Institute of Medicine.

Katz, D., & Kahn, R. L. (1966). *The social psychology of organizations.* New York: John Wiley & Sons.

Lemieux-Charles, L., & McGuire, W. L. (2006). What do we know about healthcare team effectiveness? A review of the literature. *Medical Care Research and Review, 63*(3), 263–300.

McPhee, S. J., Lo, B., Saika, G. Y., & Meltzer, R. (1984). How good is communication between primary care physicians and subspecialty consultants? *Archives of Internal Medicine, 144*(6), 1265–1268.

Medsker, G. J., & Campion, M. A. (1997). Job and team design. In P. Carayon (Ed.), *Handbook of human factors and ergonomics in healthcare and patient safety* (pp. 450–489). Boca Raton, FL: CRC Press.

Morgan, B. B., Salas, E., & Glickman, A. S. (1993). An analysis of team evolution and maturation. *Journal of General Psychology, 120*(3), 277–291.

Organisation for Economic Co-operation and Development. (2013). *Health at a glance 2013: OECD indicators.* Retrieved from http://www. oecd.org/health/health-systems/health-at-a-glance.htm

Pham, H. H., Schrag, D., O'Malley, A. S., Wu, B. N., & Bach, P. B. (2007). Care patterns in Medicare and their implications for pay for performance. *New England Journal of Medicine, 356*(11), 1130–1139.

Pronovost, P., Needham, D., Berenholtz, S., Sinopoli, D., Chu, H., Cosgrove, S., . . . Goeschel, C. (2006). An intervention to decrease catheter-related bloodstream infections in the ICU. *New England Journal of Medicine, 355*(26), 2725-2732.

Saltman, D. C., O'Dea, N. A., Farmer, J., Veitch, C., Rosen, G., & Kidd, M. R. (2005). Groups or teams in healthcare: Finding the best fit. *Journal of Evaluation in Clinical Practice, 13*, 55–60.

Sibbald, B., Laurant, M., & Scott, A. (2006). Changing task profiles. In R. B. Saltman, A. Rico, & W. Boerma (Eds.), *Primary care in the driver's seat? Organizational reform in European primary care.* Berkshire, England: Open University Press.

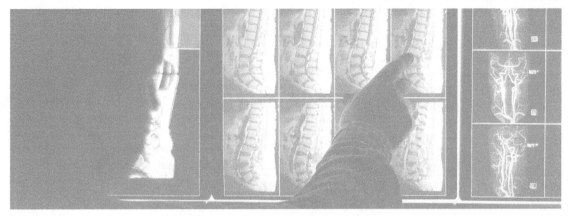

CHAPTER 13

FUTURE DIRECTIONS OF THE PHYSICIAN ASSISTANT PROFESSION

RODERICK S. HOOKER ■ JAMES F. CAWLEY ■ CHRISTINE M. EVERETT

"The empires of the future are the empires of the mind."

— *Sir Winston Churchill*

Remarkable changes are underway with the increased use of physician assistants (PAs) globally. Examining these changes and the way in which they took place provides some perspective that can shed light on the future of PAs. The origin of PAs in the United States, Liberia, and Ghana in the 1960s was a grass-roots activity, with doctors employing PAs scattered around the country. Social and political change was occurring simultaneously. Eventually, the laws regarding scope of practice were changed at the state level. In other countries, however, this process at times was different; legislation may precede innovation in some instances. Enter the PA of the new century. She or he belongs to a robust profession with legislative battles largely in the past. Yet extraordinary changes loom for all societies, and the PA is one more player in a world where severe medical shortages and generational shifts signal a variable healthcare environment.

SUCCESS OF THE PHYSICIAN ASSISTANT CONCEPT

The role of the PA in the new millennium is a product of medicine that enjoys unparalleled success among the health professions. Born in the 1960s, nurtured in the 1970s, and grown in the 1980s, the PA role emerged in the 1990s as a major player in health policy in the United States. By the new century, the PA had become a global phenomenon; by 2016, there were more than 100,000 PAs worldwide. How did this development come about? Was it due to the right person at the right time with the right vision? A fluke development? A well-planned evolution in the division of medical labor in the US health system being taken up elsewhere?

Various explanations have been advanced as to why the PA concept is so successful. Clearly, PAs fit well in the entrepreneurial US healthcare system, where their economic advantages, clinical flexibility, and dependent practice stance are considered the factors most likely for their success. Yet it is other countries that are building on the success of this model, making the future of the global PA look bright. With a worldwide shortage of 4.5 million doctors (according to the World Health Organization, 2013) and an inadequate number of medical schools (approximately 2000 globally), the sheer weight of the population growth demands more medical personnel and resources. Couple these factors with the aging of the population, improvements in childhood survival measures, and the control of archaic diseases that have remained unchanged over thousands of years (e.g., malaria, tuberculosis, dengue fever, smallpox, polio) and the result is that people will live longer and more comfortably than their parents. Technological advancements are limited only by logistics of delivery to remote populations. The percentage of elderly people who are living longer and more productively means a large cadre of health workers are needed. Without more doctors and nurses, the next group of providers to look to is PAs.

A broad sociological explanation for the success of PAs in the United States is that they (and nurse practitioners [NPs]) represent an evolution in the division of medical labor. Medicine and the delivery of healthcare have become infinitely more complex over the past several decades. The required knowledge base to practice medicine is enormous and has led to greater levels of specialization and subspecialization. The once-vaunted supremacy of doctors over health and medicine has given way to a sharing of diagnostic and therapeutic tasks, in part because modern physicians cannot know everything and do everything in a field so vast. In the 20th century, new diagnostic technologies and therapeutic approaches led to the evolution of new professions, such as radiological technology, physical therapy, and genetics. The expansion of medical activities and capabilities necessitates the inclusion of additional trained personnel who share the domains that once were in the exclusive possession of physicians.

Other reasons for success of the PA profession in US medicine include the major social forces thought to have influenced the PA movement:

- **Changing lifestyles.** The new practice preferences of physicians grew out of the 1960s. Doctors, along with others, realized they did not want to work as hard as their predecessors and needed help.
- **Gender shift.** Women in all professions entered the workforce in a major way, with many seeking a career in healthcare. Many were trying out careers that had been traditionally occupied by men and found them to their liking. For a young woman, a career as a PA is a shorter route than some other professions and a sterling profession to adopt. It also provides an opportunity to raise a family and remain employed.
- **Physician dependency.** The commitment to being a dependent profession that is closely associated with doctors allowed for widespread acceptance of the PA by organized medicine.
- **National competency.** The early establishment of program accreditation and a national board to oversee the specific skills and competency expected of PAs allowed for enabling state legislation.
- **Primary care.** A national emphasis on training primary care generalists grew when projection models showed there were inadequate numbers. Enter PAs and NPs with their primary care training.

The profession also succeeds in part because of the personal and career attributes of PAs. The first two generations in particular saw themselves as change agents in the health system and believed they had a mission to prove that individuals trained in the PA model could practice medicine safely and effectively. The profession has been and continues to be one of the most exciting careers in the 21st century.

In looking forward, key questions that arise are:

- What does the future hold for the PA profession?
- Will the demand for PA services continue to increase, or will it plateau or decrease?

- Does the past predict the future?
- How will the changing face of various healthcare systems have an impact on the PA profession?
- Will a PA educated and certified in Utrecht, The Netherlands, for example, be able to work in Mt. Isa, Australia (and be as effective)?

Two phenomena are shaping PAs and their futures: (1) the change of human societies and (2) the change of healthcare delivery. By examining these directions and then seeking a convergence point, one can make some predictions that apply to PAs in all settings and in all countries.

THE FUTURE OF SOCIETIES

Forecasts are not so much meant to be predictions but instead glimpses of what is likely to (or should) happen. For many futurists, projections are intended to provoke thought and inspire action. The world literature offers some emerging thoughts on what the years ahead may portend for healthcare in general and PAs in particular:

- **World populations.** World populations are growing larger than predicted due, in part, to people being healthier and living longer than before. Despite declines in fertility, the increase in longevity contributes to population growth. The United Nations increased its forecast for the global population to 11.2 billion by 2100 (Table 13–1).
- **Demographics.** Population characteristics are shifting in ways unexpected only a few years ago. The aging of America will alter society, with one in five individuals being retired by 2030. This factor will change the labor force and economy, straining employment-intensive services, such as healthcare, transportation, and food services. Medicare, the US healthcare entitlement for the elderly, will not be adequate to meet demand, and few good ideas have been promoted to address this shortfall. More years in retirement may diminish resources for children and working

TABLE 13-1
World Population Milestones

WORLD POPULATION REACHED		
1 billion in	1804	
2 billion in	1927	(123 years later)
3 billion in	1960	(33 years later)
4 billion in	1974	(14 years later)
5 billion in	1987	(13 years later)
6 billion in	1999	(12 years later)
7 billion in	2011	(12 years later)
WORLD POPULATION MAY REACH		
8 billion in	2028	(15 years later)
9 billion in	2054	(26 years later)
11 billion in	2100	(74 years later)

Data from the United Nations Department of Economic and Social Affairs, Population Division. (2015). *World Population to 2100.* New York: United Nations.

adults. Special pressures on the elderly will emerge in areas where they are concentrated, such as Arizona, Nevada, and Florida (Figure 13–1).
- **Unrealistic expectations of generations X and Y.** Roughly 50% of American high school seniors plan to continue their education after high school and obtain a bachelor's degree. This trend is in contrast to 20% of seniors in 1976. However, reality differs from those expectations; only one-quarter of high school seniors actually obtain a bachelor's degree, suggesting young people may have unrealistic expectations about the future. Among those who do obtain a bachelor's degree, less than 2% accomplish this task in less than 4 years, and the majority now take 4 or more years to complete tertiary education and graduate.
- **Government.** Burdened by programs that assist society (such as Social Security, medical research, support for the needy, and the courts), government will be strained by a revenue base to respond to the demand for increasing services. People may outlive their savings, having planned for a shorter life span.
- **Education.** Blended learning, virtual classrooms, and online courses will replace a significant portion of the classroom. Medicine

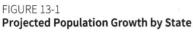

FIGURE 13-1
Projected Population Growth by State

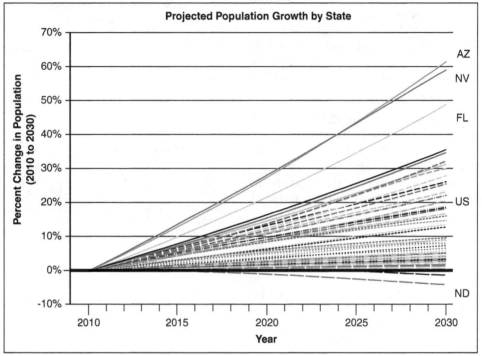

will be taught using visually stunning graphics and creative courses. New software will portray virtual blackboards and model diseases. As a result, fewer students are likely to work with real cadavers. Massive open online courses (MOOCs) are blending classrooms with computers where graphics enrich structure and learning goals, at the same time promoting the reuse and remixing of resources.

- **Human knowledge capability.** This factor is the quantity of available knowledge that continues to multiply each decade. The doctor, PA, nurse, and health worker of tomorrow will have access to knowledge in ways that are only rudimentary now. Best practices, evidence-based medicine, and the patient's genetic profile will drive standard-of-care templates for a particular patient. Experiences in medicine will enhance knowledge capability by making it more interesting and engaging than just memorizing facts.

- **Decisions by nonhumans.** Electronically enabled networks will make financial, health, educational, and even political decisions. The power of statistics to make complex decisions based on probability will dictate many new behaviors. In one example, partnerships of Apple, Epic, and IBM emerged in 2015 as one entity to address healthcare. Another example, *UnitedHealth-Optum* has partnered with a wide variety of institutions. Both of these organizations are building and adding to immense databases intended to make highly reliable predictions of medical responses to medications and outcomes of care. Such massive data systems will create healthcare decision-making that is far more advanced than even a group of internists standing around a patient's bedside.

- **Outsourcing.** Development of many products available electronically, including education and medical care, are from outsourced systems. Some predict that statisticians in India will analyze large databases for firms and healthcare systems in Europe to drive best-fit services. Workers in many parts of the world will input data into large systems to fuel these engines. Global systems will be connected seamlessly to enhance all products.

■ **Technology.** New drugs and devices will save and extend lives. They will be delivered by improved communications and technology, and no place on the planet will be logistically isolated. For example, drones are able to deliver vaccines to remote villages where an Ebola virus outbreak has occurred. In addition, the elderly will provide a growing market for medication and equipment to overcome or manage their disabilities. Understanding senescence may extend lives, creating more demand for healthcare services and technology.

The ways in which these societal changes will benefit healthcare delivery systems is not fully understood. However, individual patient care is certain to change as a result of these transformative systems and the globalization of healthcare. For example, giant linked database systems, such as those of Kaiser Permanente and Optum, will help to determine on-the-spot optimal treatment for an individual encounter based on such patient factors as age, gender, comorbidities, and genotype. These complex systems will permit customization based on the expectations and experiences of similar cohorts in an effort to identify the required treatment and dose for optimal benefit. More likely than not, the experiences will be globally merged to be as refined as possible and as predictable as possible.

THE FUTURE OF HEALTHCARE

Many experts believe that innovation in every aspect of patient care will be nothing less than astonishing as the century unfolds. The accelerating pace of technology will bring together healthcare providers who have the ability to adapt to change quickly and adroitly. Futurists have identified some of the technological advances that will likely shape and inform the next generation. They range from fundamental advances in computing and administration, research, nursing, and patient care delivery to minimally invasive surgery, biomolecular therapies, bionics, and beyond. Other advances in technology will emerge in the next decade that existed only in the realm of science fiction.

The Pew Health Professions Commission predicted that a number of forces will interact to produce a US healthcare system that will be different from the one to which we are accustomed. The obvious changes in healthcare will be:

■ More managed care with better integration of services and financing
■ More accountability to those who purchase and use healthcare services
■ More awareness of and responsiveness to the needs of enrolled populations
■ An ability to use fewer resources more effectively
■ More innovation and diversity in providing healthcare
■ Less focus on treatment and more concern about education, prevention, and care management
■ Orientation to improving the health of the entire population
■ Reliance on outcomes data and evidence

Other changes that will shape how healthcare is delivered—and with it, the fate of the PA—will take place in the next decade. Some of these anticipated changes are already underway.

Epidemics

Obesity, osteoporosis, diabetes, heart disease, dyslipidemia, arthritis, and dementia are some of the diseases associated with an aging population. These conditions will be contained and even put into remission due in part to early recognition and early treatment, contributing to the longevity of populations. Viral epidemics such as poliomyelitis, Ebola, Marburg, Lassa, Zika, Crimean-Congo hemorrhagic fever, human immunodeficiency virus, hepatitis C, and others will be eradicated (or, in theory, can be eradicated if people are willing to be immunized). Guinea worm will join polio and smallpox as diseases of the past.

Imaging

The ability to image the body's metabolism in real time will drive new pharmaceuticals and early aggressive treatments to augment disorders associated with an aging population.

Human BRAIN (Brain Research through Advancing Innovative Neurotechnologies) Initiative

The human BRAIN project is a $3 billion investment by the National Institutes of Health, partnered with many other US agencies, to better understand neurocognition, physiology, and brain disease. Inaugurated in 2013, the program involves thousands of scientists, more than a hundred institutions, 24 countries, and a dozen research areas. Its goal is to fill major gaps in the current knowledge of the brain. The initiative provides unprecedented opportunities for exploring exactly how the brain enables the human body to record, process, utilize, store, and retrieve vast quantities of information, all at the speed of thought.

Neuroanatomy Repair

The neural processes, long an enigma to researchers, are now being repaired, enhanced, and modified. Cell division and stimulation allows for replacement of neurons and growth of more complicated structures. Already, a mouse has survived a head transplant. Such advances will expand the horizons for neuroanatomy repair in humans.

Robots

Surgeons are now using robotic instruments and wireless technology as tools to improve surgical outcomes. New technology using robots has allowed surgeons to feel and visualize areas of surgery more fully while performing delicate procedures using high microscopic fields and micromanipulators of instruments. In 2013, more than 12,000 robotic operations were performed with excellent outcomes.

Nutraceuticals

The range of food and supplements to enhance wellness and prevent disease is increasing. Vitamin D, more of a hormone than a vitamin, is reemerging as an important food supplement because of the long periods in which people remain indoors and attempts to avoid excessive solar radiation. Enriched foods are being engineered to improve the ability to obtain the minerals and vitamins needed for aging organs, such as bones, that are needed for long lives. Adding vitamin A to rice has stemmed the developed of ocular diseases in some countries.

Interventional Radiology

The imaging of tiny vessels in healthy, injured, and diseased organs allows new surgical techniques to interrupt the growth of tumors and repair damaged tissue. Using ultrafine lines of polyethelene and other materials, the interventionist can coil these in remote organs to choke off blood supplies to the neoplasm.

No-External-Wound Surgery

Natural orifice transluminal endoscopic surgery (NOTES) involves inserting a fiberoptic scope through a natural body opening (such as the mouth, rectum, urethra, or vagina) rather than via an external incision. The most frequently used technique involves inserting the endoscope through the mouth and then through the stomach wall to access the abdomen and remove and repair organs. This approach allows surgeons to remove a diseased gallbladder, appendix, or kidney without an external scar.

ARTIFICIAL ORGANS AND PROSTHETICS

The development of eyes, ears, limbs that can sense touch, kidneys, livers, hearts, pancreases, and other organs are nearing perfection.

Microelectrodes, the size of a human hair, implanted into a human brain allows robotic/prosthetic arms and legs to move with only casual thinking. The cost of such technology will be high initially but will plummet as the manufacture of parts is outsourced and economy of scale produces efficiency.

Xenographs

New animals created through the process of cross-species gene transfer are called *xenographs*, and the transplanting of organs across species is called *xenotransplantation*. Genetically engineered animals are being developed as living factories for the production of pharmaceuticals and as sources of organs for transplantation into humans.

Genetics and Genomics

The understanding of genetics, epigenetics, and proteomics has produced unparalleled growth in new biologically engineered drugs for management of rare conditions. Diseases such as rheumatoid arthritis and lymphoma can now be controlled with genetically engineered proteins not previously known to nature.

Humans differ from each other by less than 0.1% genetically. The phenotype and genotype of individuals will merge, and single nucleotide pairs that make up the differences between individuals will be known. This task can be accomplished using genome-wide association studies (GWAS) of hundreds of thousands of people to find rare genes of interest. The HapMap Research Initiative will accelerate treatment to be tailored to the individual, not to the response of populations.

Vaccines

More than 25 vaccines are currently approved for human use, with more on the way (Box 13–1). One vaccine prevents cervical, oropharynx, and anal neoplasm from human papillomavirus, another from hepatitis B; both are stunning advancements in the war on cancer. Other vaccines in development include those for malaria, tuberculosis, HIV,

BOX 13-1
Vaccines Available (or in Development) for Various Diseases

Avian influenza
Anthrax
Cholera
Dengue
Diphtheria
Ebola
Encephalitis, viral
Hepatitis A
Hepatitis B
Hepatitis E
Haemophilus influenzae type b (Hib)
HIV/AIDS
Human papillomavirus (HPV)
Influenza (seasonal)
Japanese encephalitis
Malaria
Measles
Meningococcal meningitis
Mumps
Pandemic influenza
Pertussis
Pneumococcal disease
Poliomyelitis
Rabies
Rotavirus
Rubella
Smallpox
Tetanus
Tick-borne encephalitis
Tuberculosis
Typhoid
Varicella
Yellow fever
Zika
Zoster (Shingles)

rheumatoid arthritis, Chagas disease, Ebola, and lymphoma.

Rural Healthcare Advances

High-technology monitoring tools will continue to expand expertise to patients in rural intensive care units (ICUs), allowing patients to be under the electronic gaze of specialists at bigger, distant facilities. This process involves a bundle of sensors and software, thus creating an electronic ICU. Preliminary testing in more than 100 hospitals has demonstrated that this technology is enabling some facilities to cut length of stay and probably save lives.

Healthcare Finance

Forecasting the changing picture of healthcare financing necessitates understanding policy changes at federal and state/provincial levels as well as movements in the employer and consumer markets. It also requires tracking long-term shifts in demographics and technology. Changes have been underway for some time, and government priorities tend to expand medical coverage for more Americans. The healthcare reform that is developing from the Affordable Care Act of 2010 requires an adjustable workforce component. These policy changes increase demand on a healthcare system that is struggling with labor costs. PAs offer an opportunity to provide this care at less expensive salaries. The substitutability of PAs for traditional physician services means they are likely to be used in more ways to help fill the gaps in the demand for healthcare access.

Fee-for-service and cost-based reimbursements have been largely replaced with per diems, case rates, and percentage-of-billed charges. New, life-saving technologies and treatments have entered the market, adding to the cost of staffing and equipment. Many stand-alone hospitals have become horizontally integrated systems. Small, autonomous physician practices have, in some markets, given way to large group practices with prescribed treatment protocols. Decades-old challenges continue, including high costs, medical errors, and the complex issue of insurance coverage.

The New Healthcare Consumer

Telecommunications via the Internet is only one example of how the new consumer has fundamentally changed many industries—and healthcare is included. Newly empowered patients (and their children) are demanding more accountability of their healthcare dollar. However, in the United States, this demand is not well balanced because of the tiered health insurance system. Those with good paying jobs have excellent healthcare coverage compared with those without the benefit of a generous employer. The heavy users of healthcare services are, on average, older, poorer, and less knowledgeable about health than the mainstream baby boomers. As a result, the disenfranchised have less access because those with coverage receive preferential treatment. So it is unclear exactly who the new healthcare consumer will be and how quickly the healthcare marketplace will change. Increasingly, those who staff healthcare systems are turning to PAs as a solution to meeting the demands of shifting healthcare consumers.

Healthcare Delivery Systems

For many consumers and physicians, managed care was not the panacea that was predicted. New organizations and relationships in healthcare delivery systems will continue to be built. At the core of each new experiment will be healthcare providers. Increasingly, health systems realize that diversity of the workforce means not only gender and ethnic diversity but also various types of providers, such as PAs, NPs, midwives, and others. Generally, people want and demand choices, and this transcends to providers such as such as PAs, NPs, and certified nurse-midwives.

Sociodemographic Trends and Health Status

There is a growing realization that medical care alone does not equal a positive health status, and new demands for healthcare are emerging. For example, empowered consumers are demanding new types of health services, such as "complementary and alternative" medicine. On top of this demand will emerge different philosophies about health spending and different ideas as to what contributes to health outcomes. Technological developments in electronic information and communication (including the Internet) and new modalities (such as telemedicine) will require a new array of appropriately trained individuals to not only institute new processes and procedures but also to evaluate the outcomes of these advances on patient access to and the quality of care.

THE FUTURE FOR PHYSICIAN ASSISTANTS

What does the future hold for PAs? How blue are the skies for the next generation of PAs? Is this a profession that will continue to attract young, bright, and capable people? Although these questions are usually answered in the affirmative, the evidence to support a prediction of a rosy scenario is a mixture of probabilities based on current trends and conjecture. The most solid evidence is that the PA profession is growing in its acceptance and incorporation into the health systems of the world, and its demographics are changing.

Between 1990 and 2012 in the United States, the number of physicians increased by 50%, while the entire healthcare labor force doubled and the number of NPs and PAs grew fivefold. The American PA profession is predicted to see a growth in annual graduations from 7,500 in 2015 to 12,000 in 2025, just based on the number of institutions that have applied for PA program accreditation. As of 2016, the ratio of clinically active American PA/NPs to clinically active physicians is 1:3. Further expansion in the participation of PAs and NPs is embedded in the long-term projections that physician supply will remain inadequate for the changing demographics in many countries. Similar to the United States, Europe is expected to see a larger presence of PAs by 2025.

Supply and Demand

Economic modeling—drawing from an understanding of scarcity of resources relative to human behavior—suggests that, if supply exceeds demand, then price goes down. Conversely, if demand exceeds supply, price increases. The following is an examination of these two fundamental principles as they apply to the future of PAs.

Supply Side

As of 2016, there were 218 accredited PA programs in the United States and approximately 40 or more in development. Outside of the United States, there are at least 25 PA programs in operation and more than 30 in some stage of planning. These programs have produced an increasing supply of PAs that is projected to continue (Figure 13–2). By the end of 2016, more than 7,500 new PAs entered the US workforce and another 400 PAs entered the workforce in other parts of the world; approximately three-quarters of these new graduates are women. Since the new century, the PA workforce in the aggregate has been largely composed of women and likely to stay that way in the near future.

FIGURE 13-2
Supply Projections of US PAs: 2010 to 2025

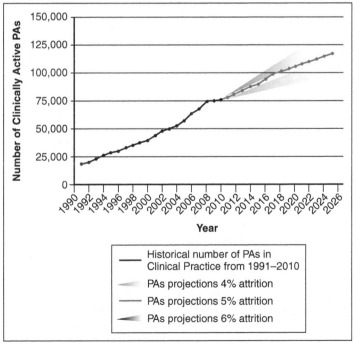

Proportionally fewer men are applying to PA schools, and the men in the workforce are at least 5 years older than their female counterparts.

A swelling of the ranks is expected until at least 2025, when the number of US PA programs in the pipeline may reach their maximum output. By 2025, there will be an estimated 150,000 clinically active PAs in the US workforce, with an estimated 12,000 US PA graduates per year and 2,000 graduates per year outside of the United States. These numbers take into account retirements of male and female PAs, who are being replaced by more young women than men. The historical 3% annual annulment of the US PA cadre is not likely to change anytime soon (Figure 13–3). By 2025, the ratio of PAs and NPs to physicians is expected to reach 1:2.

Shifts in gender from historical ratios to new ones may create different work habits. In the United States, doctors' workweeks are down from 55 hours in 1990 to 50 hours in 2003 and predicted to be 45 by 2020 (Table 13–2). In other countries, the workweek is shorter than 40 hours

and is not likely to increase. The 45-hour workweek for US PAs has remained fairly steady since 1995. Annual leave varies but for most is 5 to 6 weeks. In the federal system, the annual leave is 4 weeks, with 12 holidays. Maternity leave for doctors is 6 to 12 weeks in the United States but is typically more in resource-rich countries (Figure 13–4).

Other influences are at work to expand the supply of PAs. For example, the Council on Graduate Medical Education (COGME) and the Advisory Group on Physician Assistants and the Workforce (AGPAW) developed a list of recommendations addressing PA education, PA practice characteristics, practice obstacles, and current and anticipated demand. AGPAW called for the following actions:

- Increasing federal support for PA educational programs to expand the supply of PA graduates
- Increasing National Health Service Corps scholarships and loan repayment programs that support PA students

FIGURE 13-3
Average Career Duration of US PAs

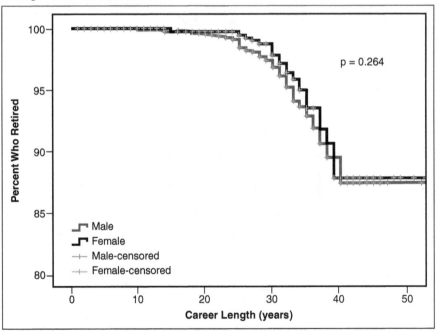

Source: Coombs, J. M., Hooker, R. S., & Brunisholz, K. D. (2013). What do we know about retired physician assistants? A preliminary study. Journal of the American Academy of Physician Assistants, 26(3), 44–48.

TABLE 13-2
Work Hours per Specialty

Specialty	Lifestyle	Average Income, $ in Thousands	Average Work Hours per Week	Years of Graduate Medical Education Required
Anesthesiology	Controllable	225	61.0	4
Dermatology	Controllable	221	45.5	4
Emergency medicine	Controllable	183	45.0	4
Family practice	Uncontrollable	132	52.5	3
Internal medicine	Uncontrollable	158	57.0	3
Neurology	Controllable	172	55.5	4
Obstetrics and gynecology	Uncontrollable	224	61.0	4
Ophthalmology	Controllable	225	47.0	4
Orthopedic surgery	Uncontrollable	323	58.0	5
Otolaryngology	Controllable	242	53.5	5
Pathology	Controllable	202	45.5	4
Pediatrics	Uncontrollable	138	54.0	3
Psychiatry	Controllable	134	48.0	4
Radiology (diagnostic)	Controllable	263	58.0	4
Surgery (general)	Uncontrollable	238	60.0	5
Urology	Uncontrollable	245	60.5	5
Average for the above specialties	Not applicable	208	53.9	4

Data from: Dorsey, E. R., Jarjoura, D., & Rutecki, G. W. (2003). Influence of controllable lifestyle on recent trends in specialty choice by US medical students. *Journal of the American Medical Association, 290*(9), 1173–1178.

FIGURE 13-4
Pregnant Doctor

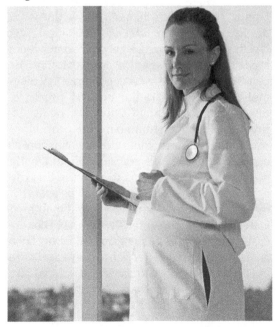

- Developing federal policy to support and encourage increased representation from racial and ethnic minorities in the PA profession (Figure 13–5)
- Including PAs in national and state health workforce planning activities
- Encouraging states to provide a more uniform regulatory climate for PAs

Demand Side

The demand side of the equation is more difficult to predict and relies on data from other sectors of the healthcare field. However, the expansion of PA use will likely continue. The demand for healthcare services is expected to exceed supply through 2025, even with a supply of 150,000 clinically active PAs. In fact, the Bureau of Labor Statistics' career outlook projections for healthcare professionals indicate increased demand specifically for PA services through at least 2024 (Quella et al., 2015). State survey data of practicing PAs suggest a

FIGURE 13-5
Occupational Health Physician Assistant

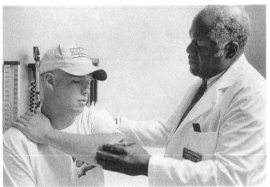

Courtesy of American Academy of Physician Assistants

similar trend. The wild card is the role US healthcare reform will play in the demand for PA services.

Doctor-centered care continues to be a labor-intensive business. The fact that doctor-centered care is expensive alone bodes well for the demand for the PA profession in the short run. Managers increasingly recognize the value of PAs as a skilled but mobile labor force, able to shift from one area of demand to another. Demand will continue for a while; a slow but steady rise in programs will continue and, by 2025, the supply of PAs is expected to double what it was in 2010. Many welcome this expansion, but the greatest threat to the PA profession is the fickle marketplace. As salaries increase, the cost-effectiveness of PAs will diminish under this invisible hand—pricing oneself out of the market. If PA wages continues to increase then cost, value, and productivity differentials will influence who is hired. Eventually, there may be more PAs than opportunities, and relationships with physicians may suffer. The marginal cost of the PA is what it costs to have an extra PA (salary and benefits). The marginal value of an additional PA is the savings from not having to pay salary and benefits for an additional physician.

In the short run, hospitals will increasingly employ PAs and NPs, as more intensive services demand that a permanent, salaried house staff be present 24 hours per day. The number of acute care beds in the United States is near one million, but the number of doctors and nurses to tend to those bed patients is not adequate to meet patient needs. Teams of hospitalists (physicians, PAs, and NPs) will manage inpatient populations that require highly skilled personnel because only the very ill will be hospitalized for any significant period. In many teaching institutions, residency program directors have already incorporated PAs (as well as NPs) in resident-substitute roles, in part because of mandated cutbacks in hours worked by residents. There is every reason to believe that this trend will continue.

Significant increases in the role of PA and NP use in managed medicine, such as health maintenance organizations (HMOs), will be augmented by the degree to which physicians can be persuaded to hire them. Ambulatory care, where most PAs work, will continue to employ more PAs as physicians become more familiar with PA skills and services and the demand for PAs increases. In the nonprimary care arena, advances in technology will create more and more need for skilled providers such as PAs to aid in the application of the technology. This trend is already occurring in areas such as emergency medicine, dermatology, ophthalmology, neurology, nephrology, cardiothoracic surgery, and many other medical and surgical subspecialties.

Other emerging new roles for PAs that will help to sustain their demand are wellness and disease prevention; clinical, biological, and health services research; legal professions; genetics; toxicology; and medical administration. Expanded roles for PAs exist in geriatrics, oncology, molecular biology, radiology, and protracted disease management. PAs may also be used to provide effective, humane, and economical care to the millions of individuals with chronic disease. PAs and NPs are probably in a better position than physicians to provide this care because patients will increasingly be absorbed by managed care organizations, and their medical care will require intensive efforts to contain costs through innovative forms of labor. There is also unrealized potential for PAs in the delivery of clinical preventive services. It has long been hypothesized that PAs could become providers that deliver not only medical care services (physician-substitutive) but also clinical preventive services (physician complementary) (Ritsema et al., 2014).

Another phenomenon will be the demand for PAs to work globally. The ability to work in another country and experience the culture and diversity of another healthcare system, as well as an adequate salary, will make employment in different countries more attractive—and not just in English-speaking countries. Because the shape of the global healthcare workforce is so uncertain, the fundamental question of how many PAs will be enough remains unanswered.

A proposed gloomier side of the demand curve is that the number of PAs in the workforce could result in too many clinicians. For example, PAs are in direct competition with NPs and, to a lesser extent, with nurse-midwives. The majority of NPs are in primary care, and the number of clinically active NPs is more than the number of PAs. Such NP activity may prevent a growing presence in the primary care arena for PAs. Physician workforce experts believe that the continuing shortage of physicians will be real and that the nation will require the contributions of both PAs and NPs to meet the demand for medical care services (Sargen et al., 2013).

One of the nagging issues facing the profession is the appropriate number of PAs to train. How many PAs should there be in the United States? When considering this issue, one must also ask: How many primary care physicians should be available to the population and in what ratio? Should PAs, NPs, and midwives be considered part of the equation? Unlike some countries that have developed prescribed physicians/population ratios (e.g., Canada, England, Australia, and The Netherlands), the United States has largely allowed the markets to dictate how many physicians there should be. The governor of physician supply is the number of medical and osteopathic schools and their ability to turn out graduates if international medical school graduates are to be discounted. In 2015, the number of US medical/osteopathic school graduates was approximately 19,000 annually (and the number of US PA graduates 7,500). Both are predicted to grow. However, constraints are in the making. In 2015, the US residency match was the largest on record, with more than 41,000 applicants vying for approximately 30,000 residency positions in 4,756 programs.

There are various responses to the question of how many providers is enough. Some believe there is a surplus of physicians and that PAs and NPs are redundant. This argument is based on counting physician heads and comparing ratios of physicians to populations and comparing these numbers with those of other countries (the head count of licensed physicians in 2015 is 950,000, but the actual number of clinically active physicians is something less than 720,000). Others believe there are not enough primary care physicians and that many communities go underserved in terms of access to primary care services. Still others believe The Bureau of Health Professions should mandate primary care quotas in residencies and reduce specialized residencies. Finally, some believe that it is unrealistic to expect that physicians in any appreciable numbers will by themselves reverse the trend of professional specialization. If this notion holds true, doctors will continue to avoid primary care practices. Moreover, it remains doubtful that established specialist physicians will convert to generalist roles in any appreciable numbers. But as previously observed, PAs appear to be emulating this trend of greater specialization, creating doubt with regard to the future role for PAs in primary care.

The continuing decline in interest in primary care and generalist practice careers among young physicians has not yet been reversed, and it will take decades to do so in a way that would affect service delivery—even if the number of medical graduates choosing primary care significantly increases before adjustments in graduate medical education outcomes. This prospect raises the question of which type of healthcare personnel will provide primary care now and in the future. As physicians become increasingly specialized, moving further away from primary care, PAs (and NPs) are likely to assume a greater profile in delivering primary care services. This is particularly true in settings such as HMOs, other types of managed care systems, and organized healthcare systems, such as Veterans Affairs (VA) hospitals, state and federal correctional systems, and the military.

One veteran workforce observer believes that physicians are no longer in the primary care business and that PAs and NPs, working with physician "managers," may be the best providers to meet future primary care needs. In 1992, Dr. Meikle was a lone voice in recommending increasing PA educational output and using PAs in primary care roles (Meikle, 1992). As a keen health workforce observer, many believe Meikle was right. Some free market economists advocate that as many PAs should be graduated as the market will bear because, in the end, competition produces a public good in distributing products and driving down costs.

In 2012, 46.1 primary care physicians and 65.5 specialists were available per 100,000 populations. Of this number, 53% of primary care physicians employed a PA or NP. Again, looking just at the population of patients seen by PAs and NPs, approximately one-third of all patients are younger than 18 years, suggesting the physician is delegating a great deal of healthcare to these providers (Hing & Hsiao, 2014).

In the future, the demand for PAs and other health professionals is likely to be determined by political, economic, and legal factors that affect the evolution of their roles in relation to those of physicians. As the US healthcare system changes from one encompassing a disease-oriented and economically open-ended structure to one stressing a more preventive, patient-centered, and cost-conscious direction, PAs or NPs will assume a higher profile than in the past (Spetz, 2016).

The further evolution of the professional roles of PAs and NPs in US healthcare will be determined by changes in the division of medical labor, higher public expectations in regard to physician response to societal healthcare problems, population-based needs, patient satisfaction, and outcome evidence. One forecast is that the interdisciplinary team approach to healthcare may become the standard while Americans' demand for accountability from their health professionals increases. This new accountability will require adjustments in the educational preparation of medical and healthcare providers.

Approaches will need to extend the biomedical model to encompass the population-based and behavioral sciences.

Decline in Physician Influence

In 1975, Rick Carlson wrote a book titled *The End of Medicine*. At the time, the author (a lawyer) and his thesis were regarded as being on the radical fringe of healthcare policy. In this futuristic polemic, he asserted that eventually the medical profession, partly because of its arrogant stance of self-regulation, the rise of consumerism and preventive care, and the corporatization of healthcare delivery, would become obsolete. Although actual physician obsolescence is unlikely, it is clear in today's health system that the medical profession is not what it used to be in terms of power and prestige. Medicine's power and prestige reached its zenith in the 1960s, the so-called Golden Age of Medicine, and has since declined substantially. Over the past decade in particular, physician influence over the health system has eroded to the degree that the number of applicants to medical schools is off once-peak levels. State medical boards are now led by a wide assortment of professionals, attorneys, physicians, and consumers. In the midst of this transformative change, NPs are asserting their roles as independent providers of primary care services. PA autonomy is likely to follow.

A multitude of reasons explain the decline in physician influence over the health system but, without question, an important consequence has been the steady growth over the past quarter century in the numbers and clinical activities of PAs and NPs. Medical sociologists who assert a decline in the power and prestige of the medical profession in the United States refer to this trend as "deprofessionalization" (Hafferty & McKinley, 1993). McKinley in particular is among the more outspoken of the deprofessionalization theorists and observes that the growing corporatization and bureaucratization of medicine has resulted in effectively eliminating physician self-employment and reduced physician autonomy. As the medical workplace becomes more and more bureaucratized, physicians are increasingly subject to the rules and systems of hierarchical structures that are not of their own making. Physicians are no longer professionally dominant because traditional elements of classic professionalism have been lost. Prerogatives such as control over training content, work autonomy, and the means and remuneration of labor have eroded. Today, the federal government, insurance companies, and consumer groups now hold considerable sway over medical training and practice and the methods by which physicians are paid for their work.

Another important factor in the decline of medicine as a profession is that physicians no longer have a monopoly over medical knowledge. Health consumers and a wide variety of other providers now approach or even exceed physician knowledge in specific areas. The days of the all-knowing, paternalistic physician dispensing medical directives to a subservient patient are gone. As they have become more sophisticated, patients as consumers now view medical care much as they view other services and are demanding more control, choice, and convenience (Figure 13–6).

Delivering medical services in a manner convenient to the patient is a relatively new concept to many physicians. Understandably, accustomed as they are to dealing with life and death situations, physicians in the past have not placed a high priority on customer service

FIGURE 13-6
Physician Assistant and Patient

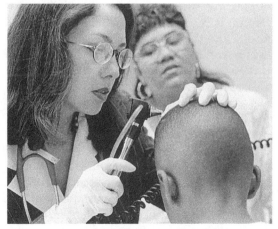

Courtesy of American Academy of Physician Assistants

and convenience considerations. Yet such adjustments may be required in the future healthcare delivery market. The nature of physician roles in medical work is also changing. It is now clear that health providers such as NPs and PAs can deliver a wide range of medical services as effectively and safely as physicians and at a lower cost. PAs and NPs may be equally knowledgeable in certain clinical disciplines (e.g., primary care) and have been shown to be as capable as physicians in performing technical procedures in a number of specialty areas, such as cardiac catheterization and colonoscopy.

Consumers and others have come to the realization that physicians may be overtrained for the tasks they perform most of the time. Advances in technology now permit great accuracy and precision in diagnosis, placing less emphasis on physician differential diagnostic and cognitive capabilities. Washington health pundit Daniel Greenberg once said that the system of medical education in the United States was akin to putting all bus drivers through astronaut training. The point is that it might not require 12 years of expensive and federally subsidized education to prepare the medical practitioner of the future, and perhaps this is particularly true in primary care. Physicians have reverted to a movement toward increasing specialization and appear to be abandoning primary care to other providers. In 2015, fewer US medical school seniors chose primary care residency positions than in the preceding years. Among internists, the hospitalist movement has become increasingly popular, driven in part by a desire by physicians to better control the circumstances of their work. It would be a mistake to believe that physicians as we know them are going to fade from the health delivery scene, yet it is clear that their roles are changing in the division of medical labor.

As economics and technology continue to drive medical care, portions of the work that once were exclusively in the domain of physicians will be passed on to others. Familiar examples of this trend are already evident with psychologists and psychiatric social workers working in place of psychiatrists and nurse-midwives working in place of obstetricians. It may very well be that, should such trends continue, NPs and PAs will take on an increasing share of the work of primary care. This occurrence could come about due to a combination of factors:

- Practice economics in the delivery system
- Aggressive tactics mounted by some NPs to wrest from physicians their dominance in primary care
- Physicians abrogating primary care and instead seeking inpatient and specialty roles

Possibly, such a scenario could result in physicians assuming a more medical managerial and care oversight role, with actual clinical care being provided primarily by PAs and NPs. If such a redistribution of medical work were to transpire, a key question would be to what degree would PAs be granted autonomy in their practice. As of 2016, NPs are able to practice under their own license in at almost half the states. This change came about not because physicians voluntarily granted such practice prerogatives but because nurses believe they are a stand-alone profession with the right of independence.

SELF-ACTUALIZATION

Responsibility for administering the profession belongs to the profession. When PAs emerged in the late 1960s, the laws governing the practice of medicine were amended to recognize the physician's ability to delegate tasks to supervised individuals. Most of these laws have been modified and expanded, but the power to regulate PAs has remained, with only a few exceptions, in the hands of the licensing boards, which are predominantly controlled by physicians. If PAs are to seek their own destiny, they must overcome these shortcomings in self-actualization and begin seeking avenues to educate their regulators.

However, if formal participation of PAs in the regulatory process is a worthy goal, it is not a panacea for problems that may exist between physician licensing boards and PAs. Once a PA becomes a board member or sits on a committee

that is set up to ensure the benefit of citizens, he or she assumes the role of protector of public health and safety. The responsibilities of that person are to the citizens of the state, not to the PA profession. Advocacy of professional concerns at the state level still rests with state PA associations, often aided by the national organization.

The ability of PAs to effectively identify, attract, and efficiently serve the vagaries of consumers will largely determine their professional future. Organization and financing services will be key variables in these efforts to increase the demand for PAs. Macroeconomic strategies include creative, aggressive, and effective marketing of the quality that PAs bring to society, as well as the recruitment of social scientists into education programs to undertake sorely needed research on the profession. Research must be done on the economic use of PAs and the expansion of PAs into specific client areas such as home health and genomics. These and other macroeconomic and microeconomic strategies are outlined in Table 13–3.

Another approach to self-actualization is to constantly update the knowledge base of what roles PAs play and how well they do them. Collecting demographic data is not enough; research on the healthcare workforce is constantly in demand and needs to be continuously updated. Policymakers want to see data, not opinions.

Taking Stock

After a long period during which medical leaders showed little interest in PA education, attention is now being paid to PA educational policy and the roles that PAs can play in the health workforce. A key issue is whether the PA profession should expand its output of graduates, as has been suggested by advocates of the expansion of health professions education. Medicine is counting on PAs to pick up a proportion of the slack in the workforce and the PA profession to raise the output of educational programs, similar to the circumstance underway in medical schools. In an attempt to determine the dimensions of current program expansion, the Physician Assistant Education Association (PAEA) has conducted surveys.

TABLE 13-3
Strategies for Increasing Demand for Physician Assistants

Macro (on the professional organizational level)	Micro (on the individual level)
Aggressive, creative marketing of the profession	Aggressive, creative individual marketing
Research on economic use	Creative self-employment or group employment
Creative organization and financing	Expansion of client areas and contact
Expansion of client areas and contact (scope of practice)	Use of advanced technologies
Use of advanced technologies	Inclusion in policymaking

But thus far, little has been done with the information obtained in response to calls for a greater supply of PA graduates and policy direction. Even more basic questions can be raised: Who determines PA educational policy? Is it the PA professional organizations or is it left to individual institutions? What is the role of the PAEA in shaping PA educational policy?

US history suggests that it is market forces in higher education, rather than a concerted effort by the professional organizations, that sets the course of PA education. This trend was certainly the case in the second phase of PA program expansion that occurred in the late 1990s, when the number of programs more than doubled. The PA professional organizations have tended to take a passive role by looking forward to tomorrow and refraining from taking any public positions on current program expansion. Over the years, the PAEA has traditionally shied away from taking official positions on workforce policy issues. In view of the recent challenges presented to PA education by prominent leaders in medicine, it seems that the time has come for a more assertive organizational approach. There are many reasons why the United States chooses to be a decentralized system of states' rights. However, in other countries, central planning is used to address medical workforce policy

issues that ultimately shape the direction for the profession. Perhaps a blend of decentralization and central planning might be in order.

Lessons From PA Models

As changes take place, there are lessons to be learned from other health systems that have installed assistants to physicians. Similarly, other systems can learn from the US model of PAs.

Lessons From Other Systems

In projecting the future of PAs in the US healthcare system, it is useful to consider the experiences of PAs in the medical systems of other countries. Practitioners similar to PAs have been used in a number of other nations. Examples include the *feldsher* in Russia and the Ukraine, the barefoot doctor in China, the assistant medical officer in parts of Africa, and a wide range of the variously named healthcare providers working primarily in developing countries throughout the world. As the concept of the PA expands globally, educational approaches have emerged that are different from the US system. How these compare with each other should be a prime focus of research.

The natural history and pertinent experiences of these practitioners have been examined, and compared with the American experience with nonphysician providers, it is clear that only a few parallels exist. Experience with PAs and their successful (or unsuccessful) integration into a country's healthcare delivery system are based primarily on how these providers fit into the medical, economic, and cultural systems of the nations that employ them. Rarely are experiences with these types of providers exportable to other countries. Each nation that has created and used PAs has fashioned them and their roles to meet specific needs and requirements in that country's systems. However, some overriding patterns do exist that are relevant in the assessment of the American PA.

Health practitioners are created by the existing cadre of medical providers in a country and emerge from specific perceived needs in healthcare delivery. In nearly all cases, these needs involve a shortage of fully trained physicians to provide adequate medical services to the population. This was in fact the fundamental rationale for the creation of PAs in the United States and appears to be the case in other countries.

Once health professionals enter the delivery system, evolving circumstances and changes in the system affect the roles and perceptions of these providers. As the supply of a country's physician population rises, and as experience with these providers accumulates, new perceptions of the roles that these providers can assume then develops. In some instances, there is no further need for these providers in the healthcare system. In others, the role of the new health professional changes and becomes more technically oriented. In still other systems, non-physician clinicians evolve into well-established members of a healthcare delivery team, participating with physicians in a wide variety of clinical functions. The broadest generalization that can be made is that PAs must adjust and adapt to changing forces within the health delivery system in which they work once they outlive the rationale of their initial creation. As previously discussed, this situation is what has occurred with PAs in the United States. Roles for PAs continue to expand and new employment niches appear regularly. The capability of PAs to adapt to various clinical roles has kept them on the forefront of medical workforce innovations and should continue to expand their utilization in the US system.

FUTURE ISSUES

No futurist is ever confident of his or her predictions. Making predictions is based on lessons learned; the sciences of history, economics, demographics, anthropology, sociology, and politics; and observations of changes based on technology and sociology. However, every prediction is subject to "wild cards," which are events and movements that are not expected that can produce unanticipated changes. The potential wild cards for PAs are PA licensure autonomy, doctoral degrees, and international medical graduates (IMGs). Each could change society's attitude toward PAs. The healthcare reform established by the Affordable Care Act, passed in 2010 and enacted in 2013, has already

created demand for the employment of PAs and NPs not experienced as early as 2008 (US Department of Health and Human Services, Health Resources and Services Administration, 2013).

Independence and Professional Recognition

Issues of whether PAs should seek practice independence arise from time to time—typically when there are issues about professional recognition. To some PAs, professional recognition will come only if they gain the legal right to full independence of practice, meaning they would be free to contract and negotiate for services similar to what a small number of NPs do in certain states. To some extent, this movement is already underway, as PAs find opportunities to be entrepreneurs and independent owners of healthcare systems.

Although the push for recognition comes from the PA profession, increased financial pressure on the healthcare industry is also an important substrate for change. A partial list of advantages and disadvantages of independent practice for PAs is listed in Table 13-4.

PAs, however, remain generally satisfied with their dependent practice stance. The matter has not emerged as a concern in any formal sessions of the American Academy of Physician Assistants (AAPA) or its House of Delegates. PAs have come to realize that it is an ideal circumstance to be able to assume great responsibility for patient care and medical decision-making within a dependent relationship with physicians. Physicians delegate many duties and functions to PAs, who appear to be satisfied with the balance of autonomy and responsibility that the PA role brings. The much-debated independent-dependent issue may represent an outdated paradigm, particularly for PAs who do not see being a dependent provider as an issue.

FUTURE RESEARCH

The research community continues to evaluate the effects of PA employment on quality, cost, access, and other aspects of healthcare delivery. Only by carefully documenting the capabilities

TABLE 13-4
Advantages and Disadvantages of Physician Assistant Independent Practice

Advantages	Disadvantages
■ The ability to seek employment and negotiate terms improves. ■ Supervising physician can help share the responsibility and fallout in malpractice cases. ■ PAs will have a greater say in standards of care and educational levels.	■ If physicians are not employers, jobs may not be as plentiful. ■ PAs may be seen as more vulnerable to plaintiff lawyers. ■ PAs will constantly have to improve standards of care, seek legislative changes, and improve educational levels on their own.
■ PAs can negotiate salary with more independence. ■ A PA can form a business, work for the business, and reap the rewards of one's own labor. ■ Independent reimbursement from insurance companies will improve return for work.	■ Physicians are increasingly opting for salaried work. ■ Businesses are increasingly regulated with compliance consuming large amounts of time and resources. ■ Many third-seeking reimbursement party payers may resist another group.

of PAs using acceptable research methodologies will policy analysts be able to measure the profession's ability to meet the needs of the medical marketplace. Staffing remains a function of physician attitudes, instead of administrative rationale. Not until the measured benefits and utility of PAs are reported will change take place. Radical changes in healthcare staffing are not happening (or, if they are, they are happening slowly) because the data are not available to move managers to act favorably to PA employment. Data proving that PAs can function safely and effectively in healthcare roles are slow in coming and rarely adequate for large structural changes.

Without doubt, there will be encroachments on the homeostasis of the PA in the financial, choice, and professional domains. The girders of physician support for PAs are linked to being less autonomous and more dependent, regardless of skill and outcome. Relative to PAs, economic factors will to a great extent determine future utilization patterns. Important questions remain for researchers as to how to best use PAs in various societies.

Formulating Research Questions

The essential nature of research is to create new knowledge and information about a subject that was relatively unknown. One of the ways the PA profession can effect change is to help formulate questions that will guide research in ways not only theoretically fruitful but also historically appropriate. As part of this process, the following research questions are offered:

■ **Economics:** Will the market forces remain sufficient to create a long-term demand for PAs? How can the profession document the efficacy, efficiency, and economy of PAs as primary care providers for patients?

■ **Global view:** How will the expansion of PAs globally stimulate interest in PAs?

■ **The next generation:** Should the profession try to recruit more trainees into the PA profession who are trained in economics, psychology, anthropology, and sociology who could stimulate areas of research?

■ **Organizational influences:** Should the AAPA contribute to funding research by supporting proactive, innovative studies that would enhance healthcare delivery?

■ **Leadership:** Should the AAPA help educate and nurture institutional leadership within organizations that have sufficient vision to recognize the pivotal role that PAs can play to more cost-effective healthcare delivery?

■ **History:** What should a time capsule on the profession contain?

■ **Adaptability:** How can PAs continue to demonstrate innovation, high quality, and technical sophistication in primary care medicine?

Some changes are underway that show promise. The PAEA has created a mechanism to stimulate and fund research. The PAEA Research Council is organized to use the proceedings of investments to fund small grants for research ideas that examine PA behavior and education.

SUMMARY

Growth and *opportunity* are catchwords for the PA profession as it moves along in time and space. Numerous changes are expected, along with stimulating challenges. The 21st century is an exciting time to be a PA, and it is difficult for a profession to be too concerned about the future when it is riding the wave crest of demand. Current focus is on the expansion of the profession to meet the demand of the changing healthcare environment that wants more PAs. For the first time, PAs are part of the health policy equation as planners estimate what the health workforce should be like in the years ahead.

An expanding and aging population means greater demand for services. Furthermore, an uninsured population that needs care tends to create demand for services that are unexpected. Excessive health costs, poor access for some citizens, and uneven quality of care bodes well for the PA profession because PAs can help meet this demand quickly.

However, increased penetration and the fickle nature of managed care, coupled with efforts to improve efficiency in delivery, may dampen physician salaries. If rising PA salaries come close to physician salaries, then the surge of new graduates may produce the supply side of the equation that catches up with the demand side sooner than expected. Like all waves, the crest will break, and supply will exceed demand. When this event will occur is difficult to predict.

The quality of PAs and medical care in developed countries has never been higher. If PAs want to remain in the great debate about what the medical workforce should look like, they must meet the challenge with the science that confirms they are viable players.

References

The following citations are key to supporting this chapter's content. You can find a complete list of citations for all chapters at www.fadavis.com/davisplus, keyword *Hooker*.

Hafferty, F. W., & McKinley, J. B. (Eds.). (1993). *The Changing Medical Profession.* New York: Oxford University Press.

Hing, E., & Hsiao, C. J. (2014). *State variability in supply of office-based primary care providers: United States, 2012* (National Center for Health Statistics Data Brief No. 151). Hyattsville, MD: National Center for Health Statistics.

Meikle, T. H. (1992). *An expanded role for the physician assistant.* Washington, DC: Association of Academic Health Centers.

Quella, A., Brock, D., & Hooker, R. S. (2015). Physician assistant wages and employment: 2000–2025. *Journal of the American Academy of Physician Assistants, 28*(6), 56–63.

Ritsema, T. S., Bingenheimer, J. B., Scholting, P., & Cawley, J. F. (2014). Differences in the delivery of health education to patients with chronic disease by provider type, 2005–2009. *Preventing Chronic Disease, 11,* E33.

Sargen, M., Hooker, R. S., & Cooper, R. A. (2011). Gaps in the supply of physicians, advance practice nurses, and physician assistants. *Journal of the American College of Surgeons, 212*(6), 991–999.

Spetz, J., Cawley, J.F., Schommer, J. (2016). Transformation of the nonphysician health professions. In: *The Healthcare Professional Workforce: New Directions in Theory and Practice.* Hoff, T., Sutcliffe, K., Young, G. (Eds). New York: Oxford Press.

US Department of Health and Human Services, Health Resources and Services Administration, National Center for Health Workforce Analysis. (2013). *Projecting the supply and demand for primary care practitioners through 2020.* Rockville, MD: US Department of Health and Human Services.

BIBLIOGRAPHY

AANP. (2014). *2012 NP Sample Survey (NPSS)*. Austin, TX: American Association of Nurse Practitioners.

AANP. (2015). *2013-14 National NP Practice Site Census*. Austin, TX: American Association of Nurse Practitioners.

Agarwal, A., Zhang, W., Kuo, Y., & Sharma, G. (2016). Process and outcome measures among COPD patients with a hospitalization cared for by an advance practice provider or primary care physician. *PLoS ONE, 11*(2), e0148522.

Agency for Healthcare Research and Quality (AHRQ). (2015). *2013 Annual hospital-acquired condition rate and estimates of cost savings and deaths averted from 2010 to 2013* (AHRQ Publication No. 16-0006-EF). Rockville, MD: AHRQ. Retrieved from: http://www.ahrq.gov/professionals/quality-patient-safety/pfp/index.html

Albert, N. M., Fonarow, G. C., Yancy, C. W., Curtis, A. B., Stough, W. G., Gheorghiade, M., et al. (2010). Outpatient cardiology practices with advanced practice nurses and physician assistants provide similar delivery of recommended therapies (findings from IMPROVE HF). *American Journal of Cardiology, 105*(12), 1773–1779.

Alliance for Aging Research. (2006). *Ageism: How healthcare fails the elderly*. Washington, DC: Author.

American Academy of Physician Assistants. (2006b). *Physician assistants: State laws and regulations* (10th ed.). Alexandria, VA: Author.

American Academy of Physician Assistants (AAPA). (2008). *2008 AAPA physician assistant census report*. Alexandria, VA: Author.

American Academy of Physician Assistants (AAPA). (2013). *2012 AAPA physician assistant census report*. Alexandria, VA: AAPA.

American Academy of Physician Assistants (AAPA). (2014). *2013 AAPA Physician Assistant Census Report*. Alexandria, VA: Author.

American Academy of PAs. (2016). *2016 AAPA salary report*. Alexandria, VA: Author.

American Academy of Physician Assistants (AAPA). (2016). *AAPA model state legislation for PAs*. Retrieved from https://www.aapa.org/WorkArea/DownloadAsset.aspx?id=548

American Hospital Association. (2014). *Fast facts on US hospitals*. Retrieved from http://www.aha.org/research/rc/stat-studies/101207fastfacts.pdf

American Medical Association. (2001). *Guidelines for physician/physician assistant practice*. Chicago, IL: Policy Compendium.

Arnopolin, S. L., & Smithline, H. A. (2000). Patient care by physician assistants and by physicians in an emergency department. *Journal of the American Academy of Physician Assistants, 13*(12), 39–40, 49–50, 53–54, 81.

Asprey, D., Dehn, R., & Kreiter, C. (2004). The impact of age and gender on the Physician Assistant National Certifying Examination Scores and pass rates. *Journal of Physician Assistant Education, 15*(1), 38–41.

Association of American Medical Colleges. (2012). Estimating the number and characteristics of hospitalist physicians in the United States and their possible workforce implications. *AAMC Analysis in Brief, 12*(3). Retrieved from https://www.aamc.org/download/300620/data/aibvol12_no3-hospitalist.pdf

Baker, T. (2005). *The medical malpractice myth*. Chicago, IL: The University of Chicago Press.

Baldwin, K. A., Sisk, R. J., Watts, P., McCubbin, J., Brockschmidt, B., & Marion, L. N. (1998). Acceptance of nurse practitioners and physician assistants in meeting the perceived needs of rural communities. *Public Health Nurse, 15*(6), 389–397.

Ballenger, M. D., & Estes, E. H., Jr. (1971). Licensure or responsible delegation? *New England Journal of Medicine, 284*, 330–332.

Banja, J. (2005). *Medical errors and medical narcissism*. Boston, MA: Jones & Bartlett.

Bergeron, J., Neuman, K., & Kinsey, J. (1999). Do advanced practice nurses and physician assistants benefit small rural hospitals? *Journal of Rural Health, 15*(2), 219–232.

BLS [Bureau of Labor Statistics]. *Occupational employment statistics*. Retrieved from http://www.bls.gov/oes/tables.htm. BLS code: 29-1071 Physician Assistants; BLS code: 29-1171 Nurse Practitioner

Bosch, M., Faber, M. J., Cruijsberg, J., Voerman, G. E., Leatherman, S., Grol, R. P.,... Wensing, M. (2009). Review article: Effectiveness of patient care teams and the role of clinical expertise and coordination. *Medical Care Research and Review, 66*(Suppl. 6), 5S–35S.

Brock, D. M., Nicholson, J. G., & Hooker, R. S. (2016). Physician assistant and nurse practitioner malpractice trends. *Medical Care Research and Review*, 1077558716659022.

Bunn, W. B., III, Holloway, A. M., & Johnson, C. E. (2004). Occupational medicine: The use of physician assistants and the changing role of the occupational and environmental medicine provider. *Occupational Medicine, 54*, 3145–3146.

Bureau of Health Manpower Education. (1971). *Selected training programs for physician support personnel.* Washington, DC: National Institutes of Health, Department of Health, Education and Welfare.

Caprio, T. V. (2006). Physician practice in the nursing home: Collaboration with nurse practitioners and physician assistants. *Annals of Long Term Care, 14*(3), 17–24.

Carpenter, D. L., Gregg, S. R., Owens, D. S., Buchman, T. G., & Coopersmith, C. M. (2012). Patient-care time allocation by nurse practitioners and physician assistants in the intensive care unit. *Critical Care, 16*(1), R27.

Carter, R. (2001). From the military corpsman ranks. *Perspective on Physician Assistant Education, 12*, 130–132.

Carter, R., & Thompson, A. (2008). People v Whittaker: The trial and its aftermath in California. *The Journal of Physician Assistant Education, 19*(2), 44–51.

Carzoli, R. P., Martinez-Cruz, M., Cuevas, L. L., Murphy, S., & Chiu, T. (1994). Comparison of neonatal nurse practitioners, physician assistants, and residents in the neonatal intensive care unit. *Archives of Pediatrics & Adolescent Medicine, 148*(12), 1271–1276.

Cawley, J. F. (2008). Physician assistants and Title VII support. *Academic Medicine, 83*(11), 1049–1056.

Cawley, J. F. (2013). A conversation with E. Harvey Estes, Jr., M.D. *Journal of Physician Assistant Education, 24*(2), 22–24.

Cawley, J. F., Cawthon, E., & Hooker, R. S. (2012). Origins of the physician assistant movement in the United States. *Journal of the American Academy of Physician Assistants, 25*, 1–7.

Cawley, J. F., & Jones, P. E. (2013). Institutional sponsorship, student debt, and specialty choice in physician assistant education. *Journal of Physician Assistant Education, 24*(4), 4–8.

Cawley, J. F., Rohrs, R., & Hooker, R. S. (1998). Physician assistants and malpractice risk: Findings from the National Practitioner Data Bank. *Federal Bulletin, 85*(4), 242–247.

Chalupa R., & Hooker R. S. (2016). Physician assistants in orthopaedic surgery: Education, role, distribution, compensation. *Journal of the American Academy of Physician Assistants, 29*(5), 1–7

Cherry, D. K., Woodwell, D. A., & Rechtsteiner, E. A. (2007). National Ambulatory Medical Care Survey (NHAMCS): 2005 summary. *Advance Data from Vital and Health Statistics, 387.* Hyattsville, MD: Centers for Disease Control and Prevention, National Center for Health Statistics.

Cooke, M., Irby, D. M., Sullivan, W., & Ludmerer, K. (2006). American medical education 100 years after the Flexner report. *New England Journal of Medicine, 355*(13), 1339–1344.

Coombs, J. M., Hooker, R. S., & Brunisholz, K. D. (2013). What do we know about retired physician assistants? A preliminary study. *Journal of the American Academy of Physician Assistants, 26*(3), 44–48.

Coombs, J., & Valentin, V. (2014). Salary differences of male and female physician assistant educators. *The Journal of Physician Assistant Education, 25*(3), 9–14.

Cooper, R. A. (2013). Unraveling the physician supply dilemma. *Journal of the American Medical Association, 310*(18), 1931–1932.

Costa, D. K., Wallace, D. J., Barnato, A. E., & Kahn, J. M. (2014). Nurse practitioner/physician assistant staffing and critical care mortality. *Chest, 146,* 1566–1573.

Counselman, F. L., Graffeo, C. A., & Hill, J. T. (2000). Patient satisfaction with physician assistants (PAs) in an ED fast track. *American Journal of Emergency Medicine, 18*(6), 661–665.

Crile, G., Jr. (1987). Cleveland Clinic: The supporting cast 1920–1940. *Cleveland Clinic Journal of Medicine, 54*(4), 344–347.

Davis, A., Radix, S., Cawley, J. F., Hooker, R. S, & Walker, C. (2015). Access and innovation in a time of rapid change: Physician assistant scope of practice. *Annals of Health Law, 24*(1), 286–336.

Deal, C. L., Hooker, R. S., Harrington, T., Birnbaum, N., Hogan, P., Bouchery, E., Klein-Gitelman, M., & Barr, W. (2007). The United States rheumatology workforce: Supply and demand, 2005-2025. *Arthritis Rheumatism, 56*(3), 722–729.

Dehn, R. (2013). PA-Is PA residency training worth it? Clinical advisor. Retrieved from http://www.clinicaladvisor.com/pa-is-pa-residency-trainingworth-it/article/116919

Dehn, R. W. (2002). Does experience count? *Clinical Advisor, 5*(1), 98.

DeMots, H., Coombs, B., Murphy, E., & Palac, R. (1987). Coronary arteriography performed by a physician assistant. *American Journal of Cardiology, 60*(10), 784–787.

Dhuper, S., & Choksi, S. (2009). Replacing an academic internal medicine residency program with a physician assistant–hospitalist model: A comparative analysis study. *American Journal of Medical Quality, 24*(2), 132–139.

Dial, T. H., Palsbo, S. B., Bergsten, C., Gabel, J. R., & Weiner, J. (1995). Clinical staffing in staff and group-model HMOs. *Health Affairs, 14*(2), 168–180.

Dill, M. J., Pankow, S., Erikson, C., & Shipman, S. (2013). Survey shows consumers open to a greater role for physician assistants and nurse practitioners. *Health Affairs, 32*(6), 1135–1142.

Donnellan, F., Harewood, G. C., Cagney, D., Basri, F., Patchett, S. E., & Murray, F. E. (2010). Economic impact of prescreening on gastroenterology outpatient clinic practice. *Journal of Clinical Gastroenterology, 44*(4), e76–e79.

Dracup, K., DeBusk, R. F., De Mots, H., Gaile, E. H., Sr., Norton, J. B., Jr., & Rudy, E. B. (1994). Task force 3: Partnerships in delivery of cardiovascular care. *Journal of the American College of Cardiology, 24*(2), 296–304.

Essary, A. C., & Coplan, B. (2014). Ethics, equity, and economics: A primer on women in medicine. *Journal of the American Academy of Physician Assistants, 27*(5), 35–38.

Essary, A. C., Green, E. P., & Gans, D. N. (2016). Compensation and production in family medicine by practice ownership. *Health Services Research and Managerial Epidemiology, 1*, 3.

Essary, A., Wallace, L., & Asprey, D. (2014). The relationship between physician assistant program costs and student tuition and fees. *Journal of Physician Assistant Education, 25*(1), 29–32.

Estes, E. H. (1993). Training doctors for the future: Lessons from 25 years of physician assistant education. In D. K. Clawson & M. Osterweis (Eds.), *The roles of physician assistants and nurse practitioners in primary care.* Washington, DC: Association of Academic Health Centers.

Everett, C. M., Thorpe, C., Palta, M., Carayon, P., Bartels, C., & Smith, M.A. (2013). Physician assistants and nurse practitioners perform effective roles on teams caring for Medicare patients with diabetes. *Health Affairs, 32*(11), 1942–1948.

Fan, V. S., Burman, M., McDonell, M. B., & Fihn, S. D. (2005). Continuity of care and other determinants of patient satisfaction with primary care. *Journal of General Internal Medicine, 20*(3), 226–233.

Fréchette, D., & Shrichand, A. (2016). Insights into the physician assistant profession in Canada. *Journal of the American Academy of Physician Assistants, 29*(7), 35-39.

Freeborn, D. K., & Hooker, R. S. (1995). Satisfaction of physician assistants and other nonphysician providers in a managed care setting. *Public Health Reports (Washington, D.C. 1974), 110*(6), 714–719.

Freeborn, D. K., Hooker, R. S., & Pope, C. R. (2002). Satisfaction and well-being of primary care providers in managed care. *Evaluation & The Health Professions, 25*(2), 239–254.

Gamm, L. D., Hutchison, L. L., Dabney, B. J., & Dorsey, A. M. (Eds.). (2003). *Rural healthy people 2010: A companion document to healthy people 2010.* Volume 1. College Station, TX: The Texas A&M University System Health Science Center, School of Rural Public Health, Southwest Rural Research Center. Retrieved from http://www.srph.tamhsc.edu/centers/rhp2010/Volume1.pdf

Gandhi, T. K., Sittig, D. F., Franklin, M., Sussman, A. J., Fairchild, D. G., & Bates, D. W. (2000). Communication breakdown in the outpatient referral process. *Journal of General Internal Medicine, 15*(9), 626–631.

Gillard, J. N., Szoke, A., Hoff, W. S., Wainwright, G. A., Stehly, C. D., & Toedter, L. J. (2011). Utilization of PAs and NPs at a level I trauma center: Effects on outcomes. *Journal of the American Academy of Physician Assistants, 24*(7), 34–43.

Gofin, J., & Cawley, J. F. (2004). The physician assistant and community-oriented primary care. *Perspective on Physician Assistant Education, 15*(2), 126–128.

Goldman, M. B., Occhiuto, J. S., Peterson, L. E., Zapka, J. G., & Palmer, R. H. (2004). Physician assistants as providers of surgically induced abortion services. *American Journal of Public Health, 94*(8), 1352–1357

Gore, C. L. (2000). A physician's liability for mistakes of a physician assistant. *Journal of Legal Medicine, 21*, 125–142.

Graeff, E. C., Leafman, J. S., Wallace, L., & Stewart, G. (2014). Job satisfaction levels of physician assistant faculty in the United States. *Journal of Physician Assistant Education, 25*(2), 15–20.

Hafferty, F. W., & McKinley, J. B. (Eds.). (1993). *The changing medical profession.* New York: Oxford University Press.

Halpern, N. A., Pastores, S. M., Oropello, J. M., & Kvetan, V. (2013). Critical care medicine in the United States: Addressing the intensivist shortage and image of the specialty. *Critical Care Medicine, 41*(12), 2754–2761.

Hankins, G. D., Shaw, S. B., Cruess, D. F., Lawrence, H. C., III, & Harris, C. D. (1996). Patient satisfaction with collaborative practice. *Obstetrics and Gynecology, 88*(6), 1011–1015.

Hedden, L., Barer, M. L., Cardiff, K., McGrail, K. M., Law, M. R., & Bourgeault, I. L. (2014). The implications of the feminization of the primary care physician workforce on service supply: A systematic review. *Human Resources for Health, 12*, 32.

Henning, G. F., Graybill, M., & George, J. (2008). Reason for visit: Is migrant healthcare that different? *Journal of Rural Health, 24*(2), 219–220.

Henry, L. R., & Hooker, R. S. (2014). Caring for the disadvantaged: The role of physician assistants. *Journal of the American Academy of Physician Assistants, 27*(1), 36–42.

Higgins, R., Moser, S., Dereczyk, A., Canales, R., Stewart, G., Schierholtz, C., et al. (2010). Admission variables as predictors of PANCE scores in physician assistant programs: A comparison study across universities. *Journal of Physician Assistant Education, 21*(1), 10–17.

Hing, E., Hooker, R. S., & Ashman, J. (2010). Primary healthcare in community health centers and comparisons with office-based practice. *Journal of Community Health, 36*(3), 406–413.

Hing, E., & Hsiao, C. J. (2014). *State variability in supply of office-based primary care providers: United States, 2012* (National Center for Health Statistics Data Brief No. 151). Hyattsville, MD: National Center for Health Statistics.

Hing, E., & Hsiao, C. J. (2015). In which states are physician assistants or nurse practitioners more likely to work in primary care? *Journal of the American Academy of Physician Assistants, 28*(9), 46-53.

Holmes, S. E., & Fasser, C. E. (1993). Occupational stress among physician assistants. *Journal of the American Academy of Physician Assistants, 6*(3), 172–178.

Holt, N. (1998). "Confusion's masterpiece": The development of the physician assistant profession. *Bulletin of the History of Medicine, 72*, 246–278.

Hooker, R. S. (1993). The roles of physician assistants and nurse practitioners in a managed care organization. In D. K. Clawson & M. Osterweis (Eds.), *The roles of physician assistants and nurse practitioners in primary care.* Washington, DC: The Association of Academic Health Centers.

Hooker, R. S. (2002). A cost analysis of physician assistants in primary care. *Journal of the American Academy of Physician Assistants, 15*(11), 39–48.

Hooker, R. S. (2004). Physician assistants in occupational medicine: How do they compare to occupational physicians? *Occupational Medicine (Oxford, England), 54*(3), 153–158.

Hooker, R. S. (2009). Assessing the value of physician assistant postgraduate education. *Journal of the American Academy of Physician Assistants, 22*(5), 13.

Hooker R. S. (2015). Is physician assistant autonomy inevitable? *Journal of the American Academy of Physician Assistants. 28*(1): 18–19.

Hooker, R. S., Benitez, J. A., Coplan, B. H., & Dehn, R. W. (2013). Ambulatory and chronic disease care by physician assistants and nurse practitioners. *Journal of Ambulatory Care Management, 36*(4), 293–301.

Hooker, R. S., Brock, D. M., & Cook, M. L. (2016). Characteristics of nurse practitioners and physician assistants in the United States. *Journal of the American Association of Nurse Practitioners, 28*(1), 39–46.

Hooker R. S., & Cawthon E. A. (2015). The 1965 White House conference on health: Inspiring national policy and the physician assistant movement. *Journal of the American Academy of Physician Assistants, 28*(10). 46-51.

Hooker, R. S., & Cipher, D. J. (2005). Physician assistant and nurse practitioner prescribing: 1997– 2002. *Journal of Rural Health, 21*(4), 355–360.

Hooker, R. S., & Freeborn, D. K. (1991). Use of physician assistants in a managed healthcare system. *Public Health Reports (Washington, DC: 1974), 106*(1), 90–94.

Hooker, R. S., Hess, B., & Cipher, D. (2002). A comparison of physician assistant programs by national certification examination scores. *Perspective on Physician Assistant Education, 13*(2), 81–86.

Hooker, R. S., Klocko, D. J., & Larkin, G. L. (2011). Physician assistants in emergency medicine: The impact of their role. *Academic Emergency Medicine, 18*(1), 72–77.

Hooker, R. S., Kuilman, L., & Everett, C. M. (2015). Physician assistant job satisfaction: A narrative review of empirical research. *Journal of Physician Assistant Education, 26*(4), 176–186.

Hooker, R. S., & Muchow, A. N. (2014). Supply of physician assistants: 2013-2026. *Journal of the American Academy of Physician Assistants, 27*(3), 39–45.

Hooker, R. S., & Muchow, A. N. (2014). The 2013 census of licensed physician assistants. *Journal of the American Academy of Physician Assistants, 27*(7), 35–39.

Hooker, R. S., & Rangan, B. V. (2008). Role delineation of rheumatology physician assistants. *Journal of Clinical Rheumatology, 14*(4), 202–205.

Hooker, R. S., Robie, S. P., Coombs, J. M., & Cawley, J. F. (2013). The changing physician assistant profession: A gender shift. *Journal of the American Academy of Physician Assistants, 26*(9), 36–44.

Hooker, R. S., & Warren, J. (2001). Comparison of physician assistant programs by tuition costs. *Perspective on Physician Assistant Education, 12,* 87–91.

HRSA. (2014). U.S. Department of Health and Human Services, Health Resources and Services Administration, National Center for Health Workforce Analysis. Sex, race, and ethnic diversity of U.S. health occupations: Technical documentation. Rockville, Maryland: Author.

Hudson, C. L. (1961). Expansion of medical professional services with nonprofessional personnel. *Journal of the American Medical Association, 176,* 839–841.

Hyams, A. L., Shapiro, D. W., & Brennan, T. A. (1996). Medical practice guidelines in malpractice litigation: An early retrospective. *Journal of Health Politics, Policy and Law, 21*(2), 289–313.

Institute of Medicine. (2001). *Crossing the quality chasm: A new health system for the 21st century.* Washington, DC: Institute of Medicine.

Isberner, F. R., Lloyd, L., Simon, B., Joyce, M. S., & Craven, J. M. (2003). Utilization of physician assistants: Incentives and constraints for rural physicians. *Perspective on Physician Assistant Education, 14*(2), 69–73.

Jalperneanmonod, R., DelCollo, J., Jeanmonod, D., Dombchewsky, O., & Reiter, M. (2013). Comparison of resident and mid-level provider productivity and patient satisfaction in an emergency department fast track. *Emergency Medicine Journal, 30*(1), e12.

Jones, I. W. (2015). Should international medical graduates work as physician assistants? *Journal of the American Academy of Physician Assistants, 28*(7), 8–10.

Jones, P. E. (2008). Doctor and physician assistant distribution in rural and remote Texas counties. *Australian Journal of Rural Health, 16*(2), 12.

Kark, S. L., & Kark, E. (1983). An alternative strategy in community healthcare: Community-oriented primary healthcare. *Israel Journal of Medical Sciences, 19*(8), 707–713.

Katz, D., & Kahn, R. L. (1966). *The social psychology of organizations.* New York: John Wiley & Sons.

Kaups, K. L., Parks, S. N., & Morris, C. L. (1998). Intracranial pressure monitor placement by midlevel practitioners. *Journal of Trauma, 45*(5), 884–886.

Kimball, A. B., & Resneck, J. S., Jr. (2008). The US dermatology workforce: A specialty remains in shortage. *Journal of the American Academy of Dermatology, 59*(5), 741–745.

Kindman, L. A. (2006). Medical education after the Flexner report. *New England Journal of Medicine, 356*(1), 90.

Kohn, L., Corrigan, J., & Donaldson, M. (Eds.). (2000). *To err is human: Building a safer health system.* Washington, DC: National Academies Press.

Krasuski, R. A., Wang, A., Ross, C., Bolles, J. F., Moloney, E. L., Kelly, L. P., et al. (2003). Trained and supervised physician assistants can safely perform diagnostic cardiac catheterization with coronary angiography. *Catheterization and Cardiovascular Interventions, 59*(2), 157–160.

Krein, S. L. (1997). The employment and use of nurse practitioners and physician assistants by rural hospitals. *Journal of Rural Health, 13*(1), 45–58.

Larson, E. H., Coerver, D. A., Wick, K. H., & Ballweg, R. A. (2011). Physician assistants in orthopedic practice: A national study. *Journal of Allied Health, 40*(4), 174–180.

Larson, E. H., Palazzo L., Berkowitz, B., Pirani, M. J., & Hart, L. G. (2003). The contribution of nurse practitioners and physician assistants to generalist care in Washington State. *Health Services Research, 38*(4), 1033–1050.

Lauftik, N. (2014). The physician assistant role in Aboriginal healthcare in Australia. *Journal of the American Academy of Physician Assistants, 27*(1), 32–35.

LeLacheur, S., Barnett, J., & Straker, H. (2015). Race, ethnicity, and the physician assistant profession. *Journal of the American Academy of Physician Assistants, 28*(10), 41–45.

Lemieux-Charles, L., & McGuire, W. L. (2006). What do we know about healthcare team effectiveness? A review of the literature. *Medical Care Research and Review, 63*(3), 263–300.

Lo Sasso, A. T., Richards, M. R., Chou, C. F., & Gerber, S. E. (2011). The $16,819 pay gap for newly trained physicians: The unexplained trend of men earning more than women. *Health Affairs, 30*(2), 193–201.

Makinde, J. F., & Hooker, R. S. (2009). PA doctoral degree debt. *ADVANCE for Physician Assistants, 17*(3), 30–31.

Marsters, C. E. (2000). Pneumothorax as a complication of central venous cannulation performed by physician assistants. *Surgical Physician Assistant, 6*(3), 18–24.

Marzucco, J., Hooker, R. S. & Ballweg, R. M. (2013). A history of the Alaska physician assistant: 1970–1980. *Journal of the American Academy of Physician Assistants, 26*(12):45–51.

McCarty, J. E., Stuetzer, L. J., & Somers, J. E. (2001). Physician assistant program accreditation— history in the making. *The Journal of Physician Assistant Education, 12*(1), 24–38.

McDaniel, M. J., Hildebrandt, C. A., & Russell, G. B. (2016). Central Application Service for Physician Assistants (CASPA) ten-year data report 2002–2011. *Journal of Physician Assistant Education, 27*(1), 17–23.

McPhee, S. J., Lo, B., Saika, G. Y., & Meltzer, R. (1984). How good is communication between primary care physicians and subspecialty consultants? *Archives of Internal Medicine, 144*(6), 1265–1268.

Medsker, G. J., & Campion, M. A. (1997). Job and team design. In P. Carayon (Ed.), *Handbook of human factors and ergonomics in healthcare and patient safety* (pp. 450–489). Boca Raton, FL: CRC Press.

Meikle, T. H. (1992). *An expanded role for the physician assistant.* Washington, DC: Association of Academic Health Centers.

Miller, W., Riehl, E., Napier, M., Barber, K., & Dabideen, H. (1998). Use of physician assistants as surgery/trauma house staff at an American College of Surgeons–verified level II trauma center. *Journal of Trauma, 44*(2), 372–376.

Moore, M., Coffman, M., Cawley, J. F., Crowley, D., Bazemore, A., Cheng, N., Fox, S., & Klink, K. (2014). *The impact of debt load on physician assistants.* Washington, DC: Robert Graham Center.

Moran, E. A., Basa, E., Gao, J., Woodmansee, D., Lamenoff, P. L., & Hooker, R. S. (2016). PA and NP productivity in the Veterans Health Administration. *Journal of the American Academy of Physician Assistants, 29*(7), 1-7.

Morgan, B. B., Salas, E., & Glickman, A. S. (1993). An analysis of team evolution and maturation. *Journal of General Psychology, 120*(3), 277–291.

Morgan, P. A., Abbott, D. H., McNeil, R. B., & Fisher, D. A. (2012). Characteristics of primary care office visits to nurse practitioners, physician assistants and physicians in United States Veterans Health Administration facilities, 2005 to 2010: A retrospective cross-sectional analysis. *Human Resources for Health, 10*(1), 42.

Morgan, P., Everett, C. M., & Huminick, K. (2016, February 4). Scarcity of primary care positions may divert physician assistants into specialty practice. *Medical Care Research and Review.* Advance online publication.

Mundinger, M. O., Kane, R. L., Lenz, E. R., Totten, A. M., Tsai, W. Y., Cleary, P. D, et al. (2000). Primary care outcomes in patients treated by nurse practitioners or physicians: A randomized trial. *Journal of the American Medical Association, 283*(1), 59–68.

Murray, R. B., & Wronski, I. (2006). When the tide goes out: Health workforce in rural, remote and indigenous communities. *Medical Journal of Australia, 185*(1), 37–38.

Nabagiez, J. P., Shariff, M. A., Molloy, W. J., Demissie, S., & McGinn, J. T. (2016). Cost analysis of physician assistant home visit program to reduce readmissions after cardiac surgery. *The Annals of Thoracic Surgery, 102*(3), 696–702.

National Commission on Certification of Physician Assistants. (2014). *National Commission on the Certification of Physician Assistants. 2013 Statistical profile of certified physician assistants.* Johns Creek, Georgia: Author.

National Commission on the Certification of Physician Assistants (NCCPA). (2015). *2014 Statistical profile of recently certified physician assistants: An annual report of the National Commission on the Certification of Physician Assistants.* Retrieved from http://www.nccpa.net/uploads/docs/recentlycertifiedreport2014.pdf

National Commission on Certification of Physician Assistants. (2016). *2015 Statistical Profile of certified physician assistants: An annual report of the National Commission on the certification of physician assistants.* Retrieved from http://www.nccpa.net/research

O'Callaghan, N. (2007). Addressing clinical preceptorship teaching development. *Journal of Physician Assistant Education, 18*(4), 37–39.

Ogunfiditimi, F., Takis, L., Paige, V. J., Wyman, J. F., & Marlow, E. (2013). Assessing the productivity of advanced practice providers using a time and motion study. *Journal of Healthcare Management, 58*(3), 173–185.

Ohman-Strickland, P. A., Orzano, A. J., Hudson, S. V., Solberg, L. I., DiCiccio-Bloom, B., O'Malley, D., et al. (2008). Quality of diabetes care in family medicine practices: Influence of nurse practitioners and physician's assistants. *Annals of Family Medicine, 6*(1), 14–22.

Oliphant, J. (2014). *How you can help during the ebola crisis.* Retrieved from https://www.aapa.org/twocolumn.aspx?id=3389#sthash.vJfVJhWr.dpuf

Organisation for Economic Co-operation and Development. (2013). *Health at a glance 2013: OECD indicators.* Retrieved from http://www.oecd.org/health/health-systems/health-at-aglance.htm

Oswanski, M. F., Sharma, O. P., & Shekhar, S. R. (2004). Comparative review of use of physician assistants in a level I trauma center. *American Surgeon, 70*(3), 272–279.

Pedersen, D. M., Chappell, B., Elison, G., & Bunnell, R. (2008). The productivity of PAs, APRNs, and physicians in Utah. *Journal of the American Academy of Physician Assistants, 21*(1), 42–47.

Perry, H. B., III. (1977). Physician assistants: An overview of an emerging health profession. *Medical Care, 15*(12), 982–990.

Pham, H. H., Schrag, D., O'Malley, A. S., Wu, B. N., & Bach, P. B. (2007). Care patterns in Medicare and their implications for pay for performance. *New England Journal of Medicine, 356*(11), 1130–1139.

Phillips, R. L., Jr., Bazemore, A. M., & Peterson, L. E. (2014). Effectiveness over efficiency: Underestimating the primary care physician shortage. *Medical Care, 52*(2), 97–98.

Philpot, R. J. (2005). *Financial returns to society by National Health Service corps scholars who receive training as physician assistants and nurse practitioners.* Unpublished doctoral dissertation, University of Florida.

Physician Assistant Education Association (PAEA). (2014). *Twenty-ninth annual report on physician assistant educational programs in the United States, 2012–2013.* Alexandria, VA: PAEA. Retrieved from http://www.paeaonline.org/index.php?ht=d/sp/i/243/pid/243

Pronovost, P., Needham, D., Berenholtz, S., Sinopoli, D., Chu, H., Cosgrove, S., . . . Goeschel, C. (2006). An intervention to decrease catheter-related bloodstream infections in the ICU. *New England Journal of Medicine, 355*(26), 2725-2732.

Quella, A., Brock, D. M., & Hooker, R. S. (2015). Physician assistant wages and employment, 2000–2025. *Journal of the American Academy of Physician Assistants, 28*(6), 56–63.

Record, J. C., Blomquist, R. H., McCabe, M. A., McCally, M., & Berger, B. D. (1981). Delegation in adult primary care: The generalizability of HMO data. *Springer Series on Healthcare and Society, 6,* 68–83.

Record, J. C., McCally, M., Schweitzer, S. O., Blomquist, R. M., & Berger, B. D. (1980). New health professions after a decade and a half: Delegation, productivity and costs in primary care. *Journal of Health Politics, Policy & Law, 5*(3), 470–497.

Record, J. C., & Schweitzer, S. O. (1981a). Staffing primary care in 1990: Effects of national health insurance on staffing and costs. *Springer Series on Healthcare and Society, 6,* 115–127.

Record, J. C., & Schweitzer, S. O. (1981b). Staffing primary care in 1990—Potential effects on staffing and costs: Estimates from the model. *Springer Series on Healthcare and Society, 6,* 87–114.

Ritsema, T. S., Bingenheimer, J. B., Scholting, P., & Cawley, J. F. (2014). Differences in the delivery of health education to patients with chronic disease by provider type, 2005–2009. *Preventing Chronic Disease, 11,* E33.

Roblin, D. W., Howard, D. H., Becker, E. R., Adams, E. K., & Roberts, M. H. (2004a). Use of midlevel practitioners to achieve labor cost savings in the primary care practice of an MCO. *Health Services Research, 39*(3), 607–626.

Roblin, D. W., Becker, E. R., Adams, E. K., Howard, D. H., & Roberts, M. H. (2004b). Patient satisfaction with primary care: Does type of practitioner matter? *Medical Care, 42*(6), 579–590.

Roblin, D. W., Howard, D. H., Ren, J., & Becker, E. R. (2011). An evaluation of the influence of primary care team functioning on the health of Medicare beneficiaries. *Medical Care Research and Review, 68*(2), 177–201.

Rodriguez, H. P., Rogers, W. H., Marshall, R. E., & Safran, D. (2007). Multidisciplinary primary care teams: Effects on the quality of clinician-patient interactions and organizational features of care. *Medical Care, 45*(1), 19–27.

Rohrer, J. E., Angstman, K. B., Garrison, G. M., Pecina, J. L., & Maxson, J. A. (2013). Nurse practitioners and physician assistants are complements to family medicine physicians. *Population Health Management, 16*(4), 242–245.

Rosenberg, C. E. (1987). *The care of strangers: The rise of America's hospital system.* New York: Basic Books.

Roy, C. L., Liang, C. L., Lund, M., Boyd, C., Katz, J. T., McKean, S., & Schnipper, J. L. (2008). Implementation of a physician assistant/hospitalist service in an academic medical center: impact on efficiency and patient outcomes. *Journal of Hospital Medicine, 3*(5), 361–368.

Sadler, A. M., Jr., Sadler, B. L., & Bliss, A. A. (1972). *The physician's assistant: Today and tomorrow.* New Haven, CT: Yale University Press.

Saltman, D. C., O'Dea, N. A., Farmer, J., Veitch, C., Rosen, G., & Kidd, M. R. (2005). Groups or teams in healthcare: Finding the best fit. *Journal of Evaluation in Clinical Practice, 13,* 55–60.

Sargen, M., Hooker, R. S., & Cooper, R. A. (2011). Gaps in the supply of physicians, advance practice nurses, and physician assistants. *Journal of the American College of Surgeons, 212*(6), 991–999.

Schafft, G. E., & Cawley, J. F. (1987). Geriatric care and the physician assistant. *The physician assistant in a changing healthcare environment.* Rockville, MD: Aspen.

Scheffler, R. M., Waitzman, N. J., & Hillman, J. M. (1996). The productivity of physician assistants and nurse practitioners and health work force policy in the era of managed healthcare. *Journal of Allied Health, 25*(3), 207–217.

Schneller, E. S. (1978). *The physician's assistant: Innovation in the medical division of labor.* Lexington, MA: Lexington Books.

Schulman, M., Lucchese, K. R., & Sullivan, A. C. (1995). Transition from housestaff to nonphysicians as neonatal intensive care providers: Cost, impact on revenue, and quality of care. *American Journal of Perinatology, 12*(6), 442–446.

Shi, L., Samuels, M. E., Ricketts, T. C., III, & Konrad, T. R. (1994). A rural-urban comparative study of nonphysician providers in community and migrant health centers. *Public Health Reports, 109*(6), 809–815.

Sibbald, B., Laurant, M., & Scott, A. (2006). Changing task profiles. In R. B. Saltman, A. Rico, & W. Boerma (Eds.), *Primary care in the driver's seat? Organizational reform in European primary care.* Berkshire, England: Open University Press.

Sigurdson, L. (2007). Meeting challenges in the delivery of surgical care. *Clinical & Investigative Medicine, 30*(Suppl. 4), S35–S36.

Silver, H. K. (1971). The syniatrist. A suggested nomenclature and classification for allied health professionals. *Journal of the American Medical Association, 217*, 1368–1370.

Simmer, T., Nerenz, D., Rutt, W., Newcomb, C., & Benfer, D. (1991). A randomized, controlled trial of an attending staff service in general internal medicine. *Medical Care, 29*(7), JS31–JS40.

Singh, S., Fletcher, K. E., Schapira, M. M., Conti, M., Tarima, S., Biblo, L. A., & Whittle, J. (2011). A comparison of outcomes of general medical inpatient care provided by a hospitalist-physician assistant model vs a traditional resident-based model. *Journal of Hospital Medicine, 6*(3), 122–130.

Smith, D. T., & Jacobson, C. K. (2015). Racial and gender disparities in the physician assistant profession. *Health Services Research, 51*(3), 892–909.

Spetz, J., Cawley, J.F., Schommer, J. (2016). Transformation of the nonphysician health professions. In T. Hoff, K. Sutcliffe, & G. Young (Eds.), *The Healthcare Professional Workforce: New Directions in Theory and Practice.* New York: Oxford Press.

Starr, P. (1982). *The social transformation of American medicine.* New York: Basic Books.

Stead, E. A., Jr. (1967). The Duke plan for physician's assistants. *Medical Times, 95*, 40–48.

Stead, E. A., Jr. (1971). Use of physicians' assistants in the delivery of medical care. *Annual Review of Medicine, 22*, 273–282.

Stecker, M. S., Armenoff, D., & Johnson, M. S. (2004). Physician assistants in interventional radiology practice. *Journal of Vascular and Interventional Radiology, 15*(3), 221–227.

Studdert, D. M., Yang, Y. T., & Mello, M. M. (2004). Are damages caps regressive? A study of malpractice jury verdicts in California. *Health Affairs, 23*(4), 54–67.

US Congress, Office of Technology Assessment. (1986). *Nurse practitioners, physician assistants, and certified nurse-midwives: A policy analysis* (Health Technology Case Study 37). Washington, DC: Government Printing Office.

US Department of Health and Human Services, Health Resources and Services Administration, National Center for Health Workforce Analysis. (2013). *The US health workforce chartbook.* Rockville, MD: US Department of Health and Human Services.

US Department of Health and Human Services, Health Resources and Services Administration, National Center for Health Workforce Analysis. (2013). *Projecting the supply and demand for primary care practitioners through 2020.* Rockville, MD: US Department of Health and Human Services.

US Department of Health and Human Services, Office of the Inspector General. (2010). *Adverse events in hospitals: National incidence among Medicare beneficiaries* (OEI-06-09-00090). Retrieved from https://oig.hhs.gov/oei/reports/oei-06-09-00090.pdf

US Department of Labor, Bureau of Labor Statistics. (2013). *Occupational employment and wages, May 2013: 29-1071 physician assistants.* Retrieved from http://www.bls.gov/oes/current/oes291071.htm

US Department of Labor, Bureau of Labor Statistics. (2014). *Occupational employment and wages, May 2014, 29-1071 physician assistants.* Retrieved from http://www.bls.gov/oes/current/oes291071.htm

Van Rhee, J., Ritchie, J., & Eward, A. M. (2002). Resource use by physician assistant services versus teaching services. *Journal of the American Academy of Physician Assistants, 15*(1) 33–38, 40, 42 passim.

Weitz, T. A., Taylor, D., Desai, S., Upadhyay, U. D., Waldman, J., Battistelli, M. F., & Drey, E. A. (2013). Safety of aspiration abortion performed by nurse practitioners, certified nurse midwives, and physician assistants under a California legal waiver. *American Journal of Public Health, 103*(3), 454–461.

Wick, K. H. (2015). International medical graduates as physician assistants. *Journal of the American Academy of Physician Assistants, 28*(7), 43–46.

Will, K. K., Williams, J., Hilton, G., Wilson, L., & Geyer, H. (2016). Perceived efficacy and utility of postgraduate physician assistant training programs. *Journal of the American Academy of Physician Assistants, 27*(3).

Wilson, I. B., Landon, B. E., Hirschhorn, L. R., McInnes, K., Ding, L., Marsden, P. V., & Cleary, P. D.

(2005). Quality of HIV care provided by nurse practitioners, physician assistants, and physicians. *Annals of Internal Medicine, 143*(10), 729–736.

Woodin, J., Mcleod, H., McManus, R., & Jelphs, K. (2005). *Evaluation of US-trained PAs working in the NHS in England. Final Report.* Birmingham, England: Health Services Management Centre, Department of Primary Care and General Practice, University of Birmingham.

Wright, K. A., Cawley, J. F., Hooker, R. S., & Ahuja, M. (2009). Organizational infrastructure of American physician assistant education programs. *Journal of Physician Assistant Education, 20*(3), 15–21.

Wright, W. K., & Hirsch, C. S. (1987). The physician assistant as forensic investigator. *Journal of Forensic Science, 32*(4), 1059–1061.

Yang, W., Williams, J. H., Hogan, P. F., Bruinooge, S. S., Rodriguez, G. I., Kosty, M. P., et al. (2014). Projected supply of and demand for oncologists and radiation oncologists through 2025: An aging, better-insured population will result in shortage. *Journal of Oncology Practice, 10*(1), 39–45.

Youngclaus, J., & Fresne, J. A. (2013). *Physician education debt and the cost to attend medical school: 2012 update.* Washington, DC: Association of American Medical Colleges.

INDEX

Page numbers followed by "f" denote figures; those followed by "t" denote tables; and those followed by "b" denote boxes